The PATIENT Doesn't Come First... YOU DO

A GUIDE FOR HEALTH CARE WORKERS TO TAKE CARE OF THEMSELVES

SHANNON HART, RN, BSCN

ISBN: 978-1-7388394-0-7 (print)
ISBN: 978-1-7388394-1-4 (ebook)
Library of Congress Control Number: 2023900296

First print edition 2023
Cover and Interior Design: Jennifer Federico Stimson

Social media: shannonhartauthor

Acknowledgements

I would like to thank all of the people who helped me bring this book to fruition. To my family, friends, and coworkers, thank you for being a part of my journey.

To my editor, Val, thank you for your hard work and thoughtful contributions to making this labour of love a reality.

I dedicate this book to my DI family. Thank you for being there during times of laughter, as well as times of tears. I have grown so much from the time I started in the department, and I cherish each and every moment. Thank you for helping me become the person I am today.

Contents

Foreword

As I write this, we are dealing with the fallout of the COVID-19 pandemic. We have watched as our world has changed radically into something we don't quite know how to handle.

From a layman's perspective, we are winding down. From a health care worker's perspective, we are still very much in combat. Beaten up, exhausted, demoralized, we nevertheless walk into our jobs every day, suit up our PPE armor, and engage in battle with everything this virus has created. While some of our experience is directly related to the virus itself, much of what we are dealing with is the ripple effects it has caused. Consistently short-staffed prior to the pandemic, our hospitals are now bare bones. Staff are dropping like flies, either from exhaustion, prolonged illness, or leaving the profession altogether. Our initial surge of encouragement from the public in 2020, being hailed as "Health Care Heroes," has extinguished, despite the fact that we are still very much engaging in the same stressors as we were at the beginning. Now, in 2023, we are dealing with even less staff, less resources, and less strength to continue.

During this three-year period, we have endured fear of an unknown virus with no vaccine at the beginning of it to protect ourselves; rationing equipment and working with a lack of PPE (some of it stolen by our own colleagues); working extremely short-staffed, working extended shifts, without meals or bathroom breaks; overwhelming grief and loss from the deaths of thousands of people; becoming surrogate families to our patients, as they were unable to have visitors; dealing with aggressive and even violent families while having to enforce policies we did not create; fearing for our safety from anti-vax protesters as we went into our place of work; watching before our own eyes our units crumbling from the pressure to sustain what our system was never capable of sustaining. We were put in the horrifying position of deciding between what was morally right and what was physically viable.

How are we still showing up, amid the burnout, threats, and lack of support?

We are showing up because we care. We care about our patients. We care about the families of our patients. We care about our colleagues. And we care about society as a whole.

But we have reached a tipping point.

According to the International Council of Nurses website, nurses were the most impacted group in health care by the pandemic, with over two thousand nurses in over fifty countries having died of COVID, and 1.6 million of them contracting the virus by the end of 2020.[1]

The impact of the virus did not just affect us physically. A recent survey in the U.S. of nurses working during the pandemic stated that "more than 50% of respondents experienced symptoms of depression and anxiety and close to one-third had symptoms of post-traumatic stress disorder."[2] The secondary trauma as a result of COVID due to our feelings of helplessness is taking its toll, and the cracks are starting to show in our critically short-staffed hospitals.

Our world changed in 2020, and when we health care workers were needed, we rose to the occasion valiantly. The effects of the pandemic will leave lasting symptoms, and we will need support to make sense of everything that has happened to us. This requires us to stop and take stock of how *we* are coping, physically, mentally, and emotionally. This is something we as health care workers are not used to doing.

Ignoring our mental health will have an effect on our health care system now and in the future. Dealing ineffectively with the traumas that we have acquired during this stressful time may result in continued psychological distress, may lead to increased substance use, and may cause health care workers to leave the profession.[3] What is more, the younger generations will be less likely to opt into a career in health care, as they will be well aware of the poor working conditions, long hours, and possible risk to their wellbeing. Who would choose this the way things are right now?

As we are already facing these outcomes, it is time to do something about it. Health care has been in crisis for a long time; the pandemic has simply shone a spotlight on it. While there have been numerous studies and undertakings to fix how health care operates, very little has improved, and in fact, it has gotten worse. We need a radical overhaul in how we approach health. We are holistic beings, not just bodies. Treating the patient physically is only treating part of the issue. While we know this empirically, we are not exercising this knowledge in our practice.

As our patients look to us for knowledge, we need to be leading the way. We encourage our patients to put their health first. We can only be setting an example for them if we are actually doing it ourselves. Putting our own needs above others' is something that we in health care are not used to. It feels uncomfortable to think about it, but if we are to glean anything from the last three years, may it be that our needs have been long neglected—and only we can do something to change it.

"(Health care workers) must know that self-care is not selfish, but smart. The effects of distress are cumulative. It must be understood that if a provider is not well, it becomes challenging to heal others without doing further harm to oneself."[4]

Right before the pandemic began, I was very close to leaving nursing. We were working short with daily overtime long before I had ever heard of the new coronavirus, and I was burned out.

Then the pandemic hit. I sat, frozen, as I watched the world slide into lockdown and deaths around the world began to rise. Could I walk away from the career that, while causing me stress, was also filled with the people that I call family? Would I walk away from nursing in the time I am needed most?

I couldn't. I couldn't do it, because, while I have goals and aspirations outside of nursing, at my core, I am a nurse. I am there to help others in their time of need. And this is the definition of time of need, right now.

I want to make it very clear: I made a choice. I willingly chose to go back to the place that was burning me out. I willingly picked up shifts whenever they needed me. I made a choice, because I was lucky enough to have that choice.

You also have a choice. Every day you walk into work, you have a choice whether or not you show up, and how. While it may be uncomfortable to think about, you also have the choice to cut back, say no to overtime, or seek other options. How you choose to spend the hours of your day is completely up to you, even if it doesn't always feel that way.

Often, we feel we do not have a choice. As I watched the pandemic slowly take our freedoms away from us, it became glaringly obvious that we in society had a lot more freedom than we thought we did.

My intention for this book is to give you hope, to help you realize that you do have the power to make change. You do have a choice. The fallout of the pandemic is exposing what is actually, truly vital. Life is heartbreakingly short for some of us. Knowing that we are important, valued, and cherished is vital to being fulfilled— and accepting anything less just isn't worth it anymore.

If you want to make a change in your life, in your department, in your career, know that it is possible. The tools and exercises I have included here are ones that I use on a regular basis. Take what resonates, leave what doesn't. You are not broken; there is nothing wrong with you. Yet, I know for myself that dealing with unhealthy environments for so long caused me to question my worthiness, and I didn't know that I deserved more until I started working on myself. If you have been feeling disempowered, apathetic, frustrated, then my hope is that this book will provide you with some tools to address and overcome these feelings.

But it starts with having the courage to put your needs first—above your patients, above your colleagues, and above your family (yes, I said it). We are not capable of taking care of others if we are not taking care of ourselves. While this has become cliché, few of us are actually embodying this perspective. When we sacrifice our sleep, our meals, and our bodily functions in order to get the work done, we are sacrificing ourselves—and the patient does not truly benefit from this. Ask yourself: Who are you truly doing this for? If we let ourselves believe it is for the patients, we are woefully ignorant in thinking it benefits them when we are running on nothing but fumes. Ditto for the family members we are sacrificing our time without.

I have a confession: While I love my patients, I love my colleagues more. I realized early on that while I went into nursing to help my patients heal, my true calling was to help those who help the patients. I am in awe of people in health care. The dedication, the caring, the over and above my colleagues engage in with their patients truly blows me away. It's in the little things—going down to the first floor because a patient really wanted ice chips, or wheeling them down to the door to meet a family member, or downloading children's TV shows to their phone just because they know it might make a pediatric patient smile. The way they show up and give 100 percent of themselves, knowing that some type of adversity awaits them, whether it be a palliative oncology child or a 450-pound abusive paraplegic, is nothing short of magical to me. I deeply admire and respect all health care workers, and this book is a true labour of love I have for each and every one of you.

Health care workers rise to the occasion every day, and this pandemic is no different. It is just who you are and what you do. You are the true heroes of our society, and my hope is that once you read this book, you will believe it as much as I do.

CHAPTER 1

Pee Break

"If you gotta go, you gotta go."

We were at a busy skating rink in downtown New York. I was visiting my friends over the Christmas holidays, and we had been in line to rent skates. We had a few hours, but it was getting close to the time I was going to have to leave for the airport back home. We'd had a couple coffees beforehand, and I needed the washroom. The lineup for the washroom extended outside the building and was moving at a snail's pace. It became clear that I either had to choose the washroom or skating. I contemplated holding it in and skating anyway, but knew I wouldn't make it. I apologized to my friends profusely as they waited in the bathroom line with me.

Both of them looked at me bizarrely and questioned why I was apologizing for having to go to the bathroom.

And it dawned on me.

It wasn't normal to hold your bladder for hours. It wasn't normal to deny your bodily functions so you could do something else.

It. Wasn't. Normal.

Both of my friends, being yoga instructors, were well-practiced in being in tune with their bodies. I, on the other hand, had ignored mine so much I was basically offline from the neck down. I realized that this was just what I did in my profession—it's what all of my coworkers did—on a regular basis.

As I looked wistfully at the happy people skating, I knew there was something deeply wrong.

Having been a nurse for fifteen years, putting others' needs above my own was just part of the job description—everyone in health care does it. You do what you gotta do to get the job done. Long hours, going without breaks, overtime, returning to work on call-back—it was what was expected of us, and so nobody questioned it. We may have complained (!) but we never questioned it. This was what we signed up for. This was our calling.

I may have been a nurse for fifteen years, but I have been taking care of people my whole life. I grew up in a dysfunctional household, with my parents both suffering from substance abuse issues. From a young age, I was not only basically taking care of myself, but I was also taking care of them, as well as my younger

---

sister. Being in a volatile environment most of my childhood, I quickly learned what I could and couldn't say or do. I learned how to read my parents very well, as it was required to help me survive. One wrong move around either of them when they were drinking would mean punishment for me—physically or emotionally. I learned how to pick up on nonverbal cues, figured out the right thing to say at the right time, and learned when to stay away from them altogether.

Despite their abuse issues, they were still my parents, and I loved them. They provided me my basic necessities, and I still craved their affection. I learned early on that if I was a "good girl," I would get some positive attention, thus igniting my people-pleasing behavior. As a child, it was all I knew to earn affection from my parents, as my high marks in school would grant me their praise. Unfortunately, I adopted this strategy to survive well into my adult years, and it was exploited both in my personal life and in my career.

How many of you have similar stories? Experiences of being abused, neglected, not accepted? Feelings of not being enough? Inner dialogue of negative self-talk? Do my words echo yours of growing up? Can you see yourself in this scene?

My belief is that my story isn't unique. Many people with a background of abuse go into helping professions. Our desire to help others while they are in a vulnerable state is indicative of our powerful gift of empathy. We know what it is to feel pain, and so we wish to help others who are enduring their own form of pain in an attempt to ease their suffering.

Career Move

It was only natural for me to go into nursing, as I had already been caring for people and was quite adept at it. Being able to read people was a great asset when assessing my patients for pain or stoicism, and the abuse I received from patients (and staff) didn't faze me—I'd been used to it my entire life.

As I advanced in my career, from a NICU nurse to a more schedule-friendly job in diagnostic imaging, I just kept using the same survival plan that had served me as a child: *Give, give, give, and you will be rewarded. You will be liked. You will be admired. You will feel like a good person.*

But I didn't. I didn't feel like a good person. Having come from a broken home and endured bullying as a kid, I felt like there was something inherently wrong with me. People-pleasing at work and in my personal life only made me feel good for so long, until I became overstretched. I noticed I started feeling resentful when others asked for things, and that I seemed to be the one who they were always asking. I would feel anger at times, being overworked and overused, but I wouldn't feel like I was justified in my anger, so I would stifle it. I always needed to be doing, and I was always in a hypervigilant state, yet I didn't know it at the time.

Nursing made me feel like a good person. Whenever I met someone and they asked me what I did, I was always so proud to say I was a nurse. You never got a bad reaction from it (as opposed to my friends and family members who are lawyers—sorry, guys!). People were always grateful and marvelled at how I could do such a demanding job, and I wore that like it was a badge of honor. Long hours, wearing heavy lead, middle of the night calls—I knew I was working really hard. This made me feel good about myself, and knowing I had put in the effort meant others would directly benefit. To most people in my department, it wasn't really working hard, it was doing what was expected. And if that meant working ten, twelve, fourteen hours and being called back in for a middle-of-the-night procedure, that was just what you did—it was what we all did. Emergencies happen, and someone needed to be there—that meant us.

Yet I couldn't help but notice my health was starting to suffer. I was exhausted after coming home, even if it was only an eight-hour shift. I would sit on the couch and wait until it was a reasonable hour so I could go to bed. I didn't have many hobbies; I was too tired to do anything after work. I dreaded any after-work class or activity I did sign up for, as I knew I would be too tired to participate. I envied my friends who weren't nurses, as they always had a ton of energy. I wasn't a Mom, and I don't think I could have been with that low of energy. I don't know how my coworkers, after a long day, would rush home to make dinner before whisking off their children to dance class or hockey practice—it made me tired just thinking about it.

Again, I looked inward, thinking something was wrong with me. I had my doctor check my bloodwork. I was eating healthy and exercising when I had the energy to do so ... so what could it be?

Again, many people in our department were suffering from something. Shoulder injuries, plantar fasciitis, chronic illness, constant flu and colds going around. Everyone else seemed to just manage, or at the least put up with it. So I sucked it up, too.

I chalked my lack of energy up to stress in my personal life. I had lost my father when I was twenty-five to cancer and my mother when I was thirty to opioid overdose. I knew my stress was a factor. But a full year after Mom's passing and dealing with the estate, I felt like I had "dealt" with the grief, too—so why was I still so exhausted?

After my half-brother and aunt both had heart attacks in the same month a couple years later, I realized I was right back in my hypervigilant state—I had probably never left it, truly. I decided to take time off of work to fully deal with all I had gone through in the last seven years. I hadn't ever dedicated time to healing for myself, despite being in a profession where I supposedly help others heal. This is typical of a health care worker—putting others first. I decided it was time to put me first, as I clearly wasn't coping.

These experiences all occurred before the pandemic, before burnout was becoming commonplace. It was the hardest thing I had ever done, admitting I wasn't okay and that I needed help. I had always been the "strong one"—for my parents, then my sister, to my friends and family. Now they would know I was a fraud, and that really, I wasn't able to handle it all. I knew I had to do it anyway, and my doctor was more than sympathetic and placed me on stress leave, writing me a note for six weeks off.

The time I had off was instrumental to my healing. Being away from work gave me the ability to look at things clearly—I had been neglecting myself for a long time. Getting professional help, learning skills to help me cope with people-pleasing and boundaries, I felt certain that I was going to go back and be healthier, more assertive, and happier. I had the skills to say no now! What could go wrong?

But as I began to become more of myself—more assertive, surer of my needs—I realized I was fighting a very uphill battle.

Having been the instigator of change for several projects in the department, I was now taking on the big task of asking for more staff in one of the busiest areas, Interventional Radiology. With the new procedures and increased acuity in the hospital, our workload (and overtime) had increased dramatically, and we were drowning on a daily basis. We were also doing double the amount of on-call shifts because nurses from the floor were no longer accompanying the patient. These changes came in very close together, yet there had been no increase in staffing. We were burned out. Staying late nearly every day, the cases becoming more complex, the patients more acutely ill, it was taking its toll on all of us. I proposed a trial to have an extra nurse in the department to help with break relief, turning over rooms, and generally helping out to make us more efficient and less chaotic.

Despite my new skills I had acquired around boundary setting, I was falling into similar patterns as before. My need to fix (stemming from the people-pleasing and perfectionistic tendencies) was still happening. I also learned the painful lesson that just because I asked for help didn't mean I was going to get it. I recall mustering up the courage to ask some of my colleagues for support with the task I had already agreed to take on of proving we needed more staff in the department, and I was met with crickets. It was one of the more painful silences I had ever experienced. I had thought naively that if I had the courage to ask for help (probably the hardest thing on the planet for me to do), I would receive it. Bueller? Bueller? Anyone?

Yet the need for change was there. There was more and more work being piled on us, we were staying for more and more overtime, and we were expected to do it with the same amount of staff. And, while perhaps my own people-pleasing nature was manifesting itself in this way, I wasn't alone. My colleagues were bending over backwards to fit cases in, the phone was ringing nonstop, and the radiologists were surrounded by staff physicians demanding we "do" their patients that day. We were all suffering from trying to do too much in one way or another. And we were taking out our stress and frustration on each other. As I was beginning to open my eyes to how "normal" this had become, I realized how unhealthy the environment was that I was placing myself in every day.

We had to fight for everything, from new lead that wasn't falling apart to cleaning products that weren't carcinogenic. Coming from an Irish background, I am used to being feisty—it's in my blood. But I was tired of fighting for things that should be a given. And unfortunately, many of my colleagues had resigned themselves to just putting up with it, counting down their days to retirement.

The Paradigm Shift

I couldn't control it. I couldn't control the workload, I couldn't control the lack of staff, and I couldn't control upper management's lack of support. I realized (finally) that the only thing I could control was my reaction to it—and, inevitably, my participation in it. I started making changes that I could actually control—and my life began to shift.

I stopped picking up extra call shifts. I went to the bathroom when I needed to, not just timed in between cases. I eventually quit my position and picked up shifts as a casual staff member, as it meant I didn't have to do call anymore. When I began to focus on what was best for me instead of fighting for the inequities I witnessed, things really shifted. I noticed I was calmer and happier as I went into work, and had more energy when I left it.

Things may have stayed the same for others, but they were better for me. It was hard seeing my colleagues struggling with the same issues as before (and even harder not to get sucked into the drama), but despite things being relatively the same for others, I felt like I was finally in charge of my own life. I did have to endure some snarky comments and some side glances as I began to say no to overtime at the end of the day, and I'm sure that there were some underlying thoughts that I was no longer a team player. It was really hard coming to the realization that as I was putting myself first, some of the colleagues I knew and loved were still overstretching themselves. I had to shift my focus from this, as it caused me anguish to see, and instead concentrate on the fact that I felt happier and freer than I had in years.

I had tried being an advocate for my colleagues through projects, perfectionism, and people-pleasing—it may have gotten some results, but it left me drained and bitter in the process. Once I let go of this, I became a happier person, which, if I looked really closely, was probably the best thing I could do for the people around me. Being happier allowed me to focus more clearly on my work, on my patients, and on my colleagues. I was more laid back, and I handled stress better.

It all started with putting my needs above everything else. I needed to heal, I needed to learn new skills, and I needed to reflect. Once I gifted myself with that, I had the clarity to make better decisions, ones that positively impacted my life.

Soul Purpose

It is why I am writing this. I am passionate about sharing what I have learned and helping others who are seeking guidance around these issues. Those of us in health care know we are in crisis. It has been long coming, and the pandemic has only expedited what we knew would occur. Health care workers are leaving the bedside in droves. The American Nurses Foundation found that the pandemic is causing 92% of nurses to consider leaving the workforce, with nearly half citing insufficient staffing as one of the primary reasons.[1] If we want to continue working in health care, we have a long road ahead of us. We need a paradigm shift.

My intention for this book is to help you along the path that I walked, hold your hand as you go through your own healing journey, and give you the tools and guidance that I found the most helpful as I navigated my own path to healing.

To be clear, I don't have it all perfect. I still actively work on many of the topics listed here every day. I used to think that if I read enough books or took enough courses, my problems would magically be solved. Unfortunately, that's not how life works. Despite having done a lot of work, I still have days where I forget what I've learned (or don't care) and fall back into my old habits. The goal isn't perfection—it's having the awareness and some tools to deal with the bad days as best we can. What I do have is a lot of life experience, some that has helped me write this book. And I want you to learn from my mistakes.

My hope is that you, the reader, start to see yourself as your own priority. That the tools listed here help you as you navigate putting yourself first. That it gifts you knowledge and comfort as the uncomfortable feelings and situations that inevitably arise from doing so occur. Putting yourself first is one of the most difficult things you can do in life, *especially* as an empathetic person. It means disappointing people who are closest to you—for this shift will not only affect your work life, it will affect all aspects of you—not something easily done. But as we continue to battle the pandemic with as much courage and perseverance as we can muster, I have no doubt in my mind that courage is not an issue for you—you walk into work every day with a bravery that only few can claim they possess.

To get the most out of this book, I highly encourage you to complete the exercises listed. It will immerse you further into your own healing, and will help solidify the content so that it sticks. I know, I know—you have a lot on your plate (you wouldn't be reading this if you didn't), and it's easy to simply breeze through the pages. But like a yogi cannot stretch themselves further by simply looking at poses, neither can we embody what we have learned unless we act on our knowledge.

As a serial devourer of self-development texts, I can tell you that a few months later I might only remember a few lines from what might have been a book chockfull of wisdom. Even the ones that had exercises in them, if I neglected to partake in this step, I would soon forget what I had uncovered. What I did retain became easier the more I participated in the exercises listed. Some of them were uncomfortable; some were just a pain in the ass. However, it helped me not only remember what I had read, but it also helped move me forward in changing whatever it was I was looking to change.

If you feel you won't have the time, I promise you, doing these exercises will help you in being able to make more time for yourself. The time you invest in yourself now will pay off later. Give yourself permission to go through each chapter thoroughly and complete the exercises as you go. Try not to read ahead unless you have completed the exercises.

I have nothing but respect, compassion, and a deep sense of dedication for my health care workers. My vision for us is that we shift the paradigm of health care. That we go from taking care of not just others, but ourselves—first and foremost. That we begin to see that by neglecting our own needs, we inevitably neglect others, because we become too tired to participate in the career we have dedicated our lives to.

I hope to see a revolution in health care in my lifetime. As we commit to taking care of ourselves first, it sets in motion a significant shift in how health care operates, and forces the system to make the necessary alterations we on the front lines know have to be made.

May you feel empowered and more in control of living the life you want to be living. Now go pee, and let's dive into the next chapter.

EXERCISES

1. If you don't already have one, purchase a journal. It will be a convenient place to complete the exercises listed in this book, and it may spark the habit to continue journaling once you have completed it.

2. Think about what prompted you to choose your career. What life experiences did you have that may have influenced this decision?

3. Where do you believe you are facing challenges in your career today? What do you think you need in order to overcome these challenges? Write down a few ideas.

CHAPTER 2

The Patient Doesn't Come First, *YOU DO*

"For someone to develop genuine compassion towards others, first he or she must have a basis upon which to cultivate compassion, and that basis is the ability to connect to one's own feelings and to care for one's own welfare ... Caring for others requires caring for oneself." – The Dalai Lama

"Who comes first?"
"The patient!"
"Whose fault is it?"
"The nurse!"

This was a chorus we replied many times to my nursing instructor, Jacque, during our clinical rotation on a busy surgical unit in my second year of nursing school.

Jacque was intelligent, perceptive, and engaged with his students. His experience on the floors, ICU, and as an instructor was invaluable to me as I practiced for the first time in a hospital setting. He impressed upon us much responsibility in the hopes of guiding us to be credible, accountable nurses when we graduated.

Hearing that mistakes that occurred on the unit were often the responsibility of the nurse was nothing new. It was drilled into our heads that physicians who ordered the wrong dose for a medication would not be held liable, as it was the nurse who gave it. This became conditioning for us as we heard over and over that we were accountable for advocating for the patient, that the onus was on us, and that we would not be supported if we screwed up. Well-meaning faculty members warned us that we needed to practice defensive charting ("Not charted, not done!"), and we "wouldn't have a leg to stand on" if a situation went to court and we didn't chart thoroughly. They stressed that the physicians would not have our backs if they made an error and would try to pin it on us. We were warned our governing professional body was not there to support us but to protect the patient, and that we would have to be vigilant at all times to protect ourselves.

All of this came down on us while trying to adjust to shift work, remember how the spleen functioned, and maintain our sanity as we attempted to eliminate air bubbles from an IV line. It was a lot for us to endure in our education.

We were conditioned very early on that in order to survive, we had to practice nursing guardedly. While our well-intentioned faculty members were only trying to caution us about how the real nursing world functioned, it also instilled defensiveness and fear of retribution. This is very much how it operates today, yet I wonder how much of this culture exists because it was planted there.

I remember having a charting audit, and the phrase, "If this ever went to court …" kept coming up. Exasperated, I thought, *How many times do these things actually go to court? And how much are we attracting this mentality by operating under the threat of it happening?*

Unfortunately, there are cases arising in the United States that are proving my educator right. There are nurses who are being charged criminally for adverse patient outcomes. What's more, neither the hospitals nor the health authorities are supporting these nurses. They are facing every nurse's nightmare, and they are doing so without any backing. They become the scapegoat that only verifies our fear of punishment for our errors and our need for hypervigilance.

Think of how differently you would practice if you weren't afraid of being punished. It isn't just an occasional thought; it is ingrained into everything that we do. If a patient makes a complaint, we offer to fix the situation, not only for our own peace of mind, but out of fear that he or she will complain to patient relations, our managers, and our directors.

I once had a patient make a complaint against my colleague and me. She was mentally ill and under stress due to her prolonged illness. Her statement was full of inaccuracies, claiming that she didn't consent to the procedure she underwent despite signing the form, that we were unprofessional with her, etc. My manager knew that the patient's report wasn't accurate, yet she implored us to contact the patient and apologize, for fear that she would escalate it to patient relations. I got to practice my humility that day as I apologized to the patient, yet I wondered how much power we were giving her to repeat this performance with someone else.

Again, as the patient comes first, we obviously endeavor to ensure that every need is met, despite the damage it might be doing. While I am not saying that it was wrong to apologize to this patient, it caused me to stop and think about how we all are conditioned to the patient always coming first, even when the patient is making false claims. Even in higher-up positions in management and administration, the perspective is that we do all that we can so we don't sacrifice patient care.

Yet while our health care organization is claiming this, they are also sacrificing frontline health care members in the process. They may not close beds, but they will cut staff ratios in an effort to cut costs. They may not decrease wait times for procedures, but they will slash or alter quality of supplies in an effort to save dollars.

The pandemic did nothing but attack all of our areas of potential weakness. What we were barely sustaining is currently crumbling in the wake of COVID. This virus has exposed not only a weakness in our immunity, but in the very structures that are meant to confine and heal it.

While we as health care workers (HCWs) are decrying these actions, we are also working harder with less in order to get the job done. We also don't want to sacrifice patient care, so we sacrifice ourselves in order to give the same quality of treatment to our patients. Fitting cases in, trying to juggle full emergency rooms, and having over-capacity units while we struggle to get through our day—all of this is a result of attempting to put the patient first. Our conditioning has worked so well, that we do put the patients first.

And we put ourselves last.

All of us operate under this paradigm, from nurses to physicians to management to our government. The patients have always come first.

Well, I am here to challenge this perspective.

Putting Ourselves First

Nurses make up the largest group of workers in the health care field, at more than twenty million worldwide.[1] We are the backbone of health care—what occurs in our profession directly affects patient care. And what affects our profession often rolls into other health care professions—positively or negatively.

There is also a worldwide shortage of nurses, and has been for many years, due to reasons such as high rates of retirement, turnover, and a sicker population.[2] There is not enough effort executed on increasing retention, and therefore, we are leaving the profession in droves.

We, along with our allied health counterparts, our health care aides, our technologists, our respiratory therapists, our physiotherapists and occupational therapists, our dieticians, our pharmacists, our lab techs, have been sacrificing ourselves since the beginning of the profession. Being female-dominated, those in our field have learned to care for others, often neglecting our own care. This has been occurring for generations, within the profession of nursing and allied health care, as well as in our homes. We are often natural caregivers, and we feel good when we care for others.

This is a wonderful ability to have, yet it is also our weak spot. In caring for others, we can neglect our own needs for so long that we ourselves become unwell. Self-care becomes nonexistent when we become wrapped up the care of our patients, our kids, and our extended families.

When we neglect our own needs, slowly but surely, the cracks begin to show. And where the crevices run deepest is in our health care systems. We have done much to try to remedy this, to no avail. We *must* have a paradigm shift if we are to actually, effectively change the trajectory of health care.

Beneficence

It starts with putting our own needs above all else. Selfless dedication and sacrifice were expected of health care workers in the old days—we have come a far way in engaging our managers and employers to prevent exploitation. However, it still exists where a HCW who does the bare minimum of what is expected of them is met with raised eyebrows and judgement. We are not required to be martyrs, yet there is still an underlying expectation that we go above and beyond every time.

Beneficence is defined as promoting someone else's good or welfare — "do no harm." With the state of health care as it is, this is becoming murkier and much more difficult to navigate. There is a difference between doing something we would prefer not to do (taking care of that bedbug patient) versus working past our ability to work safely. Our sense of duty is not always clearly defined. In the absence of our superiors creating a safe environment for us with which to practice, we need to start declaring it for ourselves.

I come first. I do. Before my patient.

My needs come first. I am a human being, and I have needs. I go to the bathroom when I need to, I take my breaks, I don't stay overtime (unless I actually want to). I don't rush, I don't try to lift a patient without adequate staff, I don't pull meds while doing another task. We all know that rushing leads to mistakes being made, yet we, in an effort to accommodate all of our patients, have a tendency to rush in order to get everything done. We stay late so a patient doesn't have to wait longer for a procedure. We pick up OT so our coworkers don't work short. We sacrifice ourselves every single day in order to achieve what is becoming an insurmountable goal. And because we are still technically functioning, this demonstrates to everyone that it is manageable.

By putting others first—yes, including the patient—we have contributed to an environment that is toxic. Busy units with understaffing create toxicity. The patients are upset, the staff are snapping at each other, and administration is deaf to our concerns. We are walking into a warzone of our own making. Each time there is a cut of any kind on a unit, from staffing to supplies to procedures, the fact that we continue to function, that we continue to make it work, only signals to management that they were right to make the cut—that obviously, the unit is still functional. Which then prompts the question, "Where else can we cut from?"

I don't mean to say that management and the higher administration have an easy time of it—of course, they don't want to cut from their units if they don't have to. But if we continue to allow it to happen, if we start cutting corners ourselves, this will just show that we can function with less. And we have been doing this for ages. There is a reason nursing is targeted when fiscal restraints are introduced. We have been lowest on the totem pole because this is the example we have created in our health care system. By putting the patients first, we are putting ourselves last. And when nursing takes a hit, the other health care staff are not far behind.

Shifting the Paradigm

In his book *Us vs Them: The Failure of Globalism,* Ian Bremmer discusses what happens to a population that has reached its limit:

"Why do Palestinians throw rocks? To attract attention? To improve their lives? To make progress toward creation of a Palestinian state? They throw rocks because they want others to see that they've had enough, that they can't be ignored, and that they can break things. Voting isn't helping them. Outsiders don't care. Where are the opportunities to bring about change? There is nothing left but to throw rocks. In that sense, there will soon be Palestinians all over the world."[3]

When we put ourselves last, so does everyone else. Frontline workers are at the point now where we are throwing rocks because we don't have any hope that anyone will listen. We know that cutting HCWs only affects patients in the long run, yet the government and health authorities can continue to claim that they have not compromised patient care. They can claim this because we are just working harder to keep the status quo. And it is putting us in jeopardy. Our licenses are on the line each time there are cutbacks. Then, when things get bad, we leave the profession, we strike, we demand better working conditions and better pay. And sometimes this is granted—we are in this stage right now, and we were back in the '90s. And things get better for a while, until they decide to cut again. This cycle has been occurring for years and years. And I for one, am fed up with it.

Instead of throwing rocks, however, I decided to put myself first. The only way we can take back our power is to put ourselves first.

This concept will probably stir up a lot of emotions and fears. Yes, the idea is nice to put ourselves first. But how do we justify this when we have been called to a profession that involves taking care of others? Many of us are bound by a code of ethics for our professions that govern how we practice. Yet, with how the health care system has deteriorated, the ability to follow our Code of Ethics often conflicts with our morality and our own needs. How do we provide quality care when there are not enough resources? Do we take each patient and give 100% for them, leaving nothing for our other patients? Or do we do the bare minimum for all of them, knowing that each patient will receive suboptimal care? Our Code of Ethics, while ideal, is becoming more of a figurehead for us instead of an actual governing rule in the health care system we have. Instead of blindly following it, we need to re-evaluate what this code means for us and our own health, not only our patients'.

Nursing ethics can be referred to as "the expressed norms of the nursing profession: the values, virtues, and principles that are supposed to govern and guide nurses in everyday practice. It can also be referred to the moral dimension of nursing where various issues are analyzed, discussed and debated."[4] For nurses, the Canadian Nurses Association (CAN) and the American Nurses Association (ANA) both have a code of ethics that provides a knowledge base for the policies and laws that govern our practice.

Each health profession has a code of ethics that creates criteria through which the profession can evaluate members. They provide guidance for members about their own conduct. The code of ethics continually makes revisions to reflect how health care evolves, therefore, "codes of ethics cannot address all issues, and cannot provide complete guidance."[5] We use this as a model, not as a rule. "As important as they are, codes, policies, or laws cannot take the place or eliminate the need for ethical decision-making. For one thing, they are bound to be vague or silent about many ethical issues that arise ... Even when they are explicit, the answer that was once simply doing what was mandated by a code, policy, or law is never enough to satisfy the demands of ethical accountability."[6]

Unilateral decision-making affects the ability to provide quality care, and many health care workers are not educated in how to combat this. Policies become implemented without our input in order to cut costs, and this brings up concerns for patient safety. We unfortunately have taken a passive role when we face these changes, unsure of how to navigate policy reform without knowing the stakeholders who implemented them. This could be due to being a female-dominated profession, being oppressed and unable to affect working conditions, and fear of being reprimanded or shunned for speaking up. This contributes to our complicity and our subsequent feelings of powerlessness.

Moral Autonomy

The distribution of power in how health care is organized outlines many of the ethical issues we face. Through our actions or passivity, we can influence matters for good or bad. Becoming autonomous means being accountable for what we do (or fail to do). Reflection is essential to this process. According to Yeo, et al., blindly following authorities, professional expectations, the law, or our peers is pre-reflective reasoning.[7]

As we begin to examine the situation we have inherited, we question what is and what is not feasible, and our practice reflects this. In taking responsibility for what we believe is the "right" thing to do, and not simply blindly following policy, we become more confident in our values and we practice integrity. Health care is rapidly changing; our policies often do not keep up with these changes. What is more, policymakers are often out of touch with the current weather of health care, and following policy blindly is not always possible—it just isn't. Having people in places of authority enforce these policies (and reprimand those who are not following it) is detrimental to the staff, the patients, and the organization. With bureaucracy impeding the ability to change policy quickly (it can take years to simply update an existing document), we are buried in red tape and effectively powerless to prompt change when necessary.

But, as we witnessed in the pandemic, this is not always the case. Daily policy changes occurred as health authorities seemingly made it up as they went. Policy can and does change quickly when it needs to. Do we wait for policymakers to exact necessary change, or, having witnessed that this process can be streamlined, do we take it upon ourselves to make change that better suits the needs of the department, the patients, and the staff under the conditions of crisis that we are currently witnessing? Unquestioning obedience (something a "good" nurse was once expected to be) is inconsistent with moral autonomy.

The Beneficence of Putting Ourselves First

When we shift our responsibility to ourselves first, many things occur.

First, we become clearer, calmer, and more rested. We are able to do our work from a grounded perspective, which helps us prioritize better. We have more energy, get more enjoyment out of life, and the people in our personal and professional lives benefit because we are more present.

Second, changes happen as a result of our refusal to sacrifice ourselves. When we become aware of our worth, we stop putting up with unsafe working conditions and maltreatment. The uncomfortable part of this is that we can see in real time that patient care begins to deteriorate. Obviously, I am not including emergencies in this example, and of course if a patient's life is at risk, we address it. I am talking about nonurgent tasks that are involved in patient care, tasks that we deal with on a daily basis and often put before our own needs. Medication administration, dressing changes, transfers, mobilizing, hygiene—all aspects of care that we provide that the patient relies on us for. Care that we are struggling to manage, as we have so many patients to look after. Care that has become more complex as the patients' needs have increased. Care that we are rushing through to get to the next task in a never-ending list of tasks.

The truth is, patient care is already unsafe—we've just managed to keep the balls up in the air. If you look at the cuts to patient care over the years, the quality we are able to deliver has been deteriorating for a long time. Because it has happened gradually, we haven't noticed. I graduated from nursing school in 2007, and, over the course of my fifteen years as a nurse, the amount of time I spent with each patient decreased every year. I cannot recall any change that was ever made that was better for patient care (unless it was a result of something bad happening); it all had to do with cost. So, whether we allow patients to suffer now or suffer later, the end product is the same. And we are more burned out as a result.

It is no coincidence in my mind that as we HCWs become more stressed and unhealthier ourselves, the health of our patients deteriorates as well. We are sick people taking care of sick people. How can we expect our society as a whole to improve their health when our own is suffering? How can we claim to be adept at taking care of others when we don't know how to take proper care of ourselves? If *we* aren't eating, sleeping, and resting properly, how can we expect our patients to?

By shifting the focus from the patient to ourselves, we not only become healthier and better equipped to give, the gap in patient care will have to be addressed from another standpoint. Think of what would happen if all HCWs decided to come to work and address their own needs before tending to the patients. They would work at a reasonable pace, take care of a reasonable ratio of patients, and take all of their breaks in a timely manner. If we refused to accept all of the unacceptable working conditions all at once, it would be pandemonium. If we stood united in putting ourselves first and refused to do things to compensate (e.g., staying OT, working short, missing our breaks), it would quickly become apparent to everyone involved that we have a broken system—something frontline staff have known all along.

The scope of practice has expanded, we have regulatory standards and a code of ethics to guide decision-making, and we are accountable for our decisions and actions. We raise concerns when we receive orders that we do not believe are in the patient's best interest. "When collaboration and discussion have not resolved the difference of opinion, nurses are not obligated to follow orders that they believe are harmful to patients."[8] While this was meant for such instances as medication orders, it can also apply to other aspects of care. When there is a discrepancy that cannot be resolved with the staff involved (e.g., a doctor reprimanding a nurse who refused to follow an order), regulatory colleges and employers should have guidelines in place about what the next steps are. We are not forced to do anything, even if it sometimes appears this way.

When patients' needs compete with the employers', we can feel trapped. We should not accept the role of being powerless, and we have a moral obligation to address these issues. An example is assignment refusal due to workload—refusing to take on more than what is feasible puts us in a difficult moral dilemma. Activism in this respect can be difficult for us to navigate, and nearly impossible if we work alone—we need other like-minded colleagues to take these concerns to professional, regulatory, and labour organizations. To not do so is actually turning our backs on our ethical commitments. This can also be in circumstances where our ability to practice safely is compromised due to performing tasks outside of our scope. This could include menial tasks that take us away from the level of care we should be performing, or expecting us to perform tasks that we lack the knowledge, skill, or judgement to provide the expected level of care in order to practice safely.

Where there is a concern for safety, such as when dealing with aggressive/violent patients, there is also expectation to care for these individuals. We have the right to say no in these situations, however much our managers, directors, or health authorities may have us believe otherwise. They are not going to swoop in and save us if we are practicing in unsafe working conditions unless we speak up. We must be strong advocates for ourselves, and this involves being proactive in finding ways to change what has become the norm. We have the education, we have the research, and we have the professional organizations (such as unions) that have our backs. Action, such as campaigns and educating the public, can be taken. We simply need to care about ourselves as much as we care about our patients.

It's time.

The employer is responsible for adequate staffing, adequate training, and adequate resources. They are the ones who are liable for failing to provide these to us. It is time the onus falls on the people it was meant to. We as frontline workers have done our best to make things work, out of compassion for our patients, our colleagues, and ourselves. We are no longer able to control what was never supposed to be our responsibility. We need to be brave in holding the proper parties accountable.

During a pandemic, we must be provided with a safe environment, and this evidently did not always occur. We are entitled to high-quality equipment. In specific regards to working through a pandemic, "When (HCWs) are not supported through enough education, communication systems, and infection control departments, and lack a safe environment, they are justified in withdrawing care."[9]

Obviously, before doing so, we should be advocating for improvements and offer recommendations. "The nurse's health and welfare is a priority. When they face serious risks, nurses are justified in exercising moral autonomy to protect their health. In doing so, nurses are enacting professional integrity because they have assumed control over and accountability for their professional lives."[10]

When we say no, which is within our ethical power to do, it forces our superiors to investigate other ways of doing things. We have been carrying their load, trying to make things work, for too long, to our detriment.

When we refuse to perform unsafe work, we feel we may be putting the patient at risk. In actuality, we are becoming the first step to making things BETTER for the patient. By declaring that we are ethically enforcing our right to protect ourselves, we ARE protecting the patient—and it requires the stakeholders who make the decisions that affect the departments to make better ones. Management and above would be forced to investigate other avenues. They are well aware that they cannot allow the patient to have unsafe conditions, and when we refuse to submit to unsafe policies, they must create different ones—this is their scope, their jobs on the line now. Now we have involved them at a level that requires them to participate actively instead of from the ethers. Then real change could start occurring, and we could start putting funding into primary rather than tertiary care, prevention rather than putting out fires (where all of the money is currently going). If we forced them to look elsewhere instead of targeting frontline workers, perhaps they would finally listen. The prescription of prevention would keep costs low and our patients healthier. We do have the power to make radical change—and it starts with putting ourselves first.

The tension between morals and reality has long been a recurrent theme in ethics. When these situations arise, we feel powerless unless there is collaboration between us and administrators and policy-makers. We also feel fear being the person who stands up for ourself and our patients. "(HCWs) who blow the whistle can suffer a range of serious physical and mental health problems."[10] Despite many of our employers having whistle-blowing policies in place to protect the person who has spoken out, we are still suffering the effects of doing so – so we say nothing. Instead of waiting for our moral distress to get the better of us (or our licenses to be in question), many of us are choosing to leave the profession instead. By shifting the perspective to putting our needs above others (and actually carrying it out), we will begin to see the shift in the health of our patients. Having the courage to sit with the discomfort that the first stages of this paradigm shift will create (like any other type of change) will allow real, lasting change to occur. Using our superpower, which is empathy, on ourselves, we will allow that change to happen.

Society has conditioned us to put others' needs above our own for generations. The hard-working ethic that we have grown up admiring, the respect of our parents' and grandparents' generations, has done wonders for our economy. Work hard or be considered lazy. Be kind and courteous, give of yourself, desire less. Don't ask for more than you need—for this is greed. If you put yourself first, you are being selfish. Whether it be from a nobility or religious standpoint, we are rewarded for being "good"—usually meaning being "selfless". Society rewards us when we work hard, when we do for others, when we give.

How convenient this viewpoint is for the economy—it creates a people who work more with less. Perfect. Having a good work ethic not only makes us good people, it makes us good employees. Many of us in health care who support this principle are now running on empty. Our system is now reliant on us overworking ourselves in order to function. Depends on that person who works all of the overtime. Sets store by our caring nature to sacrifice our own needs in order to provide adequate patient care.

Newsflash: We shouldn't have to sacrifice ourselves in order to provide basic care to our patients. We shouldn't be expected to forgo our breaks so our patients get their meds or dressing changes or any other routine care. We shouldn't be asked to take back our vacation because we are short, or take on higher patient loads because there are less of us.

But we are.

And other than an occasional pathetic pizza party, we aren't getting anything in return. I don't know about you, but a cold slice of Domino's looks pretty paltry compared to adequate sleep and time with loved ones.

We have been conditioned to believe that we shouldn't ask for anything in return for our sacrifice. The health care system is a narcissistic boyfriend that keeps taking while we keep giving. And it will never be enough. Because as we give more, they expect more. Our feeling that this is our calling, that it's the "right thing to do," or our genuine concern for our patients' welfare will not change any of this.

It is evident on the constantly-short units. The reasons for this are many: we are absent because we have overworked ourselves. We are either physically or mentally unable to cope with the idea of running uphill for twelve hours, so we call in sick. We are unable to work fulltime hours on a unit that drains us every day, so we go part-time or casual. We burn out on high-acuity units, and so look for other areas within the health care field, or we leave the field altogether. And the younger generation takes one look at the situation and says, "I'll pass" ... leaving us remaining to figure it out.

We feel guilty for asking for our basic needs to be met, for desiring to be comfortable instead of in a constant state of working, to have some time to ourselves. Have you ever craved some alone time, and once granted it, you felt guilty for sitting and "doing nothing"? This is conditioning—it is not customary to have time to sit and be with ourselves, and our mental health is suffering as a result. While this mindset may not have been created immediately, over time, we have eroded our sense of self, of the right to say no, of the ability to demand our basic needs be met.

Never has this position been more prevalent among health care professionals. Our tireless dedication to serving the sick and the dying has always given us a reputation that we are kind, compassionate, giving souls who have answered a calling. From the era of nuns nursing alongside physicians during wars and plagues, health care workers have been immortalized as the perpetual martyrs where self-sacrificing was their purpose in life—and they should feel grateful to be given this honor. *Don't you dare complain about being run off your feet or exhausted or simply requesting a bathroom break. You are blessed to be in the position you are in, you have your health while the poor souls you take care of are suffering. Be gracious in this gift you have been bestowed to tend to the sick and dying.* From doctors to nurses to all other allied health, it is a privilege to provide care to others.

Basically, shut up and do your job.

And generations later, we are still being told to shut up and do our jobs.

Mercifully, in the wake of the helicopter parenting and the millennial mothers who are expected to do it all and the epidemic of chronic illness (coupled with an opioid crisis) and mental health issues (coupled with record amounts of antidepressant and antianxiety prescriptions and suicide rates), self-care has entered the forefront to combat these issues.

Why the Self-Care Movement?

The self-care movement puts the power back in our court. We have the ability to make changes to our lives, to make better decisions, and to bring balance back. It starts with us. More and more of us are waking up to realize that the lives we are living aren't sustainable. That it's not that we just need to suck it up or rely on prescriptions or caffeine to get us through, but that no human can thrive in the chaotic lives we have created for ourselves, no matter how society expects us to be able to handle it.

While this movement has made strides in many areas, it hasn't quite transferred to health care yet. How ironic that a movement teaching people how to take better care of themselves hasn't extended to professions that's entire structure is based on taking care of people.

How are we supposed to take care of others if we aren't adequately taking care of ourselves? It's ludicrous. Our patients put their faith in us to take care of them. Please, let us encourage our patients to get adequate rest when in the hospital (while we miss our breaks), suggest taking time off work to heal from a surgery (while we show up to work sick), scold them for not adhering to a diabetic diet (while we scarf down whatever tidbits -Timbits?- are left in the breakroom). It's insanity.

If I hired a fitness trainer, I would expect them to be fit. How can our patients trust us with their health when we are so obviously neglecting our own? The way we neglect our needs and disrespect our bodies, we may as well be paying Homer Simpson to be our fitness coaches. If I am not putting my health first before my job, I am a hypocrite. I should not be taken seriously when I educate my patients on their health if I am not taking my own health just as seriously as theirs. And deep down, a little part of us knows this. This is why we feel so tired all of the time, depressed, anxious, like something isn't right. We know there is a spiritual discord between what we are saying and what we are doing, even if only subconsciously.

This is called cognitive dissonance, and it wreaks havoc on our health, our mental well-being, and our ability to make healthy choices. When we believe one thing (and teach others this belief), yet act out in a way that is incongruent with this belief, it takes its toll. And it looks like exhaustion. It looks like depression and anxiety. It looks like burnout.

When we act in ways that are inconsistent with how we actually feel for a long period of time, it results in inner conflict and can lead to emotional exhaustion, decreased job satisfaction, and burnout.[11] Surface acting takes its toll on us, for we deny our human feelings and expressions while delivering patient care in order to be deemed "professional"—and it is slowly killing us.

We put an emphasis on health because it is our career to do so, yet our own health is suffering. This is wrong on so many levels.

We in health care are the true unsung heroes of society. We show up every day because we want to make the world a better place. We give of ourselves because we have an inherent desire to. We believe in serving humanity, and we go to great lengths to do so. Yet we have overextended ourselves too far too long. And we work in a system that has exploited our giving nature to such a degree that we are now the ones suffering as much as our patients are. We cannot bring them back to health when we are sick ourselves. If we are our environment, and our patients are healing in an environment that is surrounded by chaos, how can we expect our patients to actually get better?

We have been using our voices for years to decry the working conditions, the risk we see patients enduring. We have tried lobbying, writing our government members, complaining to our managers, all with little effect. Any short-term wins we get do little to tide us over when we negotiate our contract or gain media attention. With us already being exhausted (that being the issue in the first place), we have little fight in us left to fight for ourselves. Which is exactly what the policymakers want: keeping us too busy. Trying to keep up at work and too concerned about our patients to make a drastic effort (like striking). This keeps us from actually making real, lasting change. Like the aforementioned Palestinians, we are at the point of throwing rocks simply because nothing else seems to be working, and it is the only way to get out frustration.

No one is coming to save us.

It's time we saved ourselves.

It's time we put ourselves first.

It might sound harsh or uncaring to make the statement no one is coming to save us or bail us out. It might feel scary, even, that we are responsible for our own well-being. It isn't meant to be. In fact, it is the most empowering thing I can tell you. If you suddenly realized that nobody holds the key to your happiness except you, you would stop wasting your energy trying to get other people to make you happy and you would just do you.

We have tried to make others see what the situation is in health care—our managers, our administrators, our government. The more focus we put on others, regardless of the intent, the less we place on taking care of ourselves. Our attention is the most powerful tool we have – where we put our attention is where the power is. We have been feeling powerless because we have not been putting our attention directly on ourselves – anywhere but. When we focus on the scarcity of resources, the suffering patients, and the ineffective management, we only see more scarcity. By focusing on our own needs and abilities to do what we can, we aren't denying that the scarcity is there – we are choosing to put our power in what we can do – and that starts with making sure our needs are met first. The more we ruminate when we go home, the less rest and recovery we actually have for ourselves. What begins as a noble effort takes its toll on our health, thereby negating any good we wish we could be doing. Our attention is a powerful tool – just look at social media platforms, our attention is the currency. We need to start focusing our attention back on to our well-being. The key to our own health lies within ourselves.

As you begin to look more closely at your own areas in need of healing, the more you will realize how much you are in need of your own self-nurturing. I promise you—once you start putting your own needs first, miraculous things will occur.

Showing up for ourselves is the only way we are going to be able to make a drastic shift in the health of our patients. By shifting our responsibility on to ourselves, our own well-being, our own mental health, we make a bold statement to those who are benefitting from us being overworked and under-resourced.

Billion-dollar tech companies know that the best way to increase productivity and quality of their products is to treat their employees well. Ample time spent in self-reflection allows for creativity to flow, and helps employees deliver superior products. The same goes for any career—we work better when we are rested, fed, and nurtured. If hospitals actually want the patients to recover quicker, they would offer care from people who are well looked-after themselves.

Our empathetic natures have put others' needs in front of our own for far too long. We know what it must feel like to be in our patients' shoes (an ability not everyone has the gift of having), and so our hearts go out to them. When we miss a break, or stay overtime, or pick up a double, it is our patients who we are thinking of. It is their needs we have in the forefront of our minds, not our own. We worry what will happen if the unit runs short, or if no one picks up that shift. We think of our other coworkers who are struggling to keep up, and our hearts go out to them, too. We have the ability to feel others' suffering at the core of us, and it pains us to think that this is so when we may have the ability to stop that suffering.

Yet we are neglecting our needs in doing so. As noble as these actions are, they are also part of the reason we are in the health care crisis we are in—and we were in one long before the pandemic. We need to start putting ourselves first. No one else is going to do it for us. We need to start taking our own health seriously, before we become patients ourselves.

Let's try an experiment. Imagine you are watching someone you love—your daughter, let's say—and they have chosen your profession. They are living the life that you have created for yourself—your job, your family, your obligations. How does this make you feel? Do you see no issue with this, because you live a balanced life? Or would you feel sad for her, watching her go through the motions of life without really having time or energy to actually enjoy it? Would it be hard to watch her be disrespected by people at work, not taking her breaks and missing meals, and coming home too tired to play with her kids?

If you wouldn't wish this lifestyle on your daughter, why is it okay for you? When you have a parent who is a nurse and she implores you not to go into nursing (as many nurses do), there is a problem.

Take all of that empathy, that compassion that you have for others, and gift it to yourself. You deserve to be living a happy, healthy life. You deserve to have balance in your life. You deserve to have your basic needs met, at work and outside of work.

You are worthy of leading the life you want. You are worthy of positive change in your life. You are worthy of asking for your needs to be met.

You are allowed to say no. You are respecting yourself and your needs when you honor them before others. It isn't selfish, it's actually what is expected of you as a human being. Your responsibility is to take care of yourself. Sometimes we see ourselves taking care of others, and we wonder who is taking care of us. I subconsciously expected there to be someone there for me when there wasn't—there was only me. You are responsible for taking care of you, and only you know what that looks like. Only you know how to get your needs met (unless you don't, and if so, this book is a great place to start). It is a paradigm shift in health care that is a long time coming: healers learning to heal themselves.

By initiating this paradigm shift in our own lives, we give others permission to do the same—our patients, colleagues, and our friends and families. By leading the self-care movement, we set an example to others that taking care of ourselves is top priority. When we refuse overtime because we recognize we are tired, it sets an example for others. When we decline attending an event because we need our rest, it plants a seed in others who were hoping to do the same, and simply needed someone else to say it first. As health care professionals, people look to us to set an example.

When we start taking our needs seriously, so will our patients, families, and loved ones. Their trust in us to do the right thing for our own health will extend to others, and we as a society will become healthier as a result.

This is, thankfully, something within our own power to do. We don't need to wait for a colleague to change units, or for our manager to retire, or for a new government to be elected. We can manage our own needs without anyone else telling us how to do it. It is something we get to define, something that belongs to us personally, something that we get to control.

It is time we take our power back.

And it starts with putting ourselves first.

EXERCISES

1. What areas of your life have you been putting others' needs above your own? How long have you been doing this, and when did it start? Who or what do you think contributed to this learned behavior?

2. Imagine what it would look like if you started putting your needs first. How do you think that would play out? What barriers do you foresee hindering you from putting your needs first?

CHAPTER 3

The Stages of Putting Yourself First

"The woman you are becoming will cost you people, relationships, spaces, and material things. Choose her over everything." – Unknown

I lost both of my parents quite young. My father died at fifty-four of esophageal cancer when I was still a new nurse, and my mother died of an opioid overdose (a suspected suicide) five years later. Losing them under those circumstances, and so close together, my grieving process was long and messy.

Despite being a nurse and learning about Kubler-Ross' stages of grief from her book *On Death and Dying* in school, I didn't have an easier time of it.[1] If anything, my knowledge was a barrier. I thought I knew how grief worked (oh, how naïve I was), and because I knew what to expect, I thought I would be better prepared. A small part of me thought that because I had read about it and had experienced death in my work that I would have a leg up. Wrong.

While I was unfortunately inundated with responsibilities with each parent's passing and didn't have time to process their deaths in the moment, I also didn't gift myself that time later. I thought that after a year of sorting out accountants and lawyers, I would have also sorted out my feelings. I didn't feel much sadness or anger; I wasn't in denial—well, not about their deaths, anyway. I was in denial of having "dealt" with my feelings, that much became clear.

It took a long time to start unraveling all of the complexities around the grief I had with losing my parents. I still don't think I have fully transcended the experience, although it is less painful to think about. The resentment, the hypervigilance, and the shame and guilt (mostly around the relief I felt when they passed)—were all wrapped up in a messy ball. It has taken a lot of reflection, working with others, and accepting my feelings for what they were, to bring me to the place I am now. Once I began working on my grief in earnest, all of the emotions that had been buried while I was focusing on estate taxes and selling belongings were waiting to be seen.

Absolutely, there was sadness. There was also anger—a lot of anger. I was resentful of many things—the burden I was put through bearing, the lack of support,

---

the unfairness of it all. Once I let a lot of it out, it developed into a full-blown depression. This happened nearly ten years after my father passed, and five years after my mother. The feelings I had ignored boomeranged back with much more force; I felt like I had been hit by a truck.

But it needed to come out.

One beautiful gift that arose out of this experience was that I realized I needed to put myself first. My parents had been unwell for most of my life (mentally and physically), and I was enmeshed in their illnesses from a young age. I felt responsible for their actions, their moods, their outbursts. My childhood-self rationalized that must mean I was responsible for when they were doing well, when they laughed, when they seemed happy. Not having them anymore created a void, an emptiness. I didn't know who I really was. I identified myself as a caregiver, a crusader, and as a victim, perhaps, of a difficult upbringing. It was a source of pain, but it was also a source of strength. I felt strong to be able to "handle" it.

That eviscerated with their passings. I was left an empty shell, one who didn't know who she was unless she was taking care of others.

While it took me a bit to catch on to this (some hypervigilance and distractions with work to fill the hole in the meantime), I eventually got the message. Why was I filling up my life with projects? And why, when things that happened outside of my control (my aunt and brother's heart attacks in the same week) did I jump into action? I couldn't relax—I knew I was neglecting parts of myself that needed attention, and I was distracting myself from dealing with them. I didn't think I was afraid, per se, but I certainly wasn't making it a priority. My people-pleasing had been a coping mechanism for ignoring what I didn't want to deal with. Once I had dealt with a big chunk of the issues, I realized I was still people-pleasing. I had gone so long placating others that I really didn't know how to prioritize myself. It was just easier to focus on someone else.

One thing I noticed when I began prioritizing my own needs is that there were striking similarities between the process of putting myself first and the process of grief.

In some ways, it makes sense. The old "me" who had been putting others first was in the process of dying. The new "me" is learning how to recognize my needs, prioritize my wants, and carry out my desires. There was no room for the new version of me if I was still catering to others all of the time.

Death of Our Identity

Putting ourselves first is a death process. When we fully embody the paradigm shift that is putting ourselves first, a lot in our lives changes. When we have not been prioritizing our needs above others, it means our whole lives need to shift in order to accommodate this. Many of us, especially women, were not brought up in this way. We were taught it is good and noble to think about others first. We live our lives based on what others need, and many of us don't even think about what we, ourselves, need. Our lives are built around serving others, especially as health care workers. For many of us, putting ourselves first means significant changes to our lives. It can seem big, daunting, and overwhelming to think about.

So we don't.

It's not until the cracks start to show that we really have to start looking at what is sustainable for us. These cracks can look like having a hard time getting out of bed. They can look like not being able to face work. They can look like our marriages being in jeopardy. They can look like a serious health diagnosis.

When we face the music that we cannot be everything to everybody, and that we will have to make significant changes to our lives in order to take care of ourselves for the first time, it can be the scariest thing we will do. And sometimes we don't know how we can fix it—all we know is that we can't keep going on like this. Being in a place where we know we can't continue, but we don't know what to do, is still further than where we were before this realization. It's okay not to have all the answers yet.

When we are ready to prioritize what is most important, it can feel like we are losing part of who we are. We miss being the person who helps others in their time of need. We yearn for the hit of serotonin we get when we solve a loved one's problem. We FOMO the shit out of all of the events we have to say no to. People around us are going to notice the old "us" isn't around as much. They are going to grieve that as much as we do.

Kubler-Ross' stages of grief come into play when we start putting ourselves first. There will be experiences and feelings that show up when we start setting healthy boundaries with others, and they will be tough at times—really tough. Unlike the traditional situational grief that often comes from something that we can't change (death, the end of a relationship, etc.), putting ourselves first can be messy, everchanging, and difficult to navigate. We technically do have a choice, whether we want to go back to our old lifestyle of over-giving, which is what makes it so challenging to keep going when difficult situations arise. Just like a new exercise program or starting a new job, change can be scary and mentally exhausting. *You* have to be the one to decide if it is worth sticking out, or if you would prefer to go back to how you were living.

Also, as exemplified in the stages of grief, the feelings/experiences might not show up in order, and we might return to feelings we experienced at the beginning of our healing path. This doesn't mean we are regressing—it means layers that have been buried are coming up. Just like anything that heals, the gross stuff has to come to the surface before it can truly begin to heal (wound care nurses, y'all know what I'm talking about). And as we know with diabetic feet, sometimes that takes a lot of time, strategies, and sometimes setbacks before we're on our way. Health care workers, don't amputate—keep going.

Stages of Grief with Putting Ourselves First

Denial

This stage is one of the most difficult to navigate. All of our lives, we have been taught to give to others, to be generous, to be "good." At work, since we have had it drilled into us that the patient comes first, we don't recognize that our needs also matter—at least, not as much as we should. There are many reasons why we might be in denial of needing to put our needs ahead of others. We probably experience this stage for much longer than a typical situational grief occurrence, since we don't often have a specific incident that we can trace—for some of us, the majority of our lives is spent denying ourselves. Our over-giving starts slowly, and builds over time. Another reason we might be in this stage longer than other situations of grief is because as HCWs, we are surrounded by others who also over-give. Whether it is out of necessity (there is no one else to take care of the patient) or learned behavior to work until the point of exhaustion, we can't always see the forest from the trees. Just because it is normal where we are does NOT mean it is okay. Sometimes, though, this keeps us in denial. We don't see a way out, we don't see a point in trying to change anything, and with others around us in the same boat, we don't investigate further. Until something sparks in us (such as a major life event), we can remain in this stage for years.

Anger

Ah, our old pal, anger. As many of us HCWs are women, many of us are not on good terms with our anger. We shove it down and repress it. We are conditioned not to be angry, ever. Angry women are hysterical, crazy, bitches. We are not allowed to announce when we are mad over something, and we in turn feel guilt or shame when we feel it. We are often gaslighted when we try to express it, even when we have righteous anger, as it is deemed unprofessional. This delays our healing process, as addressing our anger is often the gateway to being able to move on.

Harkening back to our wound analogy, how often do we say a sore looks "angry"? As someone who had serious acne as a teen, this term is not foreign to me. Reddened, painful, erupting, our wounds go through an angry phase, too. We can throw salves or antibiotics at it to "calm it" (down, zit, down!), but we need to let the body do its job—and sometimes, it has to get worse before it gets better. It knows what to do, and it's even better if we let it do its thing. In regards to our emotions, our bodies need to release the anger in order to heal whatever caused it—and this means letting it out, not trying to stifle it or explain it away.

We are completely justified in our anger—we have been putting up with poor working conditions, sacrificing ourselves, and witnessing our patients suffer, all the while keeping our mouths shut in order to prevent fear by the public or out of our own fear of losing our jobs. If anything, our frustration with our current situation is subdued—I am fucking livid that we are in the health crisis we are in, mostly because we have spoken out and have not been heard. And I believe many of us, because we have been conditioned to stifle our anger in the workplace because it is "unprofessional," don't fully express what in fact should be full-blown rage at what is happening in our hospitals, clinics, and long-term care facilities.

Our anger also might show us how we have been tolerating too much in our personal lives. When I realized how long I had been putting up with being treated poorly, I got really angry. I had pushed it down over and over because I didn't think it was justified. Then I would blow up, and I would be labeled as angry, and I would believe it, feel remorse, and then not allow it to come up when I was treated badly. Lather, rinse, repeat.

Once I realized (with the help of a therapist) that I had been putting up with too much, something I didn't know because I had been abused as a child and had just thought it was normal, I was pissed. Pissed at being born into an abusive family, pissed at others for treating me like shit, pissed at being gaslighted, and pissed at myself for allowing it to happen over and over. I had to fully feel into this—allowing myself to feel anger at others (and myself) instead of justifying all of the reasons why. Emotions are a heart process, not a brain one—they don't compute why or how, they just are, until they are processed and released. And this didn't happen for me until I saw my anger as a tool for healing instead of something to be afraid of.

If you have been repressing your anger, or if you are finding you are easily irritated or frustrated, it might be a sign that you need to work with someone. Snapping at people occasionally is understandable, especially with what we in health care are going through. But it won't go away if we haven't dealt with what is causing our anger. Working with a therapist or reading books on anger are a good start. If the idea of this causes you to feel uncomfortable, that is okay. I was embarrassed by my anger when I first started healing, having been punished for it as a child. I felt like there was something wrong with me for being angry, and the idea of telling someone I was angry caused me a lot of shame.

Anger is normal. We all have it. And it is beautiful to acknowledge and know that there is a way to work with it. The same feeling of being empowered stems from our anger—we can use it to fuel ourselves in a healthy way.

Bargaining

With traditional situational grief, bargaining can look like begging for things to go back to how they were, pleading with a partner/spouse to take you back, or praying to a higher source to return a loved one who has passed away. With putting ourselves first, bargaining often refers to the difficulty experienced when we start setting healthy boundaries. We just want the situation to be easy. We want to feel heard and appreciated, and we plead with others to make this happen seamlessly—without having to go through the process of having difficult conversations or making drastic changes to our lives.

For example, if you are in a relationship that you know isn't working out, you might try to change yourself or the other person in order to salvage the relationship. We try to change things externally without doing the difficult inner work because it seems easier. While this might work temporarily (e.g., asking for changes to occur on a unit), it doesn't actually change us. We are powerful beings, and we don't need to rely on others or external situations to assert this—pleading with others prevents us from fully stepping into our power. We are responsible for our own happiness; we are not victims. Instead of putting all of our energy into pleading with people and systems external from us—our family members, our jobs, etc.—we need to focus on ourselves, define what our needs and wants are, and figure out how to meet them.

Depression

The star of the show, the feeling we classically associate with the word "grief." Many of us have felt depression at some point in our lives, usually in our personal lives. This is socially acceptable—of course we might feel depressed if we lose a loved one or a marriage ends. I'm curious to know how many of us would admit to or recognize feeling depressed over our jobs. I know for me, this was deemed "unhealthy" to let myself get too emotionally invested in my work. If I went home at the end of the day upset about something, my friends would tell me to just "forget about it" or "don't let it get to you," and I would agree. And yes, this might be good advice for the occasional blowup or difficult day. But when every day is a day like that, it begins to take its toll on us.

We need to feel it in order to heal it. I can understand why things are the way they are in health care intellectually—people are sicker, we are stressed and taking it out on each other, the economy is struggling. Yet my emotions don't give a fuck about the why. They aren't capable of understanding why, they don't listen to logic – they just are. And when we shove them down and try to explain them away, we delay the inevitable.

Much like anger, we are uncomfortable feeling sadness for long periods of time and feel as though we should be over it after a set time frame. Just like a wound doesn't have a set heal date, neither does our sadness. I'm sad that the world is the way it is, I'm sad that my patients are suffering, I'm sad that we are all burned out and overworked. But what causes me the most sadness is that we don't know that we deserve better. I'm sad that we don't feel worthy of having better working conditions, or that we work so hard that we don't have the energy to fight for ourselves. Once I got over my anger at all of this, I realized I was truly saddened by it all—and voilà—there was another layer of uncomfortable emotion to have to deal with.

While I was sad about the situation, I was also grieving the aspects of life that I had missed out on or suffered because I was people-pleasing. Once I gave into my sadness, I realized it was about so much more than what happened at work. It became about my own coping mechanisms, how unhealthy they were, and how they affected other aspects of my life. Being too tired to go out with friends, or the relationships that ended because of my people-pleasing, and the abuse I suffered because I allowed others to treat me poorly. I deserved so much better, and when I really looked at this, the sadness came sweeping in. Depression occurs when we have been ignoring ourselves for too long.

We see a considerable amount of sadness in our daily lives. Working in diagnostic imaging, we scan hundreds of patients a day. I recall seeing a terminally-ill pediatric patient, a burn patient who had lit himself on fire in a suicide attempt, and a brain-dead patient who they were scanning to see if their organs were viable for donation—and that was just in the first hour of work. It makes sense that once we start opening up, that there will be a huge backlog of emotion to experience. While this may seem daunting, it also gives us a huge gift. Once I got through my anger and uncovered the sadness that was hiding underneath, I was no longer blaming people or circumstances for my pain—I was able to acknowledge that the pain was mine to deal with. I wasn't externalizing it any longer, I was truly in my body and able to explore more fully what I was sad about. And this led me on the path to be able to fully allow where I was.

The sadness/depression we might feel when we start putting ourselves first will also be in part to the ending of relationships. Many of us chronic over-givers have people in our lives who benefit from our over-giving. Some of these people will not be supportive of us when we begin the process of putting ourselves first, and some of them will not be there at the finish line. Let these people go. It is always sad when relationships end, whether they are friends, family members, or partners. But if we have people who are not supportive of us becoming the new version of ourselves, then we need to question whether these people deserve to be a part of our new lives, or if they were only a part of the old version of us that is in the process of dying. Let yourself grieve the old version of you, as well as the relationships that went along with the old you.

Acceptance

Once we allow ourselves to fully feel all of the emotions associated with our plight, we can begin to adjust to life from a wiser perspective. When we feel all of the feelings that we have been stifling, no matter how irrational or temper tantrummy they might seem, we can fully acknowledge where we are. Acceptance doesn't mean we have to accept the situation we are in; quite the opposite. In order to make effective change and not be triggered every time something comes up, we need to heal.

If we want to make positive changes to our hospitals, clinics, and care homes, we need to do this from a place where we are not emotionally charged. From this place, we have more clarity, and we can collaborate with decision-makers with consideration instead of criticism. When we give ourselves permission to feel all of the feels, we forgive ourselves easier, and in turn, forgive others. This is when we can truly make an impact in creating change, because we see the problem for what it is—external from us—and we can address *it* as the issue instead of the people who are involved.

Other Experiences that Might Arise

When you finally commit to putting your needs above others, it will feel empowering at first—but also scary. You might feel exhausted, scared of losing people, and very isolated. Because setting healthy boundaries is often done with the people you are closest with, they might be the same people you would turn to if you needed support. You don't need to do this alone, and I would recommend working with a therapist while you are making these changes. Some of these coping mechanisms have been with you from when you were a child, and shaking them off isn't going to be straightforward. It's easier to do if you have the support of someone you trust, and a therapist is a great source of impartial support that can help you navigate your feelings.

Other Experiences in Putting Yourself First

You will feel fear—fear of losing people, fear of not being liked, fear of being seen, or fear of being labelled as selfish. It is perfectly normal to feel fear as you are navigating new territory. Many of us believe that we should "feel" ready when we need to make a change, when in fact fear is a normal response to change. Feel the fear and do it anyway.

You won't know if you are setting a boundary or a barrier—when we first start setting boundaries, we might be too rigid (known as a door slam: when we cut people out completely), or not strict enough. You have probably gone most of your life without knowing what a healthy boundary is, so it is totally normal not to get it right the first time—you are in training. It will get easier as you practice.

You will feel guilty—the "ick," I call it – when you say no to someone and you disappoint them. For me, it feels like a cold heaviness in my stomach, and I just feel icky. Again, many of us who are starting to put ourselves first believe erroneously that we should feel good about doing it, but that is rarely the case. We have become people-pleasers often to AVOID feeling guilt, and now we are having to sit with that feeling. It is going to be expected that you feel guilty when you first start saying no—this is not a reason to say yes. Unfortunately, it is not our healthy conscience that is bugging us, it is often a fear of feeling guilt that causes us to overstretch ourselves. Sit with the ick, soon enough it won't feel so icky, I promise.

People might not take too well you not doing things for them—"You've changed" is a phrase you will probably hear from at least one person. It will sting—I'm not going to sugarcoat it. Some of you might be able to say "Hell, yes, I have!" And some of you might meet a disapproving glare with guilt or shame. I want you to know that either response is normal. Whether it be from a stern aunt who was raised to sacrifice themselves and believes all of us should, or the lazy coworker who defaults to us when they don't want to do something, it will probably not be easy to hear. And you will probably question yourself if you are being selfish, as they are implying.

Without a doubt, you are being selfish (or self-FULL, as I like to define it). Because being self-full means you are looking after your own needs before taking care of others. A truly selfish person does not take care of others' needs; they only care about their own. Someone who tends to their own needs, then focuses on others, can be seen as someone who is self-full. As I highly doubt anybody reading this has the capacity to become truly selfish from putting themselves first, I fully encourage you to embrace this term when you are met with resistance.

You won't know what to do with your time—this might sound strange, but one of the things I found difficult once I started putting my needs first was that I had extra time on my hands for self-care. It was actually really difficult to exercise the right of having time to relax. I didn't really know how to do it at first. Even when I went on vacation, I was constantly doing things, as I felt guilty just lying on a beach when I was in a new country I could be out exploring.

The guilt we feel when we do make time for ourselves will seem paradoxically overwhelming at first. Animals in captivity, once released, tend to stay in the same small area despite having the freedom to roam. We get so used to not having any free time that we don't know what to do when we do get it—and we often quickly find something to busy ourselves with to deal with that discomfort. Again, this is NORMAL. Just because we feel guilty and don't know what to do with ourselves does not mean we should become busy again.

You will mess up—you might fall back into old patterns, either because you are tired or because you didn't notice. Sometimes life is crazy, and we sacrifice ourselves for others to get things done. Totally normal. Like a healthy diet, falling off the wagon once doesn't mean we don't get back on. When you recognize you have been neglecting yourself, dust yourself off and get back to prioritizing your needs.

You will feel like giving up—as someone who has people-pleased most of her life, I can tell you putting myself first has been one of the hardest things I have done— and I've done a lot of hard things. It is difficult to figure out what our needs are, let alone ask for others to respect them, especially when we have people in our lives who take advantage of us. It can seem very daunting when life is crazy to try to make it come to a complete halt to figure out our stuff. And, once we have established what our stuff is, the strength it takes to maintain our boundaries can seem overwhelming at times. If you feel like giving up, you might just need a rest. The payoff for putting your own needs first is pretty much the best thing ever—living a life YOU want—so don't give up.

Self-Compassion

The most important component to have when we embark on this journey is having compassion for ourselves. Beating ourselves up for our people-pleasing ways is not going to help. Most of us learned this technique because it helped us survive, often in a tumultuous upbringing.

Putting ourselves first is dying to the person who put everyone's needs ahead of their own. I did this for much of my life because *it helped me survive*. Growing up in a dysfunctional household, it was the best line of attack, the best way I could get my needs met. I don't have shame for doing the best that I could at the time, and neither should anybody reading this. We behave in the ways we believe best serves us. I needed to focus on my parents more than myself because it kept me safe—my childhood-self knew what she was doing. This way of being was necessary at the time.

Having self-compassion for ourselves as we navigate through this is the best weapon we have. It gives us the courage to stand up for a better way of living, it softens the blow when we mess up, and it gives us inspiration to keep going when it all seems too much. Kristin Neff, an expert on self-compassion, outlines how we can use self-compassion to be kinder, more resilient human beings. Her studies on self-compassion have found people who practice high self-compassion are more confident, focused, and resilient.[2] Unlike their less self-compassionate counterparts, they were less focused on their mistakes and more concerned with the learning process. Practicing high self-compassion helps us navigate difficult times in our lives with grace and openness, and helps us extend that compassion to others.

Unlike other self-care activities that can sometimes take time or energy away from our lives and aren't always possible (try having a bubble bath during a twelve-hour shift!), self-compassion can be practiced in the moment. When we are in the throes of our grief, self-compassion "can be as simple as acknowledging the emotional pain in that moment (e.g., "This is hard for me right now."), reminding ourselves that it is part of human nature to struggle (e.g., "Everyone struggles."), and offering ourselves kindness in that moment (e.g., "I will love myself in this moment.")."[3]

Losing an old part of ourselves feels like dying in a way, and we grieve over that old person. But the new person, the one who is experiencing life the way she wants to, out of joy, is waiting for us. It's time to let the old part of us go, compassionately.

EXERCISES

1. Think of a time where you experienced grief. How did it play out for you? How did you move through the stages? How did it feel when you reached the acceptance stage?

2. Journal what you might feel as you go through the process of putting yourself first. What emotions come to the surface as you think about prioritizing your needs?

3. From Kristin Neff's exercises (http://self-compassion.org/), write a letter to yourself through the eyes of a compassionate friend.[4] What would you say to yourself if you could see yourself through the eyes of a fiercely compassionate loved one?

CHAPTER 4

The Wounded Healer

"The wound is where the light enters." – Rumi

I don't know how well y'all fared in your Greek Mythology unit in elementary, but I bombed mine. I can proudly say it was the first test this overachiever failed. I still remember my kind-natured sixth-grade teacher, exasperated that we all flunked, lecturing us when we weren't paying attention (let's face it, none of us did. Who the heck was Achilles, and why did we give a shit about his effing heel?).

Well, lemme tell ya. They have some good lessons, our Greek counterparts. Through their murdering and philandering and naked philosophizing, they gave us some serious stuff to ponder, even in today's seemingly unrelated world.

I'm sure most of you can reach into the recesses of your minds to recall Aphrodite or Apollo or Zeus. But do any of you modern-day healers remember learning about Chiron, the Wounded Healer?

Chiron was a gifted centaur—half horse, half man. He was born to human parents, although his dad had to turn himself into a horse to hide from angry naked philosophers. Turning into a horse during conception was the Greek god version of Accutane—it messed that baby up. Horrified that their child was a mutant, they abandoned poor baby Chiron. Luckily for Chiron, he hit the adoption jackpot. Like Maddox to his Angelina, Chiron got adopted by Apollo, one of the most widely revered Greek deities. Apollo taught Chiron everything, from archery to medicine to music. He grew up to be a gifted healer and teacher, and had many famous Greeks come to study under him.

Unfortunately, Chiron's luck eventually ran out. During an altercation (they were always having those, those Greek gods), Chiron was wounded by a poisoned arrow. Normally, this arrow would have killed its target, but because Chiron was immortal, he lived, albeit in excruciating pain. Even though Chiron was a great healer, even he couldn't heal himself. To add insult to injury (literally), it was Chiron who taught the warriors to add this poison to their arrows to make them more deadly. Oh, the irony.

Chiron continued to help others despite carrying around this wound. In discovering that Prometheus would be put to death for giving humans fire, Chiron offered up his mortality to save Prometheus. Which, you know, is nice and all, but perhaps he was just tired of living with this weeping wound for all of eternity. Can you imagine being immortal and having to be in your occupation forEVER? Never-ending ostomy bag changes? Eternal trach suctioning? Discharge planning to infinity? No thanks! I can see why Chiron peaced out.

In all seriousness, Chiron represented an archetype of a caregiver who heals others while carrying his own wounds. The word *archetype* actually originates from ancient Greek, meaning "original pattern." An archetype is a pattern or prototype on which themes are based. In Jungian psychology, this is defined as "a collectively inherited unconscious idea, pattern of thought, etc., universally present in individual psyches".[1] It is the main model of something that others tend to emulate.

Carl Jung used the concept of archetypes in his theories of human behavior.[2] He recognized twelve universal character archetypes in our unconscious psyche. They represent the motivation behind our actions. Each one of us tends to have an archetype that guides our personality.

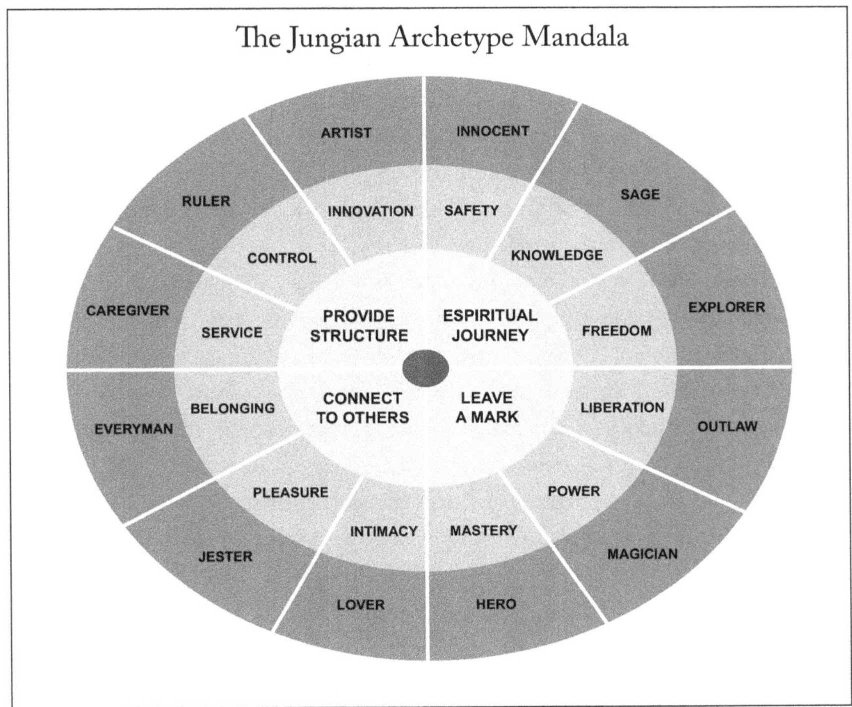

Based on this theory, we have a tendency to be drawn to a certain prototype of personality. Archetypal roles are used throughout many of our stories, from history to present day. Our books and movies give credence to the archetypes through the themes of their characters. The Hero archetype is the most obvious, as is The

Outlaw. We see The Innocent in the form of children, The Sage in our spiritual leaders, and The Jester in our comedians.

As health care workers, our obvious archetype is The Caregiver. Other names given to this archetype include The Healer, The Saint, and the Altruist. Jung coined the term in regards to psychology, theorizing that the therapist is drawn to healing arts because he himself is wounded and in need of healing. This can be conscious or unconscious, and we can project (or bleed) on to our patients. He claimed that our core wound was something we were on a path to heal, and it may take a person's lifetime to heal it, hence why we are drawn to helping others with similar afflictions.

Caregivers are noted for protecting and caring for others. Our superpower of empathy is our greatest gift to the world. Our motto is: "Love your neighbor as you love yourself" (although I wonder if we have forgotten about the loving ourselves part). While it is our greatest gift, it is also our weakness. According to Jung, our tendency to look after others can prey on our weakness of martyrdom and be exploited by others.

According to Jung, The Caregiver's greatest fear is to be viewed as selfish or ungrateful. We will do anything, including sacrificing ourselves, to prevent being seen as selfish. The discomfort we feel at being labelled as such is too much for us to bear, and so we go to extraordinary lengths to prevent it. As archetypes are mainly unconscious in their framework, the people who are drawn to the archetype they possess are often unaware of this.

Is this resonating? *Ding ding ding* … that's a hand way up in the air for me. I vividly remember being called out by my parents whenever I complained about something growing up. "You're so hard done by," was a common phrase uttered by my father. My Mum actually used the word "ungrateful" towards me a lot. They both had really difficult childhoods, and from their perspective, my sister and I had it pretty good. Which was true—compared to their childhoods, we DID have it pretty good, for the most part. So any time the word "selfish" or "ungrateful" came up, it stuck me like it was like my own poisoned arrow. It hit such a nerve growing up that I did everything I could to suppress my needs when they came up. My poor childhood-self felt guilty for asking for anything, as I feared being told I should just be grateful for what I have. It stung even more when I would ask for something that was apparently outlandish, as it might be met with mirthless laughter. Gradually, more and more I stopped asking for things, knowing I probably wouldn't get them.

As I got older, I realized the pain of being told no was becoming so much that it spilled into my relationships with friends and teachers as a kid. As an adult, being grateful for the bare minimum carried into my life personally and professionally. Being a nurse, getting targeted for lay-offs or other forms of cutbacks were just common occurrences. The role my parents and teachers had in telling me I was asking too much was replaced by my employer and the government. I was still being told to be grateful—"Be thankful that you even have a job!" "No raise in 10 years? It's selfish to even ask with this economy!" "You need to do your part, it could be worse!"

But "it could be worse" is not a reason to accept our current conditions. "It could be worse" doesn't mean an abused wife should stay ("I've never gone to the hospital from his beatings, so it could be worse!") I mean, are we crazy? Putting up with the conditions we've been putting up with for so long because "it could be worse"?

My question: Is avoiding the feeling of being selfish more uncomfortable than the extremes we go to in order to avoid it? The exhaustion, the resentment, the constant need to prove ourselves?

The Shadow Healer

There are shadow sides to our healing archetype.[3] If we are brave enough to look deeper and see things clearly (even if it means admitting we have a "weakness"), then we can begin to tackle some of the issues that are affecting our lives. Healing starts from within; we cannot change what we do not know or fully understand. The gold is there, buried beneath the things we would prefer not to look at.

Some of the issues that arise from the shadow side of a healer:

Not Caring for Ourselves—The most obvious issue is not caring for ourselves. We are so focused on others that we neglect our own needs. The shadow side of the wounded healer is that we are unwilling to look at our motives for not caring for ourselves. We give until we are burned out, and this validates our kindness and generosity. We gain satisfaction from being there for others, not realizing that the longer we don't meet our own needs, the less we will actually be able to be there for others in the future.

Feelings of Superiority—While we may not admit it or be willing to look at it, the shadow side of a wounded healer can be that our giving/profession/abilities make us feel special. We need to be needed, and healers, especially those of us with specialized training, feel validated by our ability to make people feel better—whether that is in a doctor's office or hospital or out in the community, and regardless of specialty—nurse, surgeon, psychiatrist, RT, PT. Whatever field we have trained in, we gain satisfaction from helping others on their healing journey because many of us have skills that others don't. Being the care aide that can get the difficult resident to take their pills, or the surgeon who defies all odds and successfully excises a brain tumor—we all get our hit of serotonin in some way or another in our work.

And, let's face it—there's not a lot of bonuses in our jobs (literally—give us bonuses!). So it is completely understandable that we would fixate on getting that feeling of satisfaction because we have little else in our jobs that fulfills us—it's tiring, sacrificing work. Yet when the only gravy that we get is an emphatic "Thank you!" from a patient or feeling like a hotshot for getting that IV that no one else could get, it becomes more and more necessary to have those hits on a daily basis, because we are receiving little else in fulfillment. There is nothing wrong from feeling good about helping people, but when we base our self-worth on it, it can become a problem. Some of us (me included) secretly crave the praise and admiration that we receive—and it is usually because we have been neglecting ourselves and we are using others' praise as fuel for our empty fires. It can also cause us to be overly invested in our patients and outcomes. When we feel overly guilty when we can't get the IV, or the patient doesn't make it, we know we have attached too much of ourselves to it. I have definitely seen this in myself and my colleagues, not wanting to give up poking a patient because they "need" a test, or an elderly resident being force-fed when they are no longer wanting to eat. We take the power away from our patients when we coerce them because it is "for their own good," but it is sometimes more for our own good than theirs.

Inappropriate Boundaries—This can be either not setting enough healthy boundaries for ourselves, leading to burnout, or it can involve crossing patient/family member boundaries in an effort to support them. I see this often, not necessarily with our patients, but in our personal lives. We use our knowledge and experience in the health field to help our family members with their health. We take them to doctor appointments (and are the ones asking all of the questions), we coerce them to change their eating/exercise habits due to their health, and we fuss over them in general. It is, of course, with good intentions that we do this. We obviously don't want our family members to get sick, or have a prolonged illness—we work with sick people every day, we have insight into how situations play out, and we are fearful for our family members (not to mention we also know how toxic the health care system is right now).

Think of the dread you have when you go to see a patient and the family member with them tells you they're in the medical field—you immediately straighten up a bit, because you know a) you are going to be watched like a hawk, and b) the family member will probably have a lot of questions/input.

Our shadow side is that we have a real issue with boundaries, and a lot of it is due to imbalance. We don't know how to stand up for ourselves, so we overcompensate by becoming rescuers for others. We can become so wrapped up with others (another type of unhealthy boundary) that we come off as pushy, and this can end up driving people away or causing them to exclude us from telling us about their medical issues for fear of being coerced.

What We Can Do About Our Wounds

1. *Be willing to look at them* – From our greatest weakness comes our greatest strength. If we are willing to dig down and get at the root of the issue, we can identify why our branches aren't growing, why our leaves are wilting, why we feel dried up and not able to maintain our sustenance. WHY are we feeling used up? WHY are we feeling resentful? According to Jung, our afflictions actually make us better healers, as they allow us to be partners in our patients' healing instead of being superior, allowing the patient to invoke their own "inner healer."[4]

    On the surface, it may be easy to look externally. Our failing health care system, our growing illnesses, our busy, hectic personal lives. But how did we get here in the first place? Just as we can't expect healing to occur externally, we can't expect our problems to go away from external sources. My bet is, even if we didn't have crippling health care problems, we would still be suffering as health care workers—it just might be manifesting in other ways.

    If you have issues around setting healthy boundaries, probe a bit further and ask yourself why. What is it that you're afraid of if you ask for help? Is it that you might come off as weak or incompetent? Is it that you are afraid to be a burden to others? Are you afraid that if you ask for help, you will be rejected? Or does doing it all for everyone make you feel like you matter, and might bring you praise? Be honest with yourself—you don't have to admit anything out loud to anyone. Sit with it and see what comes up for you.

    The shadow side of our giving can be traced to feelings of unworthiness, a need for external validation, and a fear of asking for help. If we are brave enough to see the shadow side of our giving as an opportunity for growth, we can begin to shift our perspective on our weaknesses and begin to see them as the gifts they truly are. Our weaknesses are nothing to be afraid of—they are there to show us where these parts of ourselves have been hidden, and begin to make us whole.

2. *Heal thyself* – Once we have identified what our shadow elements of being a wounded healer truly are (and they will look and play out uniquely for each individual), true healing can begin.

    According to Jung, the wounded healer's true purpose is self-healing. Think about it—how often do you focus on your own healing? Is it only when you have a cold or have sustained an injury? Even then, many of us will become frustrated that the healing is needing to take place in the first place, and we often ignore the signs our bodies are trying to send to us.

Think of some of the issues in the shadow healer characteristics—did any of them resonate with you? If so, which ones? When did these issues start? (Hint: they often begin waaaay before we enter the profession we are in). Can you identify some of your earliest wounds? What events have occurred in your life that have affected you as an adult? Did you have a traumatic experience? How have these early wounds shaped who you are today? Is it for the better? Did it make you more cautious? Or did it cause you to carry anxiety?

Once you are ready, I encourage you to talk about your wounds with people you trust—family, friends, a psychologist or counselor. Healers need to talk about their wounds. They spend the majority of their lives discussing their patients' wounds and so little of it giving that focus and energy to their own. Our wounds are a gift in many ways, and sharing our stories and experiences is a powerful way to initiate change in our lives.

Also, healing ourselves can promote healing in others. In a survey of nurses with depression by Caan, many nurses identified their illness as actually benefitting them in many ways, such as improved understanding (85%), empathy (78%), and compassion for others (60%).[5]

We have the power and the ability to heal ourselves. As with our patients, we don't have a magic pill that will "cure" them on a holistic level. While we are aides to their healing, we don't do the healing for them—they do it themselves, with us HCWs as facilitators to their healing. As Hippocrates stated (yep, those Greeks again), "Man does not heal, Nature does." He meant that we as health care workers are not doing the healing, but allowing our patients' bodies to do what they naturally do.

3. *Self-Care/Self-Nurture* – While much of our healing occurs from within and is more abstract, there are more practical activities that we can do to assist us in our healing. They can be physical activities, such as taking walks or hot baths, or they can be more internal, such as journaling or meditating. While we will discover more about self-care/self-nurturing behaviors in the later chapters, it is imperative to know that self-care needs to be part of the equation. It might look different for each individual, but it absolutely has to be practiced and non-negotiable in order to facilitate change.

4. *Boundaries* – Boundaries are a form of self-care. They deserve their own heading because they are imperative to our practice as healers and often are at the

root of our over-giving. What setting healthy boundaries looks like, how to implement them, and how to maintain them are a huge part of the work that we as self-healers need to examine in order to flourish and keep giving to others in the capacity we want to achieve. This will also be discussed more in depth in the chapters to come.

5. *Humility* – Healers don't heal others; we give power to our patients so they can heal themselves. We provide a caring disposition, a hand to hold, a listening ear. We sit in silence, we hug, we ask questions. We are not healing our patients' bodies, we are providing a space for them to focus on their healing, and in giving them that nourishing environment, they can begin to heal on their own. We have medicalized so much of what healing actually is, and we have forgotten our bodies' roles in the healing process. Rest, high-quality food, and a caring nature go a long way in the body's ability to heal itself. We provide support and guidance so that we give our patients the best outcome possible. The patient loses her ability to empower herself when we don't educate her or provide guidance. We as health care workers recognize that we aren't the ones healing the patient, that the patient is the one doing the healing. This requires humility, and it can be difficult when we are being put on a pedestal by our patients. When we practice humility, we don't take credit for a patient's healing journey or outcome. This is freeing—when we don't focus on the outcome, we allow grace to step in. We don't become attached to a patient's prognosis, which means we don't take credit when they overcome an illness, nor do we blame ourselves when they succumb to it. We are grateful for the wisdom we attain when we allow ourselves to learn from a patient's healing journey.

6 *Acceptance of "What Is"* – We don't control the outcomes. While we obviously desire for our patients to heal and are part of that journey, we don't have all the answers, and bending over backwards to "fix" our patients doesn't work. We need to do our best at our jobs, wish the patient the best in their healing journey, and allow nature to do what it needs to do. Letting go is an important lesson for a wounded healer, as it is part of the healing journey. Accepting what is—our own wounds, as well as our patients'—helps us live life without the worry. The anguish of going down a rabbit hole wondering what we could have done better or blaming our parents or wondering if we had just bought organic doesn't help. Embodying grace with where we are will help us to move forward in the right direction—empowered.

As we reflect on a half-horse with an affliction for poisoned arrows, I encourage you to philosophize on the following questions and see how they relate to you, your practice, and your personal life.

1. What was one of your early wounds? How does it affect you now as an adult?

2. Do you spend more of your time helping others than tending to your own needs? Explore how you might shift that balance your way.

3. Are most others dependent on you to support them in your personal life? Who can you ask for help? What would make you comfortable asking for support?

4. Do you need to take frequent vacations or trips to escape your life? How can you bring that vacation mindset to your everyday?

5. Is it hard to say no to someone that really needs you? What "obligations" can you remove to simplify your life?

6. Do you become resentful of others, or feel that others don't appreciate all that you do for them? Try to bring gratitude to mind with respect to your profession of choice, in that your nature is to care for others. Identify ways to let others be more self-reliant.

7. Would you identify yourself as humble? What are some examples of when you felt responsible for your patient's progress?

8. What is the gift you have received from your wounds? How can it help you to serve others?

CHAPTER 5

Empathy, Our Superpower (And Our Blind Spot)

"Empathy is a choice, and it's a vulnerable one." — *Brené Brown*

Empathy is the ability to put yourself in someone else's shoes and imagine what it would be like to be that person. It differs from sympathy in that it eliminates judgement or advice-giving, however well-meaning. It allows for listening. It creates a space where people can just be themselves, whatever that looks like in the moment. It doesn't preach, it doesn't tell someone to feel better, or offer suggestions. It simply states, "I hear you. I see you. You are perfectly okay to be where you are at right now." There is an excellent TED talk that Ms. Brown gave on empathy, illustrated beautifully. I highly recommend it if you haven't seen it.[1] (You can find it here: https://www.youtube.com/watch?v=1Evwgu369Jw)

In this talk, Brené describes the work of nursing scholar Theresa Wiseman and her concept of the four attributes of empathy, which are:

1. To be able to see the world as others see it;
2. To be nonjudgmental;
3. To understand another person's feelings; and
4. To communicate the understanding of that other person's feelings.[2]

"Holding space" is a term often described alongside empathy. It means to provide a safe container to be in the moment with someone, to offer your ears and heart, to accept that person's truth, no matter what.

Empathy over Sympathy

When I was dealing with my mother's illness after my father died, I was overwhelmed. When I went to friends and family members for support, what I thought I needed was advice. I would seek out their opinions on what I should do, and how I should handle certain situations. Because of this, I received a lot of sympathy and not a lot of empathy. I was offered suggestions of taking time off, of talking to someone, of working more to get my mind off of it. I was given advice to cut her out of my life, to put her in a home, or to forgive her because she is the only mother I have. Their differing opinions made me more confused than ever.

The truth was, deep down, I knew what I should do, but I was so unsure of myself that I didn't trust my gut. I went to others hoping they would give me the magic answer, when really it was me who had the answers all along. The well-meaning "solutions" made me feel more alone than ever, as I didn't really need to solve anything—this was my "fix it" brain in overdrive. I had to go through it, and no one could do that but me. While everyone was doing their best to help, what I needed most was to have someone there to walk with me. Not to do it for me, but to be there while I went through this ordeal. It was empathy I needed most that I didn't know how to ask for at the time.

It wasn't until a friend called to check in with me one day after my mother had died that I experienced true empathy. I was having a rough day—nothing seemed to make me feel better, and I was feeling really down. I fought grief for much of the time I had it, not realizing what I was doing. My friend phoned me up, and normally I would have put on a brave face and just pretended I was okay, but this time I had no energy left in me to do that.

She asked how I was. "Not okay," I said, leaving it at that.

"Okay. Do you want to talk about it?" she asked kindly.

"No."

"Okay. Do want to talk about something else?" she asked.

"No. I don't. I don't care about anything right now," I stated emptily.

"Okay. Well, do you want me to let you go?"

"…"

Truthfully, I didn't. I was so desperate for connection, for someone to just be with me. I couldn't stand the idea of making forced conversation, but I also really, really didn't want to be alone with my thoughts. And I also couldn't voice this aloud.

"Okay, well," she continued, "I'll just sit here on the phone. And if you want to talk, great. If not, I'll just sit here quietly."

And she did.

My mind was so confused as to what was going on. What was the point of this?

But there was a point. The point was that she knew I wasn't okay, and instead of letting me go, she sat there with me. She didn't offer advice, or tell me I should do x, y, and z to feel better. She just sat there with me and let me be. Eventually, I felt a tiny bit better and was able to have a conversation.

But it was in this moment that I first experienced true empathy. It left a lasting impression on me. Not right away, but eventually I realized that this one moment was so powerful, it accelerated my healing and my ability to get through one of the hardest times in my life. I didn't need to talk or pretend. I didn't need to do anything—and she was still there, just being with me. I stopped burning what little energy I had on being "strong," and I was actually able to just be.

As many of us in health care are so used to being the strong ones, I am sure you can relate. We know how exhausting being "on" all of the time can be. I didn't realize how heavy the armor I was wearing was until I was given this moment of grace. While I felt a huge sense of relief that I could take the armor off, I also felt extremely vulnerable. Sitting in silence on the phone was incredibly uncomfortable. But I experienced more healing in those moments of silence than I had done throughout my mother's illness. Being seen in that way can be absolutely terrifying, and it can be utterly freeing.

Empathy = Healing.

When was the last time you can remember someone showing you true empathy—just being there for you while you yelled, or cried, or sat in silence? No judgement, just a calm presence while you let your emotions come to the surface. What impact did that make on you in the moment? Think back to when you were a child and you fell and hurt yourself. Did it feel good for your parent to scold you for being careless? Did you want suggestions in that moment about how to tie your shoelaces better so you didn't trip? No, you wanted your parent to hold you and tell you it would be okay—and it always was. Adults need this same nurturing, yet we don't often get it.

When I'm having a bad day, I can feel like a failure, like my life is a mess. When I go to a friend with this, I don't actually want all the reasons I'm not a failure pointed out to me, I want to be *seen*. I want to feel like it's OK to feel this way, and any attempt to distract me from it just makes me feel unheard.

Empathy has the power to make a huge impact on our lives. In a world that is so focused on avoiding pain, we often create situations where we disconnect from it, and in the process, others. This makes us feel even more alone and isolated than we already are. By offering the people in our lives sympathy instead of empathy, we are indirectly stunting their healing. By rushing to make someone feel better, however altruistically, we are denying them the ability to feel their pain and go through it. What we resist, persists. If we stifle pain or ignore it or try to feel better instead of actually allowing ourselves to feel pain—and every person goes through pain at multiple points in their lives—it rebounds more intensely than before. Sympathy does not allow us to feel our pain; in fact, it supports the idea that we shouldn't be feeling it in the first place, which can do more damage than good. Toxic positivity can be attributed to statements we make that are intended to be sympathetic ("It could be worse!"), but it only perpetuates the idea that our feelings aren't valid and we shouldn't be having them.

Empathy—The World's Superpower

For those of you who are (or were—thanks, COVID) avid travellers, you will know how jarring being in another culture can be. Different races, foods, bathrooms (you can stick your hole in the ground, Indonesia!), it can be overwhelming just how diverse the same Earth is. Before I travelled, I was very naïve—and *much* more judgmental of others. Immersing myself in other cultures opened my eyes to different ways of doing things, and different ways of seeing the world. It didn't mean I came home and disowned indoor plumbing, but it humbled me, and I recognized that despite the cultural diversity, the people I met weren't that different from me. Being a guest in other countries allowed me to really see. Because I didn't speak the language, it meant I had to talk less—and witness more. This allowed me the space to watch others, and what I saw wasn't that dissimilar to what I would see back home—families going grocery shopping, children playing, crowds gathering. When I immersed myself in the culture, I was no longer focusing on the differences, but the similarities. I wouldn't have had that blessing of being more open if I hadn't been with the people who were supposedly so different from me.

Much of what the world is enduring today can be attributed to a lack of empathy. Whether looking at religion, race, culture, age, gender, socioeconomic status, or geographical location, our us-versus-them mentality causes rifts that can create wars—all because we don't understand each other. As I write this, the world has split into another us-versus-them —vaccinated versus unvaccinated. Another category to separate us.

In order to resolve any conflict, it is imperative for us to listen to each other. We don't need to agree, but healing (and therefore, positive change) cannot happen until we feel fully heard. And many of us are not allowing that to happen. It's very easy to empathize with people when they agree with us. It's much more challenging to do so for people who don't look like us, act like us, or make the same decisions as us. We can easily relate to people who have lost their jobs in health care, but what about someone who was laid off in the oil field? We females deeply feel a woman's anguish over fertility issues, but how does a man experience it? We see the devastating effect that this virus is doing in the hospital, but have we opened a dialogue with someone who is deathly afraid of the vaccine—or have we just thrown facts at them? When we talk, we are not listening. And regardless of how right we are, if we are not asking questions or allowing a safe space for others (even the "others" that have different views from our own), we will not be able to move forward.

By shifting that perspective to empathy, our true superpower, we not only establish a connection with people (our patients, families, friends), but we empower them to heal themselves. What can be more freeing than realizing you have the power to overcome something? That you don't need to rely on others for the answer, that you had the power all along?

Having people beside us to offer a safe space so we can feel nurtured and seen is one of the best things we can do for ourselves. No one needs to walk this path alone. We are so lucky to have this superpower, to be in a position where this skill is incorporated into our careers. If we focus on it, cater to it, and help it grow, we have the power to change the world, one experience at a time.

HCWs and Empathy

HCWs practice empathy on a daily basis. We are in an environment where we take care of people when they are at their most vulnerable; it is a powerful role to be in. We are in a unique position in that we practice our empathy regularly. Most careers don't revolve around doing so, and we are highly skilled at it. We know the difference between giving empty words ("At least …") versus saying something that lets the patient know that we see their pain. We know we cannot possibly "fix" a patient who has terminal cancer, and so we avoid making statements of sympathy that would create more harm than good. We know our patients need to feel like they are not alone, and we are adept at providing that comfort to them. The greatest healing we can give a patient isn't through pills or radiation treatment, it's walking with them on their journey. Holding space for them to be vulnerable, to be scared, to be seen. The healing is through the connection we give them, whether that be holding their hand during a painful procedure or sharing a joke during a dressing change.

This is where our true power lies—in understanding others. In connection.

Empathy is our superpower.

This is such an amazing gift to give to our patients who can't always fully express their thoughts or needs. It makes us excellent caregivers, as we are able to intuit what lying in a hospital bed, being in a wet diaper, or lying on a cold procedure table must feel like, even if we have never experienced it ourselves. Our considerate nature ensures our patients are getting treated the way they ought to be treated. Not everyone has the ability to do this. While it might come naturally to us, many people lack this ability. It really is a superpower.

Our Superpower, and Our Kryptonite

Empathy, while our greatest strength, can also become our biggest weakness. Because we feel so deeply, it can cause difficulty in our professional and personal lives. We feel our patients suffer, and so we want to do everything in our power to ease their suffering. The pain we feel (sometimes literally) at the thought of our patients going through a difficult surgery, of being diagnosed with a terminal illness, or of missing aspects of their care, can affect us so much that we take on their suffering. We do everything we can to minimize the pain for others, mainly at our own expense. We stay overtime out of empathy for our patients, as Mr. Jones won't get his dressing changed because they are short on the next shift. Our empathy extends to our coworkers, and we miss our breaks because Caroline is having to take a new admission by herself. We come home to our empathy, and we drag ourselves to soccer because Cayden hasn't had his parents at a game this month, Kendrick had to be dropped off at swimming by his grandparents again.

As HCWs, our superpower of being empathetic can also lead to tendencies of being too giving.

It is our blind spot—having empathy for others yet not being able to extend that empathy to ourselves.

This is true for any personality trait. Each gift we are given has a shadow side. A brilliant analytical mind can also be unfeeling. A creative person can lack structure. A feeling person may be too sensitive.

While our superpower affords us special abilities, it can also cause us to be unaware of its downfalls. Being "too" empathetic can cause us to neglect our own necessities. As with all things in life, there needs to be balance. Just as a brilliant thinker might get caught up with analysis deprived of compassion, we, too, can become overly emotional and lack logic. There are a myriad of motives behind over-giving, and it will be a main focus as we delve deeper into the chapters.

Another facet of our superpower of empathy is that it allows us to anticipate others' needs, sometimes to an almost psychic extent. Because we are able to put ourselves in others' shoes, it makes us good at guessing what others might need. This is so essential in health care, as our patients are often unable to tell us what they need. Fear, overwhelm, and altered levels of consciousness all make it difficult for our patients to communicate. With our superpower, we ensure that our patients are comfortable and cared for. This also extends to our coworkers, who benefit from our keen ability to sense when they need a break (or a latte). And our partners, children, and friends also profit from our knack of anticipating desires (especially at Christmas). It's something that is within us regardless of where we are; we can't turn it off. It makes us a considerate, thoughtful family member and friend. It's pretty nice to have a health care worker in your life.

But our ability to guess what others are thinking can also be another blind spot. Because it is so natural for us to anticipate others' needs, we forget that not everyone has this ability. It's OUR flow state, but for others, it's something that needs conscious effort—and sometimes we forget this.

Growing up, I didn't recognize this skill as something others didn't have—I just assumed everyone could do this. Being able to guess with impressive accuracy what someone must be feeling and what they might need, I took it for granted that others must be able to do this, too. I expected people to know what I wanted or needed—and they didn't.

Ever had a partner utter, "I can't read your mind!" in exasperation?

I had that partner. Because I rarely needed prompting when he needed cheering up, or when he was annoyed at me for something, or when he just needed a burger, it seemed fair that he should pick up on my subtle hints. While he tried his best, he just didn't have the same gift that I did, and it disappointed me. Insert pouting penguin meme here.

What I didn't want to admit was that I would have to ask for my needs to be met, and I really didn't want to do that. Would I be rejected? Did I even know what my needs were? As a chronic people-pleaser, I subconsciously equated not being cared for to being rejected, and so it was easier to avoid addressing what I wanted and hoping he would guess, rather than risk being disappointed. Putting that on my partner seemed easier to do ("Well you should just know!"), so that's what I did.

Our loved ones might benefit from our ability to anticipate their needs, but we can't expect them to be able to reciprocate—not in the same way. And since HCWs spend much of their time with each other (i.e., other empaths), we don't necessarily see it as a superpower; we take it for granted. We can see their inability to anticipate as a flaw, and not just typical. Which, as anyone who has been in a long-term relationship knows, leads to more conflict. If we change our perspective to recognize that empathy is something we are really, really good at and not a weakness, as it may be seen by others who it doesn't come naturally to, we achieve 1) bragging rights, and 2) compassion for others, leading to even more empathy, thus becoming even MORE superpower-y. Bam.

The Effect of Not Having Empathy for Ourselves

Our superpower of empathy has gone unchecked—the shadow side of our empathy is that we have not been granting our gifts to ourselves—and our workplaces are crumbling because of it. We are throwing sympathy around a workplace where we are neglecting our needs—and not empathy. Ignoring our needs has caused us to become anxious and depressed. Our workload causes us anxiety on a daily basis, and we wear armor as soon as we walk in the hospital door. Not having empathy for our own feelings is causing catastrophic situations in our workplace, and we HCWs are paying the price.

Our "negative" feelings crop up when there is something wrong—it is our internal alarm that something needs to be looked at. Often, we are taught that our feelings (especially negative ones, such as raising our voices in anger or tears of sadness) are unprofessional or should be suppressed. This is not only unhealthy, it is impossible. Feelings are energy, and they will come out one way or another. I wasn't conscious that my needs were going unmet, so the feeling of resentfulness was a warning sign that something needed to change. Unfortunately, I had to go through a lot of shame and guilt about these feelings, as I thought they were a sign that something was wrong with me. Because the people I was working with were also suppressing their needs and just getting on with it (as we've had to do to cope), I thought I was being a drama queen. I used my abuse as a child to push away the feelings, deeming them to be a sign of my wounding. I lacked empathy for myself, and so I judged what I was feeling as something I "shouldn't" be feeling. I gave myself the same sympathy pep-talk that I was so used to hearing ("Positive vibes only!"), and it was doing a lot of damage—to myself and others.

But I was wrong. Regardless of whether or not I "should" be feeling a certain way, the point was that I did. I did feel angry. I did feel resentful. And comparing myself to how others operated only kept me feeling ashamed and guilty for far longer than was necessary.

I think we have been lacking empathy for ourselves for a long time. I am hopeful that my experience will help those who deem themselves weak, high-maintenance, or anything else that they may truly be feeling and are shoving down. I know I can't be the only one who is feeling this way. For a long time, my feelings went unidentified and I didn't even realize there was a problem. I am hoping that you glean some insight from my experiences, the work that I have done in order to combat it, and the suggestions that I recommend, as I have personally used these methods. Simply put, they work—some of them very powerfully so.

Carl Jung's theories (whose camp I clearly belong to over Freud – no blaming Mummy here) contributed to much of what is now personality psychology. He describes one cognitive function, Extraverted Feeling, as, "What gets everyone's needs met?" As HCWs, we are very good at asking this question. Yet we are often leaving out an important factor—that the querent is part of the question. "I" am part of "everyone." I get a say. I matter.

By empowering individual health care workers, by providing them with skills to be assertive, independent, and standing up for themselves on their own, we can begin to shift this paradigm. While we weren't taught how to set healthy boundaries for ourselves in school, nor can we rely on others to stand up to inappropriate behavior or toxic workplaces, we can learn skills so that we can feel internally stronger, more self-assured, and more empowered. With more HCWs utilizing these skills in the workplace, we will begin to erode the toxic situations that are plaguing our hospitals, clinics, and patient homes.

Just as this won't happen overnight in our culture, neither will it happen overnight for you. It takes time, practice, and dedication to erase years of unhealthy learned behaviors. Be kind to yourself. Be patient. You are doing a superhero's work.

And it starts with empathy for yourself.

EXERCISES

1. Where in your life have you lacked empathy for yourself? Where do you scold yourself or try to make yourself feel better? Ask yourself, "If I was able to show myself understanding in this area of my life, what would that look like?"

2. Gift yourself some time to reflect. Find a quiet space. Think of something that has been bothering you. Have you been pushing it down, ignoring it? Use this time to sit and just be with your feelings—allow yourself to really feel what you are feeling. Is it anger, resentment, grief, fear? Do your best not to judge what comes up, and just witness. Allow tears to flow, the heaviness in your chest to rise, the anger in your throat to have a voice (yelling into pillows works great). Be patient. After, if any insights come up, write them down.

3. Think of a person/group of people whom you associate negative feelings with. It can be another culture, career field, or lifestyle different from your own. While you can easily identify differences, try to notice the similarities you might share. It can be small, or outside the box. For example, while I don't agree with much of what Donald Trump did as U.S. President (or his take on "hair"), I can appreciate that he was driven, decisive, and got shit done, unlike some waffling politicians. I also can empathize with his orange tinge, as I had a spray tan addiction myself. What this does is take the edge off of negative feelings we might be feeling towards people and groups that we may not favor, and gets our brain off of the us-versus-them track that the world has become so polarized by.

4. Taking the above exercise one step further, ask a friend, family member, or acquaintance to have a discussion about a topic you don't see eye to eye on. Go in with the intention that you are wanting to see their perspective, and don't offer yours unless asked. While it may be challenging, do your best not to judge what they say or attempt to persuade—simply listen to them. The goal is not to change their mind; it is to expand yours. It doesn't mean you will change your mind, but what it will bring about is connection, and you might be surprised by what develops.

CHAPTER 6

Establishing Your Values— Your Compass for Making Good Decisions

"Integrity is choosing courage over comfort; it's choosing what is right over what is fun, fast, or easy; and choosing to practice our values rather than simply professing them." – Brené Brown

When I came out the other end of my parents' illnesses and passings, I had no idea what to do. All that had happened to me over the course of seven years had shattered the person I thought I was. I was a shadow of a person, yet I was clinging desperately to anything or anyone that I thought could help me. I was searching for healing and was desperate to find it, whether that be through a book or a relationship. I was anxious, eager to please, and needed others to fulfill my own happiness. I was not looking internally for what could rescue me, which is obviously where the answers were.

Not having any established values was a key source of my anxiety. Having gone through major trauma, I could no longer rely on the behaviors that helped me survive in the past—I had to relearn who I was and how to navigate the world all over again, which was terrifying.

Figuring out what my values were was one of the most powerful exercises I could have done. I recognized that I was all over the place. I wasn't grounded in my career, my relationships, my health—nothing. The only value I was exercising was survival. If someone threw me a lifesaver, I grabbed on for dear life. I had little self-esteem and was willing to take anything I could get, even if it didn't truly serve me.

Once I went through a list of values and narrowed them down to what was truly important to me, I realized I had been living my life not doing any of those important things. I valued compassion, but I lacked it for myself. I valued integrity, but I was willing to sacrifice myself in order to gain approval. I valued honesty but was wearing a mask for many of my interactions. I had not been living a life true to me, and so I was suffering from anxiety and unease as a result of it, without even knowing why.

What are Values?

We aren't taught much about values in school. The phrase *align with your values* comes up often in life; we see them in businesses with mission statements or in the religious/spiritual community. We toss around the phrase "know your values" or "it doesn't align with my values," but have you ever stopped and wondered what your values actually are? Have you written a list of them down, identified why they are important to you, and acted on them? What does knowing your values actually mean?

Brené Brown (yes, her again—I'm a Brown-noser, deal with it) defines a value as "a way of being or believing that we hold most important. Living into our values means that we do more than profess our values, we practice them. We walk our talk."[1]

Personal values are the things that are important to us. They are our personality traits and behaviors that motivate us and guide our decisions. Our value system is affected by many things in life, including our parents, our social circles, our religious background, and society in general. We use our past experiences and education to develop our value system, whether we are aware of it or not. Our values are reflected in the way we behave, how we interact with people, in our activities, and the decisions we make, big or small. For example, as health care workers, many of us value kindness and compassion. We are eager to help others, and we are generous with our time and energy. We feel guilt when we are unable to help.

Everyone's values are different. Some people might value adventure, while others value security. Having the same job for twenty years might make one person feel safe while another person may feel stifled. This is where our superpower of empathy comes into play. We understand that not everyone's values are the same, and some value systems may clash with others. We have empathy for those whose value systems don't align with our own. For example, some of our coworkers might value family over their career and are less willing to work overtime than others. This might create conflict with people who value fairness, as it doesn't sit right with them that overtime work is unequally allocated. It is important that we honor each other's value systems and come up with a way to compromise when they do clash. Exercising our superpower allows us the awareness that everyone is different.

Living by your values might seem easy—I mean, it is just doing what is important to us, right? Yet so many of us don't live consistently by our values, mostly out of fear of being judged by others. Have you ever witnessed someone saying something you strongly disagree with, yet you didn't speak up and felt bad about it afterward?

While I thought I knew what my values were, in reality I had no clue. Being a people-pleaser, what was important to me depended on who I was with. This caused me inner conflict all of the time—I wasn't able to make decisions about anything and would agonize over the smallest choices because I didn't have a value system in place. The fear of missing out was real, and it caused me so much unnecessary stress. I would worry if I wasn't able to make it to a friend's birthday because it conflicted with a seminar I wanted to go to. At the time, I valued security in the form of others over my own personal development.

Why Values are Important

Values, although we can't see them, are the backbone of our lives. They define who we are, what is important to us, and how we make decisions. There are several reasons why establishing our values is important.

Values help us to be conscious and purposeful beings—Without values, we would be robots. We would be insensitive to others, we wouldn't find purpose in anything we do, and we wouldn't put effort into our actions because they would have no meaning.

Knowing our values allows us to live more consciously and gives us a sense of purpose. As HCWs, our sense of purpose in our careers may seem obvious—duh, we're there to help—yet it is not the only aspect of what we find important, nor does it define why we do what we do. There are millions of people in the health care field, and they don't all have the same values, despite having an underlying motivation of wanting to help others heal.

Values help us make decisions—Ever been stuck in a situation where you couldn't make your mind up? Eventually, you made a choice. And you probably made the choice based on your underlying values. Our values are our guides in life, they allow us to make a choice—the power we all have is to choose—and they help us do so based on what matters most to us, big or small. Whether this is which social function to attend or which career to choose, our values play a part in how we make up our minds.

This is especially critical when difficult decisions need to be made. Allocating scarce resources to those most in need is a classic example. The pandemic forced us to choose which precious supplies were given to who.

We health care workers also know, despite our fears, that our value of helping others comes at a time when it seems most unsafe to do so. While we feel afraid, we know that this is our calling. We all have the choice to continue to show up. For me, knowing that this is a choice that I have (and that it's okay to walk away if I need to) empowers me to keep showing up. While I worry about the outcomes of my patients, coworkers, friends and family, I have a sense of peace that I have this choice, and that making this choice aligns with my values. Which brings me to my next point ...

Values give us a sense of peace and fulfillment—Having a set of values that we are guided by allows us to feel a sense of peace within us. Acting on our value system consistently gives us peace that we know who we are. When we make decisions, we know that they are the right ones for us, even if we are missing out on other opportunities or disappointing others.

When you act out of alignment with your values, you are likely to feel uneasy. My personal belief is that many of us are unknowingly acting out of alignment with who we are, and this is a major reason why so many of us are suffering from anxiety and depression now more than ever. With the stress accrued from long-standing suboptimal care we are providing in health care settings, we can feel ambivalence, and in the long term, moral injury. Greenberg, et al. defines moral injury as "a long-lasting emotional, psychological, social, and spiritual effect from actions taken that run contrary to one's moral values."[2] The effects of acting out of alignment with our values can have long-term consequences, which is all the more reason to get clear on what our values actually are.

When we feel ambivalence, it contributes to a sense of not knowing—the source of much of our anxiety. Sitting down and defining what is actually important to us can help alleviate much of the ambivalence we feel in our lives. It is deeply personal—what might be important to you might not make sense to others (e.g., travel nursing instead of staying in one hospital might not work for everyone). It is important for your inner sense of peace to act in a way that is true for you. It is important to make YOU happy, and not make decisions that serve others, as difficult as that may be sometimes.

Defining Your Personal Values

There is a reason why companies have core values and mission statements—it not only tells the customer what they are about, but it streamlines the decision-making process so they can easily evaluate what matters to them and eliminate what doesn't. We humans work the same way—we can't be everything to everyone, though we certainly try. By figuring out what really, really matters to you, you will be able to see clearly what in your life is working, what isn't, and what you need to walk away from.

Where to begin with defining your values? Asking yourself what makes you feel good is a good place to start (ice cream is not a value, BTW). Does your heart sing when you do a good deed for someone? Do you love to bake? Is it yoga? Are you elated when you are traveling? What is it about the situation that makes you feel good? Is it a sense of adventure, freedom? Is it serving others? Is it connecting to your body? What is the "good" feeling you feel? Is it happiness, elation, love, belonging, spirituality? Asking yourself these questions will give you some insight into what you value most. Determining your values based on what brings you joy or fulfillment will help guide you to narrowing down what matters most to you.

On the other hand, what makes you feel very bad can also give you an indication of your values. As an example, do you feel shame or overwhelming guilt when you tell a white lie? This probably means you value honesty. While we might not be fully honest all the time, the consequences of not telling the truth may make you feel shame, guilt, or anxiety—all signs that you are acting out of alignment for you. And again, this is personal. Some people might not see anything wrong with telling a fib to save someone's feelings. That's great. For THEM. For you, it might not work.

Googling lists of values will give you an idea of what some of your values may be. There are literally hundreds of them, which can seem overwhelming at first to whittle down. Narrowing it down to five will give you the best indicator of what is the most important to you, and prioritizing those five in order of importance will also help you when you are making choices. For example, if you value family, adventure, health, honesty, and kindness, it might be difficult to choose between a steady job or work-abroad careers. But if you value family above all else, you will probably choose a job that doesn't sacrifice your family time. Ranking your values makes it easier to see what your priorities are in life, and therefore helps guide you in decision-making. For example, diet and exercise should come before everything else if you place health at the top of the list—which means working out before doing other tasks or *gasp* saying no to ice cream (the sacrilege!). If you value adventure, saving up for a trip might be more important than paying off your house.

Values as a Health Care Worker

As HCWs, we have a precious amount of energy in a day, a lot of it being directed at our careers. It is important, therefore, to prioritize what we have left to what really matters to us, whether that is our families, our health, or our sense of fun.

Our health care system is in crisis. We are not going to be able to fix it overnight. Much of the stress and anxiety we have with our jobs is that we KNOW there is a problem—and speaking out has fallen on deaf ears.

What establishing your values does is let you figure out what is most important to you and to live to your own values. We see the injustice that we and our patients suffer on a daily basis. We know the people who have made the decisions that affect us don't have to be on the front lines. We know these decisions impact us negatively, and that *we* are not being valued. We can only do what we can do. Sometimes that means being in a system that has made grievous errors in judgment.

As long as we are abiding by our own values, we are doing our best. We are not responsible for other people's values or decisions—even the ones made in health care. It is up to you if you want to continue working in this environment, or if it is worth looking at other options.

Establishing your values can be a compass for what you decide to do and how you decide to show up. As you act out your list of values and priorities, what you will learn about yourself will continue to grow.

Identifying the Why

I didn't realize how much I value a sense of humour until I dated someone who was serious, and OH … MY … GOD. I thought my soul was being crushed. It didn't make sense to me at first—he was intelligent, good-looking, and kind—all great things in a partner that I thought I put a high value on—but I couldn't joke around with him – we were just on different wavelengths. My sense of playfulness was falling flat, and I felt like I was slowly dying. My value of humour went from the bottom of the list and shot straight up to near the top (I also decided filthy rich should have its place on the list somewhere, too).

Figuring out *why* something is important to you is just as important as identifying *what*. The first time I did this exercise of identifying what my values were and why they were important to me, I thought it would be easy. Joy, Integrity, Compassion, Empowerment, and Exploration. Done.

Haha. Ha. Until I had to identify why they were important to me. Well, everyone knows it's important to be compassionate! Yes, but WHY?

I had nothing.

It took me a surprisingly long time to determine why exactly it was important to me to be compassionate, as I just found I was using synonyms of the word *compassion* (It's important to be kind! It's nice to be nice!). With some of your values that you identify, you might not be able to pinpoint what it is about it that is important other than it makes you feel good. That's okay, but doing the deep dive into why you find something important will help solidify this value and help you start not just thinking it, but living it. Was it a life experience that made you realize why something matters? Did you lose a loved one, perhaps, and know that quality time is going to be top priority from now on?

When I did the digging into my desire to be compassionate and why, I realized that it was because I hadn't felt compassion from others very much while I was growing up, and the people and situations that made a positive impact on my life were when I was shown kindness and understanding, even when I didn't feel I deserved it.

I know how it feels to be misunderstood, and I strive to go out of my way to ensure I could offer compassion to others. I am sure you as a health care worker can relate to this, and I bet many of you will list compassion or some form of it as one of your values.

How to Put Your Values into Action

Having a list of your values is great, but it won't change anything until you start living your life based on those values. How do we get a head start on implementing our values? By goal setting.

Now that you are aware of what values are important to you, and in what order, ask yourself if you are living according to your values. It will give you some insight into what might need to change. Does your career align with your values? Are you doing activities outside of work that are important to you? If you value health, are you eating right, exercising, and getting enough rest? (Hahaha—maybe it would be easier not to put health down as a value.)

It's totally normal for people who first do this exercise to see aspects of their lives they are not living in their values system. This is where goal-setting will be helpful to you to get on track.

For each value, identify things you could be doing to start living your life more aligned with that value. For example, if you value connection, making a goal of reaching out to one person per day would be an action related to that value. Or having a weekly running group, or a monthly book club, or all of these. Don't limit yourself based on practicality for now (e.g., taking a trip a year might be difficult due to time or financial constraints), but just list what comes out and observe what you come up with. Make the list of what you could be doing with your values. Then, make the goals reality, starting small with daily goals and aspiring to bigger ones.

*Disclaimer** To be clear, living by your values isn't always easy, and it may not always come naturally. For example, as a chronic people-pleaser, living with integrity was really hard for me, because it was easier to just do whatever the other person wanted instead of identifying what my needs were. But when I realized how imperative it was to my health and happiness to be fully authentic, I decided to make a concentrated effort to apply it. It is an ongoing relationship with this value, as some days I hit the mark and other days I miss it completely. Some days it's just easier to smile and nod. And that's okay. We don't have to get anything perfect here. Establishing your values is like establishing a new relationship—it takes a while to feel it out. It is a process of you finding out more about yourself.

EXERCISES

1.   Write down what is important to you in life—people, feelings, activities—don't limit it, see what comes up for you. Identify the value in these things. For example, if you listed your family, love and connection is probably the value that is important. Some might be trickier (e.g., your career), so what about this is important to you? Is it a sense of purpose? Is it ambition?

2.   List who or what inspires you. What qualities about this person/situation stand out for you? How can you begin to implement these qualities into your life?

3.   Write down what upsets you most in the world. Is it greed, pollution? Pinpoint why it upsets you so much. This might give you an indication of what you value as well. For example, I get angry when I see people being oppressed, therefore empowerment is a value that is important to me (obviously!).

4.   Do an internet search and find a list of values. Select around twenty that resonate with you. From there, whittle it down to five. You are going to resonate with many values, but identifying the five most important to you will help guide you in what is most important in your life.

5.   Once you have your list, look it over and check in with how it feels. Does it feel right? Remember this list isn't what you want others to think of you, it's identifying what actually matters to you. Maybe freedom is extremely important, or ambition. It is what really makes you feel happy and fulfilled that will help guide you in your decisions.

6.   Once you have identified your list, write out WHY each value is important. It is imperative to not only identify what is important to you, but why it is important to help you solidify it in your mind, and therefore your actions and behavior.

7.   Set goals for each value you selected. You can do this one value at a time if that is easier. Make the goals specific, time-oriented, and measurable so you can make them a reality.

8. Post the list of values somewhere you can see them (on the fridge, your bathroom mirror), and ask yourself at the end of the day if you practiced these today. If not, why not?

9. Revisit the list of values regularly. A good time to do this would be after you have met some of the goals you set out to achieve. You might realize once you have acted on your values that what you thought was important might not be so. Or, they might shift as you mature. You are an evolving human, and it's okay for your values to change over time.

CHAPTER 7

Personality-Typing

"To know thyself is the beginning of wisdom." – Socrates

When I was in my twenties, I thought something was wrong with me (I mean … I wasn't wrong). While I was social and enjoyed being with my friends, I couldn't handle being with them for long periods of time. I lived outside the city, and so I would stay over at a friend's house when we would go out. When I woke up in the morning, I NEEDED to go home. Even if I didn't have a good reason for it, I felt like I had to run out of there. It perplexed my friends, who were more than happy to hang out and have a leisurely breakfast. But for me, I felt like I needed to escape. I couldn't understand why I needed to leave so urgently, and I tried hard to ignore it.

I pushed myself to be more social because that's what you do in your twenties. I feared losing my friendships over it, so I worked hard to be at every gathering, even if I didn't feel like it. The FOMO was real. I would berate myself because I thought there was something wrong with me for not wanting to go out. Introverts hadn't yet had their moment in the sun like they are having now, so I wasn't aware of what introversion/extroversion was. I denied that aspect of myself so much and tried to fit in with everyone, that even when I took a personality test for the first time, I tested as an extrovert.

As I got older and started recognizing certain aspects of myself, I took the test again, and tested as an introvert. Once I read what an introvert was, I saw it wasn't the anti-social personality I had created in my head and I learned to truly accept myself. I learned that introverts gain their energy from doing activities alone, and often enjoy activities that are more introspective, such as reading. I learned that I needed to protect my energy and had to honor that aspect of myself.

It meant I couldn't go out as much as I would like to. I couldn't book a full weekend, because I would be drained and become resentful of not having enough time to myself. I began to learn what worked for me. And while it wasn't what seemed normal at the time, I had to respect it, for if I didn't, I wouldn't feel my best. It made sense why I was more tired than my colleagues after work—I had been around people all day, and needed more time to recharge than they did.

This was a game-changer for me. I realized that by knowing myself more, I could begin to accept aspects of myself I didn't particularly like. These aspects were my personality traits that I either was too ashamed to admit to, or completely ignored due to a lack of awareness. I couldn't make improvements to myself if I wasn't aware of them (or willing to admit them). But knowing that others like me had these personality traits as well allowed me to feel better about myself—it wasn't just me! I wasn't weird! Well, okay, I am, but now I own it.

This was so empowering. I suddenly felt a weight lift off my shoulders, as something I had been pushing against for so long was finally acceptable. And it gave me the power to work around it. I schedule in me-time now—because I need it. Otherwise, I am a pretty crabby person to be around, which doesn't help anybody. It helped me set boundaries if I was going out that let me leave early if I so chose ("Sorry, I'm an introvert! Gotta go home and recharge!"). But seriously, it allowed me to explain to others that it wasn't personal, and I just needed to be careful of my energy. Once I explained it to them, they were more understanding if I needed to duck out early.

Introversion is just one aspect of personality—there are more that we will explore later on in the chapter. But identifying that one facet of myself made an enormous impact on my life.

How Knowing Personality Type Can Help You

1. ***It helps give you awareness***—Your preferences for things can lie in your personality. Your irritation when the milk was left out, your elation at finishing a puzzle—your personality can explain those feelings. This also may be why we are drawn to certain situations or people, or why certain things stress us out that don't bother others as much. Armed with this knowledge, you can shape your world to suit your preferences, and begin to address your stressors and how to handle them better.

    Sometimes we don't recognize our tendencies until we have them explained to us, and sometimes not in a good way (e.g., a fight with your partner will probably help illuminate things for you, but you're not likely to address these issues if you're being scolded). Learning about your particular personality can shed light on your tendencies, whether subconscious or not. We can't bring about change if we don't know we have traits that could benefit from some attention, and learning more about your personality can help do that.

2. ***It helps you accept yourself***—By understanding yourself better, it helps you understand why you do the things you do, and why you think or feel a certain

way about a given situation. Knowing that you are cognitively wired to perceive the world in a certain way can help explain your thoughts, feelings, and behaviors. If other people with similar personality types share your patterns, you are probably not alone in thinking or feeling a certain way.

Once you truly accept yourself as you are, you don't have to beat yourself up for making a mistake or doing things you do (e.g., procrastinating), and you can see yourself in a whole new light. You are truly a wonderful person just as you are. That doesn't mean you can't make changes or improvements in your life. But when you see yourself from a place of acceptance and understanding, you can begin to make better decisions based on what you actually want.

3. *It helps empower you to make change*—There are certain things you have control over and certain things you don't. While you can't easily change your personality, you can make changes to your life to help you work around it. For example, if you have a tendency to procrastinate, you can set up measures to help combat that tendency (e.g., setting an alarm, putting notifications on your phone, etc.).

Knowing your personality better can help you understand how you make decisions. We each have different factors that play into our decisions that affect every aspect of our lives, from major decisions (where we live or which partners we choose) to small choices (where we shop for groceries). Knowing how you (sometimes unconsciously) make decisions can help you make better ones.

4. *It helps you with interpersonal relationships*—Knowing yourself and why you make the choices you do can help with understanding others better, too. Recognizing that everyone makes decisions differently can help you appreciate why your manager may seem rigid, why your co-worker may be flaky, or why the doctor you work with isn't in touch with his feelings. Helping you accept yourself often has the compound reaction of helping you accept others better as well. Age, culture, and childhood experience also play a role in personality, and recognizing that others may see the world differently due to these factors helps you appreciate them more. You can consciously make decisions knowing your own and others' tendencies to strengthen bonds. This may look like sticking to a schedule because you know your colleague operates that way, or toning down your chatty nature around someone who is more reserved.

This can also help you in your personal life as well. I had a friend confide in me that she got upset when she and her husband were on vacation. They would be enjoying themselves in the moment, and he would ask her at that time what they were doing next. She was hurt, believing that he wasn't having fun and needed to have something else on the agenda. With her being more of a go-with-the-flow personality, she didn't need to have that structure. Knowing that I also like to know what the plan is, I explained to her it probably wasn't that he wasn't having fun, but that he just needed to have an idea of what to expect next. Recognizing our needs that support our personalities can help prevent conflict.

As health care workers, we have been practicing this skill for most of our lives. We are already pretty in tune with others' tendencies, and we use our superpower of empathy on a daily basis. Diving a bit deeper into our own and others' personalities can help us strengthen this skill at work and at home.

5. *It helps with conflict*—Most conflict arises out of the different perspectives that others have. Knowing your personality type can help you understand your values that are being threatened and why you are feeling as strongly as you are in an argument. For example, my personality when my values are threatened is to become overly emotional, which doesn't often help. Armed with knowing this pattern in my personality, I can better articulate what I am feeling and why to the person who I am upset with ("I don't like it when you interrupt me. I feel like you don't care about what I have to say."). This often gets at the root of the issue, not what seems to be happening on the surface. This can help alleviate tension and prevent the conflict from escalating.

Knowing how others are likely to react can also give you insight into how they are feeling when they are experiencing conflict. You can then consciously choose not to behave in a way that may be triggering for them. For example, if a colleague you work with gets overwhelmed when given too many tasks, you can prevent conflict by asking others to pitch in or asking her to do the tasks in a systematic way, such as in order of priority. Taking a second to anticipate our own reactions and the reaction of others is the ounce of prevention we need to avoid "a pound of cure"—and I don't know about you, but I've got enough pounds of "cure" (namely potato chips) kicking around since the pandemic.

Personality Categorizing

There are many different types of personality categorizing. Myers & Briggs is one of the most widely used and accepted ideologies available. It has been used in a variety of specialties, from psychology classes to the corporate world.

Based on a theory from Carl Jung that included archetypes, Isabel Myers and her mother Katharine Briggs expanded on this in the 1940s. It was during the war, and many women were going to work. As many of these women had no prior working experience, Isabel, a voracious reader of Jung and psychology, created a tool to help women be placed into jobs based on their personalities. They wanted this knowledge to be readily accessible to people without having to be psychoanalyzed. They felt that people experience the world using four principal psychological functions—introversion vs. extroversion, sensation vs. intuition, feeling vs. thinking, and judging vs. perceiving—and that people use these functions in a varying degree, based on their personality type.

Criticism for Personality Tests

While it is a widely used tool, personality typing has its share of critics. It has been accused of being an unreliable and invalid instrument for measuring a concept that is very abstract. While I wouldn't rely on it as a bible, I do believe it is a helpful tool if we use it properly. Here are some common criticisms for the tool, and my rebuttal:

It is a pseudo-science and not an effective tool—While it cannot be put through a double-blind randomized study, personality typing can help give people insight into themselves and others. Most of psychology is unable to be scientifically examined the way that a clinical trial can be. While it may not hold much clout in the scientific world, it does provide value and can help people understand themselves better, which leads to better accepting of themselves and others. This is extremely valuable in the workplace, as understanding that others may not think the same as you can help with interpersonal communication and conflicts.

It puts you in a box—my INFP friend complained that this tool made her feel too structured (as a Perceiver would!). While I agree that it does need to categorize in order to type you (an ambivert may feel they are neither a true introvert or extrovert), it is a spectrum. Some people might be extremely introverted, and some, not as much.

As an INFJ, I have had the pleasure of working with other INFJs, and we are not all alike! The function of personality typing is not to put people neatly into boxes, but to give you deeper insight into who you are—your strengths, weaknesses, and tendencies—so that you can accept yourself more deeply and have the power to make conscious change. I found it massively helpful in accepting aspects of myself that I was either ignoring or too ashamed to admit to having. Once I recognized that others, like me, had these tendencies, it allowed me to accept myself and finally look at areas that I needed to look at in order to grow as a person.

You can become immersed in typing and not see the bigger picture—Do all ENFPs prefer chocolate ice cream? Seriously. If you go to the personality forums, you can see people who are so fascinated by this tool that they start looking at everything from this world. Sometimes actions don't need to be analyzed. While it is a fun tool, it is exactly that—a tool. Getting too caught up in analyzing why people do what they do can lead you down a rabbit hole that is neither effective nor healthy for living a balanced life.

The Structure of Myers & Briggs Personality Type

Expanded on Jung's work, there are four categories of personality functions with this tool: Introversion vs. Extroversion, Sensation vs. Intuition, Feeling vs. Thinking, and Judging vs. Perceiving. By selecting one in each category, we end up with four letters. For example, I am an INFJ (Introverted, Intuitive, Feeler, Judger). To get an idea of which you are, answer the following questions below:

Extroversion versus Introversion: Do you gain your energy from being around people and focusing on the outer world, or do you gain it from going mostly within?

Sensing versus Intuition: Do you prefer to collect information from what is happening (what you can see, hear, taste, touch, small), or do you tend to infer from more abstract experience?

Thinking versus Feeling: Do you tend to make decisions based on logic, or more from circumstance and how it will affect people?

Judging versus Perceiving: Do you prefer structure and routine, or do you prefer things to go with the flow?

Based on the above information, you might be able to guess which personality type you are. While we all have the capacity to be introverted and extroverted, we predominantly default to one over the other most of the time. The same can be said for the other functions. Based on which you choose in each category determines which of the 16 personalities you are.

While you may be able to guess, if you are curious, I recommend taking an online test – most are free. A number of my clients have been surprised to learn they tested differently in a category than they originally thought.

Personality Typing and the HCW

Health care workers often collaborate with a variety of people, and with this, many types of personalities. Witnessing how throwing different types of personalities together in a stressful workplace affected things was fascinating to me. Different areas tended to attract different personalities (e.g., ICUs attracting more "Type A" personalities). Different leadership styles affected the workplace (e.g., the same department in two different hospitals were run completely differently, despite having the same tasks). Staff turnover can completely transform a department (for better or worse).

When I learned more about personality typing, I definitely went through an overzealous phase. However, it strengthened my superpower of empathy—leveled it up, in a sense. I understood why my rigid co-worker had to go for break at a certain time (when we got them!). Why one of the doctors didn't seem to handle his stress well (mostly because I could also see it in myself). Why some of my colleagues had a hard time leaving work on time, as they felt they needed to complete the day's tasks before they left. It didn't excuse the unacceptable behavior I encountered, but it did give me insight into why someone might act in a certain way.

It also helped me in my daily work as well. Obviously, it helped me zero in on what I needed to work on. Being an INFJ, we have a tendency to be martyrs and can burn out easily. I knew I needed to keep this in check, and this gave me more motivation to do so.

But it also helped me play to my strengths. Doing development work, we often focus on what we need to improve on. Being aware of this is great, but we don't need to focus on it every minute of every day. Knowing your personality helps you know your gifts as well. I began to focus on my strengths more in my daily work life. Being intuitive, I often could anticipate what others might need. Being a feeler, I could empathize with my patients, which established a deeper connection with them. Being organized, I could prioritize my day well.

Knowing what my fortes were allowed me to concentrate my attention to where I could make the biggest difference. I chose tasks that played to my strengths, while forgoing others that I just accepted weren't my thing, instead of fixating on not being good at them. I actually like charting (I guess as an author it makes sense!), so I would often volunteer to do this, as most of my colleagues don't like doing it.

It is important to remember that all personality types are equal and that every type has value. Recognizing your strengths at work can help you choose tasks that you would prefer to do. Recognizing your weaknesses may give you something to work on, or identify something you would prefer not to do—we don't have to be good at everything! Recognizing that others may have a strength in a particular area will help you work with your colleagues more cohesively.[1]

1. Complete an online personality test (I recommend 16personalities.com or person-alityhacker.com). Do a thorough read-through of your type, including the listed strengths and weaknesses. How accurate do you feel it is? If you are interested in going deeper, the Myers & Briggs website does have a test available for purchase.

2. Look up famous people who have the same personality type as you. Check out their autobiographies or Wikipedia their careers and personal lives. What similarities do you notice between you? What differences?

3. If your friends/family/coworkers are interested, encourage them to take the test as well. This will give you a deeper insight into how their personality works and can really positively affect your relationships with them. By understanding their types, it helps you accept them as they are and come from a space of acceptance when you clash/disagree with each other.

4. How does knowing your personality type help you in your career? How do you think knowing more about personality types will help your patients and coworkers?

5. Now that you know a bit more about your personality, how can using your strengths help you lead a more balanced life? What weaknesses/areas for growth were noted for your personality? How can working on this help you in your career and at home?

CHAPTER 8

The Inner Child

"We don't stop playing because we grow old; we grow old because we stop playing." – *George Bernard Shaw*

Have you ever done something completely out of character when you were stressed?

Have you ever had a fear about something that seemed irrational, that you might lose your job if you made a error, but you ignored it because you thought it was silly?

Do you have a voice in your head that criticizes your mistakes or stops you from doing something for fear that it won't be good enough?

Have you ever uttered the phrase "I don't know what came over me!"?

I'll tell you what came over you—your ego. Only I want to take a different spin on the ego than what you're probably used to.

For those of us who can recall our psych rotations, the ego is defined as "a person's sense of self-esteem and self-importance."[1] While Freud meant it to mean more about separating self from non-self, the definition of "ego" often gets confused with the word "pride," so much so that it has become synonymous with it. Hurting someone's ego usually means something negative toward the person with the ego.

In spirituality, much of what the teachings revolve around is analyzing the ego and its limitations. The little voice inside our heads that tells us we aren't good enough, that causes us to fear rejection, and that keeps us stuck can be attributed to the ego. Buddhism recognizes the importance of the ego, but impresses that is an illusion. These teachings have been misconstrued in Western spirituality, where having an "ego death" is something to aspire to.

But what if we looked at our ego from a different perspective? What if we realized that it was just doing its job to survive? What if the Inner Critic was actually an Inner Child that was scared of rejection? That the hurt feelings over being excluded from something, even though it was not personal, was just our Inner Child feeling afraid that she isn't loved – and is trying to protect us?

But who is she, and why is her voice stuck in our heads?

Ego personas are different parts of ourselves that we show to the outside world. We have many different roles that we take on—spouse, parent, health care worker, etc. We have different hats, depending on the role we are assuming. These personas develop when we are young and evolve over time. We create these personas so that we can function and carry out the roles we adopt on a daily basis. They create structure and enable us to know and perform the duties that are assigned to us when we are wearing each hat. We speak differently and perhaps act differently depending on which role we are assuming in the moment (I was accused by a doctor I worked with that my "phone voice" was much more pleasant than how I spoke to him).

Sometimes, though, we get stuck in these personas because we aren't aware of our patterns. The role we embody is often created because it worked. For example, for those of us who were bullied when we were younger, we may have created a "tough" persona to stand up to the bullies. If this worked (even a little bit), then we take this identity with us until we no longer need it. The problem is that we don't always do this consciously, and we sometimes carry these unconscious personas with us into adulthood. The armor that we wore stays with us, and we use it in much the same way that worked for us back then, ready to defend when we are triggered. The issue is, we often don't need it anymore. Our conscious brains know this, but the part of us that was wounded still hasn't healed, and so our subconscious knee-jerks the same reaction when it's no longer appropriate. This can look like getting defensive when someone asks us a question (believing that we are being punished). This can also look like interrogating ourselves. That Inner Critic no longer has a bully to contend with, but we still hear her voice in our heads, telling us we should have done better or that we don't matter. We become bullies to ourselves.

So, in short, the voice in your head is you.

Isn't so scary anymore, is she?

If you've ever had an irrational thought that seemed silly (a loved one not caring about you, losing your job for making a small mistake), it probably stems from an incident an early version of you had that still hasn't healed. Our Inner Child process remains largely unconscious because it often carries painful memories that we would prefer to forget.

What if, instead of seeing that nagging voice as a nuisance, we were grateful to it? We were born with it for a reason. That part of you needs to be heard. By pushing it away, she is only going to feel more scared, more distrustful, and will get louder until she is taken notice of. This can manifest itself in your daily life, and looks like outbursts, impulsivity, insecurity, being hypercritical of yourself and others, overeating/drinking/spending, the list goes on. Basically, when you feel you are acting out of character or doing things you don't truly want to be doing or you don't feel like you are in control, this is your Inner Child acting out—because she hasn't been listened to.

You wouldn't scold a three-year-old for being sad or angry, would you? Nor would you ignore her when she is upset and trying to reach out for help. Well, by telling yourself you are being silly, or a feeling you have is unjustified, you are essentially telling an inner part of yourself that you don't matter. We wouldn't do this with our own children, yet we have a tendency to do this with ourselves, whether we are conscious of it or not.

The Inner Child metaphor has been used for a long time, developed through various psychotherapy techniques, including shadow work, the Internal Family Systems Model developed by Richard Schwartz, and Personality Hacker's The Car Model.[2] It is a common tool because it works. It gives us permission to access parts of ourselves that we ordinarily ignore. When we make the unconscious conscious, real healing can happen. It has been one of the most powerful tools I have come across in my own growth and healing, and I am excited to be able to share it with you here.

(*Woo Warning: Much of this chapter discusses psychotherapeutic concepts. If you are open to it, it can be a powerful tool. If not, carry on.)

Accessing our Inner Child can be tricky. Because many of these thoughts/feelings are unconscious, how do we communicate with these parts of ourselves?

Accessing Our Inner Child (IC)

"The cry we hear from deep in our hearts comes from the wounded child within. Healing this Inner Child's pain is the key to transforming anger, sadness, and fear." – Thich Nhat Hanh

First introduced by Jung as an archetype, the Inner Child is the part of us that hasn't matured to our actual age—and we all have parts of us that haven't. The IC is with us all of the time. She is the part of us that is playful, the part of us that is joyful for no reason. She helps us to stay present. If you have observed children, you know that they are completely in the moment, and do things for the sheer joy of it (drawing, running, and all kinds of play). The IC is also entwined with painful memories, the parts of ourselves that we suppress. She sees the world in black and white, and has difficulty acknowledging when things are in between. She reacts instead of acts in situations when under stress, and often shows herself when she is feeling defensive and doesn't want to face something. This is also where we store and carry out our emotions—positive and negative ones (e.g., anger, sadness, fear, excitement, awe). Because the thoughts and feelings of the Inner Child are often unconscious, it can affect our lives, and we may feel like we don't have control over our emotions and reactions.

One way to address this is to focus our awareness on this part of ourselves. By using our superpower of empathy, we can give understanding to the parts of ourselves that we may be ashamed of, or have a tendency to ignore. When we have "negative" emotions come up, it is often our Inner Child alerting us to something that is out of balance for us—whether our logical minds think it is justified or not.

Why Establishing a Relationship with Your Inner Child (IC) is Important

When we ignore parts of ourselves, it causes unrest within us. Much like a child trying to get our attention, it can start off with a little voice. As the child's need for attention goes unmet, it gets louder. The thing is, sometimes all that our Inner Child needs is acknowledgement. If you've been upset about something, and felt better just by saying it aloud, you will know that sometimes the inner nagging we experience doesn't need to be solved, it simply wants a voice. Ignoring that nagging feeling, however insignificant it might seem, is only going to cause our IC to get louder. In addition to silencing the nagging in our heads, there are other reasons we should develop a relationship with the Inner Child:

They are our access to our emotions — Because they are directly attuned to our emotions, (and our emotions are always valid), our IC represents an important aspect of learning about ourselves and how to handle these emotions as an adult. Without them, we wouldn't know anything is wrong. Much like we need pain receptors to keep us from bodily injury, we need emotions to keep our mental health safe – especially the uncomfortable ones.

They are our access to our authenticity — When we were young, we were clear about our likes and dislikes—what we wanted to do and what we didn't want to do. As we got older, we allowed others to influence us and cause us to change our outlook on things—our parents, teachers, and friends began to shape who we were, and in our effort to fit in, we began ignoring our IC, the key to our authenticity. When we don't act from our authentic selves, we can suffer from depression, anxiety, and apathy. Whether we gain approval or rejection from others, it is important to be ourselves. Our IC is our direct access to this, and if we ignore her long enough, health issues can arise.

They are our access to joy — Another very important reason to form a relationship with our Inner Child is because they are our access to joy. They are not only there when there is something off, they are the part of us that finds wonder and excitement in life. The part of us that remains inquisitive about everyday activities is within us, waiting to be let out. They are also our access to our creativity, as the part of us that imagines is the part still filled with curiosity about life. We give ourselves permission to act on our passion, and forget about what anyone else thinks. This is the gift our IC gives us when we nurture it. When we lose touch with our creativity, our wonder, and our excitement with how we interact with the world, we lose our joy. Our IC helps us to be carefree and present in the moment. They don't care about how many calories are in the cake, or how many steps they got in from running in the park, or what the carbon footprint is of a car ride by the sea. We adults can get so bogged down in being responsible that we lose touch with the joys of life.

I believe much of the world's apathy and depression is due to a loss of our connection with our Inner Child. Do you remember the joy you felt as a kid doing simple activities, such as coloring or playing on a playground? We didn't care if the drawing we colored was a masterpiece, we did it for the sake of doing it – it is adults who try to attach meaning to our activities. We as children had the ability to find joy in the little things, something we as adults lose the ability to cultivate. By consciously choosing to focus our attention on this aspect of our personality, we can tap into our joy. If you have been feeling sadness, anxiety, or apathy with life, I first recommend working with a professional to help get you through this. Suggesting Inner Child work with a therapist can have amazing results if you are open to the concept.

Trauma and the Inner Child

According to Robert Jackman, the author of *Healing Your Lost Inner Child,* all of us have been exposed to some type of childhood suffering (and have PTSD on some scale) when we were growing up, and how we dealt with it then was the best way we knew how to at that time.[3] However, we have a tendency to stick with what works and use the same type of protection that served us then but is no longer serving us now.

Common types of traumas that children experience, such as neglect and physical abuse, can cause unhealthy learned behaviors as an adult. For example, the child of an angry, abusive parent may have learned that the best way to survive was to stay quiet. This may have served the child well at the time, but if we don't address this as an adult, it can lead to feelings of not being heard, feeling disrespected, and resentment.

When we experience traumatic events at specific times in our childhoods, parts of us stay "stuck" at the age we were when they occurred, causing us to subconsciously act out from this perspective. Think of how you used to react at this age—what are tantrums like at age three versus age ten? A lot happened to me at the age of ten, and I really notice black-and-white thinking that a ten-year-old has when I am stressed (e.g., making a mistake at work and feeling like I am incompetent).

Some other examples that our Inner Child didn't feel safe:

- We were punished for showing our emotions.

- We were ignored or talked down to when we voiced our opinions.

- We were made to feel responsible for our parents' happiness/well-being.

We can also have trauma that we did not realize was traumatic at the time. For example, I had my tonsils out at the age of ten, and my parents did not give me the option of choosing this. What was an attempt to help me (I constantly cleared my throat because my tonsils were so big I could feel them) turned into something much bigger, although I didn't realize it at the time. I unconsciously learned that I didn't have control over my body, and this obviously led to unhealthy behaviors and perspectives as an adult.

We will always move away from what we believe is most painful, even if that belief is not conscious. If you stayed in a job or a relationship for longer than you believe you should have, some part of you believed it would be more painful to leave than to stay. If you think you are stuck or going around in circles, look into your beliefs—you might find something that even though your logical mind feels is not serving you, your Inner Child believes that it is. The unhealthy behavior you notice in your life as an adult is your IC wounding.

Much of our people-pleasing behavior can be traced back to this—if we can get people to like us through serving, it will be less painful than being rejected or abandoned. The feelings of not being in control, of being disrespected, or disempowerment is your IC bringing up something that needs attention. We as adults have a tendency to brush off much of what we experienced as a child. We think that because we are grown and have the ability to see things from a higher perspective that the hurt is no longer valid. The truth is, our past is never behind us; it is what we carry with us today. In order to deal with what we are struggling with as adults, we need to look at what we are still carrying from the "past," because it exists in the now.

Gone unchecked, the Inner Child can take over your life. The longer you leave it, the more extreme the behaviour. Some signs that you have a wounded Inner Child:

Triggering—situations where we feel unsafe, and react instead of act. This often can take the form of fight, flight, freeze, or fawn (a people-pleasing tactic). We don't feel in control of our actions, and this is a classic sign of childhood wounding.

Shame/Low Self-Worth—is the feeling that we, not our actions, are inherently flawed and unworthy. When the Inner Child suffers from shame wounding (often as a result of unhealthy parenting), she will not have the ability to own up to her mistakes because it means SHE is bad, not her actions. This often leads to more shame, and a vicious cycle ensues.

Fear/Anxiety—most of our unwarranted fears stem from childhood wounding. For example, growing up in an environment where money was scarce can lead to irrational behaviors around money as an adult. This is also common with fear of abandonment, rejection, etc.

Fear is actually a powerful tool we can use. If a fear is coming up, embrace it, as it leads to more knowledge about ourselves. The Inner Child's ability to communicate her fears to us is actually a blessing in disguise, and it means unhealed wounds have come to the surface. The best way to deal with fear is to confront it.

Self-Sabotage—is any thought pattern/behavior that stops the adult self from achieving their goals. There are two types: Self-Sacrifice and Procrastination.

- Self-Sacrifice—is putting the needs of others in front of your own, often due to the Inner Child's learned behavior of people-pleasing. This can be seen in children who grew up with neglectful/abusive parents as a way to receive love and belonging.

- Procrastination—stems from the Inner Child not believing she is worthy or capable of achieving the task she has set out to do and therefore puts it off until it is unattainable.

Guilt—is having trouble setting boundaries and feeling bad when we let others down.

Perfectionism—is having to do everything perfectly out of fear of rejection or abandonment.

Suppressing/Repressing Emotions—not feeling safe to have emotions and stuffing them down.

Substance abuse, eating disorders, gambling addictions, promiscuity—numbing out/escaping with substances or unhealthy activities.

Because we health care workers have often gone long periods of time neglecting ourselves, we are also neglecting our Inner Child. If you can see some of your behaviors in any of the above, it means your Inner Child has been trying to get your attention. If you had a child, would you go days without feeding it, making it stay up late, and waking it up early? Would you ignore it if it were crying? Then why are you treating yourself this way? The above behaviors are the adult version of crying for help. We have been ignoring ourselves for so long that our subconscious is using these unhealthy ways in order to cope with the pain of neglect. By putting others' needs ahead of our own, we are effectively abandoning ourselves, and our Inner Child feels it. It is time to pick ourselves up and nurture *us*.

Sometimes we don't know that we are doing these behaviors and the underlying reasons why. And even if we do, we have so much shame around it (some of this brought on by society) that it compounds the problem. There is nothing to be ashamed about in trying to feel better. It is normal to avoid pain—this is survival. If we have found something that gives us some reprieve from whatever we are/have experienced, this is only natural.

If you have witnessed the world operating in extreme polarities (all-or-nothing, politically becoming more extreme), this is because many people are operating from black-and-white thinking, and are unable to see that a grey zone exists. The world seems to be full of ten-year-olds right now, and much of it is due to not being conscious of the inner parts of ourselves. Because many of us were parented in a way that didn't allow us to express our emotions, we are stuck in this developmental stage—and we are playing it out now as adults.

Again, working with a therapist around the Inner Child and trauma can make a huge impact on our lives in the present. Your therapist can give you some functional tools to use instead of using your wounded ones.

From *Healing Your Lost Inner Child,* some examples of using functional tools looks like:

• recognizing the healthy choices you need to act on to get you through your day	• choosing people in your life who are good for you and encourage you
• feeling proud of yourself even when you aren't acknowledged by anyone else	• honoring yourself when you have accomplished something that was really hard, and not skimming over it or going on to the next project
• respecting yourself and your decisions	• recognizing when relationships are reciprocal and when they are not
• encouraging yourself to move forward and finding the motivation to do what is best for you	• knowing you make the best choices each day even if they aren't perfect
• encouraging yourself to move forward and finding the motivation to do what is best for you	• loving the unhealed parts of yourself and giving them extra care to heal

• asking for help from others	• getting extra rest when you need to
• being vulnerable with people you trust	• being discerning of who or what is working for you, and who or what is working against you

The more you use these tools instead of the wounded ones, the easier it gets. Wounded tools are just habits, and habits can be interrupted, but it is helpful to replace them with different, healthier ones.

Building a Relationship with the Inner Child

For those of you who are parents, you know you would be doing damage if you neglect your children long enough. We need to parent our Inner Children the way we parent our offspring. Checking in with our Inner Child gains us access to important aspects of us.

A good place to start in healing the wounded part of you that you probably haven't acknowledged in a while is to create a relationship with it. Like we have a relationship with our bodies, we can form a relationship with our inner selves. Some steps you can take:

1. *First, acknowledge that the Inner Child is there*—this is often the biggest piece of what needs to happen, as she often just needs to be heard. Who were you as a child? Were you quiet, thoughtful, loud, rambunctious, or somewhere in between? What did you like to do as a kid? Reflecting on your childhood can help you access your Inner Child. If it helps, talk to family members who knew you as a child to gain insight into that part of you.

2. *Communicate with her*—set aside time to do this. It can either be done on your own or with a therapist. It can be done verbally, or through journaling or visualization. The best question to ask her, especially in times of stress, is, what is she feeling? What is she blaming herself for? What does she need you to forgive her for?

Disclaimer—this will probably feel REALLY AWKWARD at first—I recommend working with someone initially. Later, practice silently in your head, or go to a place where you can be fully alone (your car, for instance), as talking out loud has powerful properties. As you practice this, you will get more comfortable. The most powerful healing that I have witnessed in myself and my coaching clients has come from this exercise—it really works.

3. *Recognize that your IC has a little piece of power* – accept that there are certain parts of yourself that prefer to have things a certain way, as it provides structure for your IC that she may not have gotten as a child. When she is speaking up, your IC is helping you recognize when things in your life are not okay. In essence, she helps you identify your truth when it may not be conscious for you yet. Our IC feels safest when she has a balance of consistent guidance and autonomy. She needs to feel that her opinion matters, even if your adult self doesn't necessarily agree with her.

For example, I get positively giddy when I have things in my house organized, and I'm irritable when things are out of place. Would I prefer to be able to live with clutter and not be annoyed at dirty dishes? Absolutely, especially when living with others or when I'm too tired to clean. But I recognize that I feel better when my environment is tidy. And sometimes, I tell my IC that she will have to live with dishes in the sink for a while. As long as I am clear about this by consciously declaring it (either silently or out loud), it prevents perfectionism, which I can sometimes fall into if I am not being conscious of it.

4. *Nurture her through conscious parenting*—the two things every child needs to thrive are to feel safe and to feel unconditionally loved. The wounds of the Inner Child can still be open. What is she feeling toward the adult part of you? Mistrust? Anger? Fear? It may be an ongoing journey to re-establish the relationship with that part of yourself, especially if your IC grew up in an environment where she couldn't trust adults. It may be time-consuming, but I promise you, it is the most rewarding work you can do. Reinforce this through positive self-talk (she can hear you, trust me). You can do this anywhere, but doing it while looking in the mirror can make this even more powerful.

You wouldn't ask a ten-year-old for advice on making decisions. It is not the IC's job to make grown-up choices—she sees everything in black and white and is unable to differentiate subtle nuances of life. If you grew up in a tumultuous household, you may have felt you could only rely on yourself at that time, and your IC may still think she needs to be in control. When she knows you are in charge, she will be more likely to relax, thus quieting the anxious thoughts you have.

Tell her she is safe. Give her examples of this, and do so in clear, simple language. When we are stressed, we require things to be easy to understand. Talking to that inner part of ourselves requires kind, gentle language that is easy to grasp. What does unconditional love look like to you? How can you gift this to your Inner Child?

Parenting Your Inner Child

Consciously parenting the parts of ourselves we tend to ignore is necessary for a healthy, integrated life. It helps us set healthy boundaries, reward ourselves, and troubleshoot when the "check engine" light is on. Often, when we are on autopilot, we go into automatic mode because life is busy! We only respond to the voice of our Inner Child when she is out of control. By consciously "checking in" with ourselves, this stops the tendency to have to put out fires when we ignore our own needs.

The role of parenting the Inner Child is to support them, guide them, and basically lead the parts of you that need extra support. When you are acting impulsively and you stop and do some self-reflection as to why you are acting out this way, you are consciously parenting. The message with this is that you approach your behavior from a place of compassion and kindness, exactly as you would do with an actual child. By addressing your behavior from a place of kindness and not criticism, you can fully accept yourself as you are—all of the parts of you—and begin to make positive changes in your life. When your Inner Child gets triggered, the conscious parent is the part of you that helps support them, so you never feel alone. When you make a mistake, instead of scolding yourself like you usually do, try changing the script to something kinder, knowing that there is a little person inside of you listening.

By having a practice that helps us consciously check in with ourselves routinely—it doesn't have to be every day, but it has to be consistent—we prevent the buildup of emotions and nagging feelings that we would not be able to access because they are subconscious. By journaling, going on a reflective walk in nature, meditating, etc., we connect to the inner parts of ourselves that require nurturing. This often will decrease the amount of triggering/stress we feel, because we are able to name our pain. When we don't know what is bugging us, often we do—we just haven't given ourselves the space and time to sit with it.

Some of us try to find something "out there" to comfort ourselves. Ice cream, a winning lottery ticket, a Pyxis machine that actually picks up our fingerprint on the first try? The truth is, nothing external can truly make us happy for long. As boring and cliché as it sounds, our sense of satisfaction and fulfillment needs to come from within. If we don't feel we have this, that is where we need to look—within.

Once we have identified what our Inner Child is in need of, the conscious parent, from an adult perspective, can figure out how best to tackle what has come up. If it was a colleague who snapped at you, allow the IC to tell you how it felt. If it is still bugging you the next day, you might decide (much like a real parent) the best thing to do is to say something, because you (like a child) deserve to be treated with kindness and respect. This might not have been made conscious unless you gave yourself permission to speak to that part of you that was wounded, and you might not have been willing to confront your co-worker unless you looked at the situation as you would have if you were a parent.

Dealing with Uncomfortable Emotions

Much of the reason we experience distress in our lives is our inability to deal with our emotions. We suppress them, stuff them down, deny they exist. In doing so, we deny the Inner Child the ability to be validated. Healthy children are very good at expressing emotions – and getting over them quickly. Adults, perhaps due to our parents who shamed us when we felt "negative" emotions (due to their own inability to handle their own emotions), often stifle their feelings.

Society has also not been kind in accepting us as human beings with emotions. We are shamed for our anger, deemed unprofessional for crying at work, and given products to nullify the effects of them (Botox for laugh lines, anyone?). It is no wonder, then, that we would not be adept at expressing them in a healthy way.

Emotions are energy—they need somewhere to go. If we suppress/repress them long enough, they cause distress. Think of emotions like water in our body. If we keep damming them up, they will eventually break the dam, often when we least want them to, directed at the people we least want them to be directed at. When we learn to channel the hose through conscious parenting, we do not deny the emotions are there—we acknowledge them, sit with them, and can release them in a healthy way.

One way we can work through our emotions is to LABEL them. By LABELing our emotions, we give our Inner Child a safe space to express their feelings and be truly seen.

LABEL Our Feelings

Label—Give it a name. "I feel manipulated" isn't a feeling. If you have a hard time coming up with an actual emotion, look up an emotion wheel for what it is you're exactly feeling. Most feelings can be broken down from four main emotions: happy, sad, angry, afraid (e.g., "frustrated" would be a form of anger, "anxious" would be classified as fear).

Acknowledge—Let it be there. Whatever emotion you are having. Don't analyze if you "should" be feeling it or not (you are, regardless). Your Inner Child has a reason for feeling whatever it is, even if your adult mind doesn't agree it should be there. For example, I know my friend who couldn't help me out isn't abandoning me, but the fear is there, all the same, and my Inner Child needs to know it's okay to feel. Denying it will only separate you from the feeling you are trying to deal with. Sometimes, getting to this step is enough. The feeling just wants to be acknowledged, and as soon as you acknowledge it, you might notice it fade away. Practice acknowledging what you are feeling at any given time as you go through this process.

Be with it—Sit with it. If you have named and acknowledged it and you are still feeling the discomfort, be with it. Do your best not to distract yourself or stuff it down. This is where we often go to unhealthy forms of dealing with our emotions to distract ourselves: drinking, eating, excessive cleaning, etc., in order to avoid the pain. I recommend working with someone if you are not used to dealing with your emotions in a healthy way, as they can be the person who holds space while you cry (or scream) it out.

Express it—Do what you need to do to get it out. Get creative. This can be journaling, crying, yelling into a pillow, going to a junkyard and hitting scrap metal, whatever works. Tai chi/tapping/EFT has really worked for me. Do it in a safe place, with someone safe if need be, but do it. It might feel uncomfortable/awkward at first, but believe me, you will feel a *ton* better when you are finished. It is absolutely worth it.

Let it go—This sounds challenging if you haven't done the previous steps, but often whatever needed to be released has done so by this stage. If you find yourself still thinking about whatever caused the emotion to come up after you have gone through this process, ask your Inner Child what she needs. Maybe it is to talk to the person who brought the emotion up, maybe it is to make a list of solutions. Carry out whatever you need to, and then make a conscious decision to let it go. You might not get the apology or the justice that you are wishing for, so don't be weighed down by waiting for it. You can make an affirmation statement ("I choose to let the feeling of anger towards X go"), or make a ritual of it (burning a letter, throwing a rock into the ocean), or anything that signifies closure to you. It really works, and you will come away lighter for it.

Much like when we comfort a child who has fallen down and hurt themselves, we don't try to take the pain away from them (because we can't), we don't shame them for falling, and we don't try to give them advice for not falling down in the first place. We hold them, comfort them, and provide a safe place while they cry (or yell) it out.

Inner Child work runs deep. It can be distressing to tap into, and also very rewarding. As health care workers, it is important to deal with some of the muck we have been carrying for too long, as it can contribute to harming our patients and colleagues. The stigma of going to therapy is beginning to lift, and we can be advocates for others to heal the wounds they have been carrying when we first heal our own.

E X E R C I S E S

1. What were your parents' parenting styles for you growing up? Were they authoritarian, authoritative, permissive, or neglectful? This might give you a hint as to how you might be currently parenting yourself. Research healthy parenting styles and practice using them on yourself. There is no shame—if you didn't have healthy parents growing up, how are you supposed to know what healthy parenting looks like? I learned from TV shows (thanks, Danny Tanner!). Once you have an idea as to what healthy parenting is supposed to look like, utilize these skills with yourself.

2. Can you recall difficult moments in your childhood? How old were you when these moments occurred? What was happening to you at this time? Study developmental milestones and characteristics of children at the age you were. What traits do you still carry from that time?

3. How do you react when you are under extreme stress? What do you think the message is your IC is trying to tell you? For example, I become extremely defensive and lash out. I feel like I am not good enough and feel the need to prove that I am. I show up for my IC by being consistent with my self-care (and forgiving myself when I miss a day). How can you be consistent with your IC to show her she is safe and loved?

4. What activities did you love to do as a child? Coloring? Dancing? Make a commitment to your Inner Child by doing one of these activities once a week. By being consistent, it will help gain trust and establish a rapport with this part of you. It doesn't have to be artistic (or financially lucrative), just how you express yourself. If that means making glitter headbands, go for it! Or if it means being out in nature and studying plants, that's great, too. It is imperative that you stick to this promise, as the part of you that you have been ignoring is not likely to trust you right away—those doubtful voices will subside eventually.

5. What would you do with the day in front of you if you could do anything (and I mean, AN-Y-THING)? If there were no consequences to your actions, what would you do? Would you fly, or walk through walls? Would you rob a bank and go on a trip around the world? Would you mess up your manager's perfectly coiffed head of hair? Tapping into this imaginative side is playing with your Inner Child—she doesn't care about the how or why. Don't censor yourself. While I don't recommend you do the illegal things that might come up, take a look at the list of things that do come

up—is there a theme? It will give you insight into your IC's deepest desires, and might spark some creativity within you that can help move you forward as an adult.

6. Check in with your Inner Child at least daily and ask her: What is she feeling? As the adult part of you, do your best to meet these needs if they are reasonable (obviously if she says she needs ice cream, you would parent this side of you, just like you do a child).

7. Commit to a regular self-parenting practice. Make sure it is consistent and allows time for listening to your inner voice. Revisit what came up for you the next day. If something is still bothering you, write down what the issues are and brainstorm ideas of what small changes you can make. This helps ensure your Inner Child knows they are being heard, and that you are the one in charge, so they can focus on their role of being creative and bringing joy.

8. Think of an emotion you might be burying. Use the LABEL technique to work through it. Journal about how you feel after doing the exercise.

9. Think of something that you are ashamed of about yourself. Who would you be if you didn't carry that shame? What would you accomplish, who would you talk to, what would you do with your time if you weren't ashamed of that aspect of yourself? What is one small action you could take if shame wasn't with you?

10. Write a letter to your IC. You can tell her she is okay as she is, or ask her questions, or simply write what comes up. If it helps, try to find a photograph of yourself at that age. What would she have needed to hear from you?

11. Think of a situation at work where you felt your Inner Child was being triggered. If you could go back and self-parent them, what would you say? What were they feeling at the time and what did they need from you, as the parent? Practice this inner dialogue now, as it will help you in the future when your Inner Child gets triggered again.

CHAPTER 9

People-Pleasing

"If you spend your life pleasing others, you spend your life."
– Cheryl Richardson

Throughout this book, I have described our superpower of empathy. How we as health care providers are so in tune with our patients and their suffering, we can actually feel it. Some of us were born with this ability, some of us developed it over time. I have a suspicion that some of us learned it because it was a necessary skill to survive a problematic childhood.

The Beginning of Empathy ... and People-Pleasing

Growing up with alcoholic parents, I never felt secure. My dad was prone to violence when he drank, and I distinctly remember having to hide away from him at times for my own protection. My mother, also an alcoholic and addicted to opiates, was prone to bursts of rage even when she was sober. With PTSD from living in war-torn Northern Ireland at the root of her behavior, she could be impulsive, selfish, and hurtful. She would argue with me even when I was a small child (it didn't help that I had a *definite* cheeky streak), and if I didn't behave to her liking, she would not only hit me, but ridicule me, taunt me, or insult me in any way she could to cause pain. Both of the people who were supposed to protect me were the source of my insecurity. I didn't feel safe and was always searching for a way defend myself.

In order to survive my childhood with as little abuse as possible, it became imperative for me to read my parents exceptionally well. I had to interpret their cues, their nuances, their body language, anything that would give me data. Unconsciously, I was looking for ways to detect their tells, reading any twitch or sigh that may indicate danger. Identifying the patterns kept me safe.

I became hyper-independent, knowing that I couldn't rely on them. This caused me to grow up way quicker than I should have, and I even began taking on their problems. I knew when we were struggling financially, and I would try to make suggestions to help ease the burden. Children of alcoholic parents often cope in a similar manner, and we don't give children enough credit for how ingenious they are for finding ways to survive. While there was a genuine desire to help my parents because I loved them, I also subconsciously knew that if they weren't as worried about money, I would be less likely to be mistreated by them, so it was another way to protect myself.

This was how my ability to empathize with others began. By being so attuned to my parents' behavior, I became adept at feeling other people's energy. My ability to interpret patterns developed at a young age, and I was unconsciously doing it regularly, even with people other than my parents. Being so attuned to others was a skill I needed, not knowing that I was sacrificing my ability to read myself.

Can you identify any similarities to my story in your own?

Of course, I still craved my parents' affection and love. And though they were wounded, they weren't monsters. They loved me the best way they could, given what they had been dealt with in life. Sometimes they were loving, and nurturing, and supportive. Which only fueled me more to win their affection. If I could do things that made my parents happy, their moods would improve, and they were more likely to be affectionate. I equated doing things that pleased them as love, and so I earned my affection by doing. I went out of my way to find things that would please them.

Where I learned to get the most bang for my buck was being a good student. I was rewarded for bringing home good marks, so I strove to achieve this. I created a persona of a good student, and I felt good when my parents told me they were proud of me, something they didn't often do before I started school. It brought me positive attention from teachers, which I also craved, as my parents were often in their own worlds.

My desire to help naturally led me to nursing as a career, as I was hungry to help. The perpetuation of pleasing others was very much rewarded as a nurse. My patients thanked me, my coworkers were grateful, and my manager could rely on me to stay overtime when needed. I was a good employee, well-liked by my colleagues, and I felt like I finally had my life together.

Enough was Enough

Yet, over time, I began to become resentful. Our workload was ever-increasing, my colleagues were stressed, and I didn't feel upper management appreciated anything my coworkers did for the department. I was feeling drained and started to look at the patients as procedures, not people. "Did you call for the neph tube?" Not the patient's name, the product we were placing. That was how we all referred to our cases—I was losing sight of what my patients were supposed to mean to me.

I also realized very quickly that my heroism for coming in sick, staying late, and picking up call shifts was not being rewarded the way I thought it would be. No one thanked me, I didn't get a medal—all I got gifted was feeling more resentment. I know my manager and colleagues did appreciate it, but was that enough to be sacrificing my sleep, my health, and my well-being?

My superpower of empathy was kryptoniting me. I grew up so outward-focused out of a need to survive that I never developed my ability to read my own needs. I had needed to suppress them when I was younger in order to prevent harm, and in doing so for so long, I didn't actually know what my needs were. I knew what needed to be done, I knew what *others* needed. But what did I need?

When I first started going to therapy (not realizing the real cause, just knowing that I felt resentful), my therapist would ask me what I wanted. I would list off all of the ways I wanted others to treat me, how I wanted the system to change, how I wanted better for my patients and colleagues.

"No, Shannon," she repeated softly. "What do you *want*?"

I sputtered, stumbled, and then went silent. I honestly, in that moment, couldn't give her a true answer.

I didn't know.

I didn't know what I wanted because I had always based my needs on others. Everything depended on how others treated me, how liked I was by others, how others viewed me. Everything was in my relation to other people. For me, it was co-dependency at the root of my people-pleasing behavior. My Inner Child was still using the coping skills she had learned to survive, and as an adult I hadn't been fully conscious of this. Being unable to answer a simple question of what I wanted woke me up, *big time.*

On the other end of the spectrum, I also had a problem asking people for help. Having grown up needing to be very independent, it was just easier to do tasks myself. Firstly, asking for help was hard. People could say no, and then I would feel rejected. This eventually led to me being more resentful, as people were used to me doing it all. They didn't have a problem with me doing more than my share, and then I felt used and upset.

What I had to realize was that this was a problem that I created—my loved ones and colleagues didn't ask for me to do all of the work, I took it on. While stewing, I judged them for being unhelpful, yet they weren't the ones with the problem—I was. Once I figured that out, I had the power to do something about it.

Signs of Being a People-Pleaser

There is a big difference between the desire for acceptance and people-pleasing. We all need to feel safe, secure, and accepted in our lives. A person with a healthy self-worth feels safe and secure independently of how others perceive them; they know who they are, where their values lie, and what they will and will not stand for. People-pleasers are overly reliant on others for their happiness. In her book *Worthy*, Nancy Levin writes, "When we seek validation outside ourselves, it's a sign of our desperation to feel worthy. Yet no amount of validation from others will ever work—it has to come from within."[1] People-pleasers struggle to feel worthy just for existing, which is our birthright. We feel a need to prove ourselves, either through doing good deeds, achievements, or some other form of external validation. For me, it developed as a need to survive. But we don't all require an unstable childhood to experience this—it can be from parents pushing us for good grades, scoring goals, or attending church.

Our careers have also conditioned this behavior. "Putting patients first" is the quintessential phrase of many a health authority. When I tell my non-health care friends about the events that occur at work, the abuse we are subjected to and tolerate, their eyes widen. They are in absolute disbelief at what I go through, the steps I have needed to take just to get the bare minimum, and how blasé management is to some of the complaints I have made. They marvel at how a system so dysfunctional can be responsible for the well-being of society.

I wonder how it got this bad for so long, but when I consider that our career's foundation is based on putting other peoples' needs first, it all makes sense. People who put other people first would of course be drawn to professions where we do just that. Our careers have made it almost impossible to put ourselves first because historically we have been trained to do the opposite.

If you are unsure if you have people-pleasing tendencies, ask yourself some of the following questions:

• Do you struggle to say no?	• Do you find it hard to stand up for yourself?
• Do you have a hard time accepting compliments or taking credit for your accomplishments?	• Do people often come to you with their problems, or ask you favors, because they know you will say yes?
• Do you feel guilty when you say no, and resist saying no for fear of letting people down?	• Do you worry that people will reject you or be upset with you if you do say no?
• Do you over-commit yourself frequently? Do you have a hard time setting boundaries with others?	• Do you often put yourself in others' shoes, but neglect to think about yourself?

- Do you have a strong drive to be liked by everyone? Does being criticized by someone send you into a downward spiral that takes days or even weeks to recover from?

- Do you need external validation or seek approval when you make a decision?

- Do you lack confidence in yourself?

- Is the idea of being seen as selfish too much for you?

- Do you often wonder if people are taking advantage of you?

- Do you feel resentful often, or behave passive-aggressively (being nice to someone who you feel resentful towards, but complaining about them behind their backs)?

- Do you avoid conflict, or believe that conflict is always a bad thing?

- Do you apologize quickly, even if you have done nothing wrong, because you can't stand being in conflict with someone?

- Do you avoid feeling negative feelings?

- Do you fear losing control of your emotions because you have suppressed so much that you are afraid of what might come out?

- Do you tend to only see the "good" in people, and turn a blind eye to their red flags?

Why Being "Too Nice" Can Be Dangerous

In his powerful book *When the Body Says No*, Gabor Maté explores illness that can be attributed to over-giving. [2] Known as the "nice" disease, ALS has been studied as an affliction of people who neglected themselves for too long – and their bodies gave out. MS and other auto-immune disorders can also be grouped in this category. When we are "nice" (read: repress our emotions), we may receive upfront benefits such as being well-regarded amongst our families and coworkers, but we pay the price later.

When we put others first:

1. *We let ourselves down*—by putting others' needs above our own, we are sending a signal that we are less important than others. This repeated message being sent over and over is a hit to our self-worth each time we commit this felony to ourselves. The more we turn our backs on ourselves, the more we erode our self-esteem. Our Inner Child is watching us neglect ourselves.

2. *We take on too much*—in order to please everyone in our lives, we make too many commitments, and we exhaust ourselves trying to juggle all that we have said yes

to. While we can sustain this temporarily, we cannot keep it up forever. We begin to become exhausted, snappy, and irritable. We blame others for relying on us for too much. We neglect our health, sacrificing sleep, healthy eating, and work-life balance.

3. *We get taken advantage of*—we teach people how to treat us by what we tolerate. If we are chronic yes-sayers, people have a tendency to be drawn to asking us for favors—it's just easier to ask the person who isn't likely to say no to us. Not everyone is exploitative, but we will tend to attract those types of people to us.

4. *We become controlling*—the irony of people-pleasing is that we tend to attract aggressive, controlling people to us—but people-pleasing in itself is a form of control. By always being nice and saying yes, we are manipulating others to act in a certain way (liking us, praising us). Our need to be liked trumps our basic physical and psychological needs.

5. *We suppress our emotions*—when we become tired or resentful of others, we push it down. We have bought into our own "niceness" and don't feel our emotions are justified. We are nice people, we shouldn't be feeling anger or sadness or any other uncomfortable emotion. We say one thing when we feel another. This sends mixed messages to our nervous systems, which has serious side effects. Many chronic illnesses are tied to our ambivalence, including chronic stress, anxiety, and depression.

6. *We deny others the ability to know the real us*—by appearing nice and saying yes all of the time, people don't know who we really are. In fact, if we've been doing this for a long time, WE probably don't even know who we really are. The mask we have been wearing may be hiding parts of ourselves that we would rather others not see, and many of us are afraid to show it. By avoiding self-reflection, we also avoid real intimacy with others, including our loved ones.

Guilt

Guilt is a difficult emotion to experience, and is one of the most common that comes up as we begin setting boundaries. Know that, like any emotion, it is temporary—it will pass.

People-pleasers have a real hard time with guilt. The last thing we want to be seen as is selfish, and when we experience the guilt of saying no, it is often due to a fear of being seen as self-centred. Allow yourself to acknowledge it and feel it before letting it go. Ask yourself, "Who is responsible?" when you feel guilt for not helping out. Your mother's loneliness is *her* responsibility. Your brother's financial woes are *his* responsibility. Your manager's need to staff the unit is *her* responsibility. Their problems are not your problems. You can offer compassion that they are in a tough spot without being accountable for their issues, however much they may make it seem. Put yourself first. You can acknowledge that others are in a difficult spot without becoming immersed in it.

According to Dr. Mate, if you have to choose between feeling resentful and feeling guilt, choose the guilt, every time. We can live with guilt, and the guilty feelings will fade – resentment is corrosive to us, and our relationships.

Often, we people-pleasers are enmeshed in others' lives, and so their pain *is* our pain. So it makes absolute sense why we feel uncomfortable not helping these people—we see it as not helping ourselves. Working with a therapist can help us untangle the enmeshment we might be experiencing with others.

A People-Pleaser in Recovery

The first time I said no, it was as an exercise for my coaching program. I was challenged to say no to the first person who asked me to do something for them. Not a minute after reading this homework, my sister texted me and asked me if I could send her some information on something related to her work. Mustering up my courage, I replied that I was doing a boundaries exercise, and that I couldn't do that favor for her—I was practicing saying no. She texted back, slightly confused, but accepted my response.

Whew! I thought ... *that was easier than I expected!* But then I started to worry. What if she couldn't get the info, what if something went wrong with her job? She obviously needed it! I continued to fret about it but I knew I had to stick with it. Later, I called her to apologize that I couldn't give her the info she had requested. It was something I didn't need to do, but in the early stages of saying no, I felt compelled to explain myself.

"Hmmm? Oh, yeah. No worries, I texted my friend and he sent it to me." She had already put it out of her head, but I was still ruminating hours later.

While I was relieved that she got the information, I noticed two things:

1. She didn't need me! and

2. (Gasp!) She didn't need me.

I marveled at this. Like, wow, people can get things done if I can't get to them. This was actually a source of surprise for me…but also a source of worry. If I didn't do things for her, then she wouldn't need me anymore. That thought actually ran through my head, and I was grateful to this exercise for exposing what an unhealthy belief I was carrying around. I had never had the opportunity to hear it because I usually didn't say no to people. This was a game-changer for me.

While I highly recommend working with a professional for this tendency, as there is usually a lot more to unpack, here are some suggestions for navigating interactions in a less people-pleasing way (adapted from *Worthy* by Nancy Levin):[3]

1. ***Be accountable for your own happiness***—not how you want others to treat you, or what you wish others would do for themselves. What makes you happy? What brings you joy? Identify what you want in life that doesn't involve other people. This may be tricky at first, but if you can figure out what brings you happiness that is not contingent on other people, you will be well on your way.

2. *Set boundaries*—we will go over this more in the next chapter.

3. *Tune into you*—become more inward-focused. Learn what your true likes and dislikes are, irrespective of how others might perceive them, regardless of whether it's "weird" or "useful."

4. *Positive self-talk*—"I did the best I could." "Nobody else is perfect, either." Our Inner Child is begging to hear this from us (not others). They need to know it's safe to be themselves, even when they screw up. When we hear the inner critic (and it is the Inner Child here, too) telling us we're not good enough, it's an attempt to stop us from doing something they are afraid will harm them. You can say, "Oh, you're just trying to protect me—thanks!"

5. *The world is a mirror*—ask yourself what someone who respects themselves would do in the situation in question, and *do it*. Don't think, don't hesitate, don't make excuses ("I don't feel strong enough" is a popular one). It might not feel like it's in alignment with who you are right now, but the more you act like a person with high self-worth, the more you will believe it.

6. *Get a cheerleader*—a trusted friend, a spouse, therapist. This is a big life change that you are embarking on, and you don't need to do it alone. Please reach out to people you trust.

7. *Be part of a community*—or create one (Facebook, meetups) for people-pleasers or setting healthy boundaries. This gives you a chance to not only share your struggles, but also see that you are not alone, as so many people out there have this issue. It is uplifting simply witnessing this.

8. *Do an inventory of people you have in your life*—decide who deserves to stay and who needs to go. Often, people-pleasers have very one-sided relationships. If you notice that some of your relationships involve you doing most of the giving and them taking most of it, evaluate whether or not it is worth it to have these people in your life.

9. *Recognize you always have a choice*—you might feel pressure or a sense of nobleness to help out, but realize that *you* are setting the obligation, no one else. Of course, people are going to be disappointed when you start putting your needs above others, *but will they die?* In all seriousness, the people who are worth being in your life will more than likely be supportive of you taking care of yourself, and you need to question the ones who aren't.

Remember, improving our self-worth is a gradual and life-long process. It didn't erode overnight, so it's unlikely to come back that quickly. Focus on the journey, not the destination.

The Art of Giving and Receiving

"It is more blessed to give than to receive." Acts 20:35

Many of us grew up with the edict that it's more noble to give than receive. The fact that it's in the Bible AND makes us more productive is a win-win for the receivers. And health care workers got that shit down pat. We are great at giving. This is our home, this is where we are comfortable. Casa de Giving is where we stretch out—we own the place. Need something? I got you. If there was a twelve-step program for over-giving, it would be overrun by people in health care.

But ever try to give a us a compliment, and you'll be met with shrugs, blushing, or a dismissive, "Oh, it's just what I do." While we are gracious givers, we are remedial receivers.

When we were in the throes of the COVID-19 pandemic, society was full of fear. Every day, frontline health care workers were putting themselves at risk to care for the most vulnerable. We have been gowning up and going into a war zone every day. We were scared to hug our children because we were afraid of passing on the virus to our families. We were stripping in our garages and immediately showering, or sending our families to grandma's house, or sleeping in RVs to avoid spreading it to our loved ones.

While this isn't the first pandemic most of us have worked through an infectious disease outbreak (does anyone even remember SARS or H1N1?), it is the first one during which people have recognized the sacrifice that we make on a daily basis. People realized what we actually do every day, how much we put ourselves at risk to care for the most vulnerable, the sacrifices we make, the danger we are in. People *finally* got it. While the environment might have shifted when the vaccine was introduced, there was a time when the gratitude was pouring in for "Health Care Heroes."

And we had no idea what to do with it.

A compliment, a gift, a kindness—we are uncomfortable with so much attention, and we are not really able to fully receive it.

We are so used to giving, that when it comes time to receive the appreciation and gratitude that we are *so* deserving of, we can't fully process it. Many of my colleagues were bewildered with the praise, shrugging it off. This has been part of the job description for so long, we aren't doing anything we haven't done before. Yet it is finally garnering attention from people, and we don't know how to react. Some people actually felt uncomfortable with the attention and wished it would go away. I wanted to scream from the rooftops, "JUST TAKE THE PRAISE!" We were finally getting the recognition that we deserved (however short-lived).

But I was just as uncomfortable. One day, I went across the street for lunch in my scrubs. A lady stepped in front of me as I was about to pay and tapped her card over the machine, thanking me for my service as the cashier and I looked as each other, bewildered. Instead of graciously accepting the gift of a free lunch from a stranger, I awkwardly muttered a thank you, fleeing faster than the Ikea lady could shout "Start the car!" I felt so uncomfortable with sitting with this praise because I wasn't used to it, and that is a fricking problem.

Deep down, we know what we are doing is important, we know we're making an impact on people's lives. What's more, we know that only a certain type of person can do the job that we do every day. And we do it without fanfare or fussing. What we do on a regular basis is something only special few can do. We are vital to society. Our power of empathy is more powerful than you know. And this is a power we emulate on a daily basis.

While it is important to remain humble, it is also important to know our worth. One way that we can exercise this is by getting better at receiving.

Why is it important to receive?

If we continue to slough it off, people will be less inclined to offer it again. I once had a partner that I complained never complimented me. He told me I just blew off anything nice he said, and that I didn't seem to believe him ... so he stopped complimenting me. While it wasn't the best way he could have handled that (he's an ex for a reason), I had to admit, if I was giving someone compliments regularly and they refuted what I said or dismissed it, I would be inclined to stop giving them myself.

People are telling us these things for a reason! By being bashful about it, we aren't allowing the compliment to actually get to us. We deflect it. We shrug it off. By not fully accepting whatever good comes our way—compliments, gifts, hugs, whatever—we cut off what we are so deserving of getting. These things fill us up! They may seem like small gestures, but they make a big impact to our mental well-being. If we are feeling a lack of respect or like we are being taken advantage of, we can't complain about it if we don't acknowledge when we DO receive praise or gratitude. We are being ungracious receivers!

People who know they are worthy of the praise they receive are gracious. They accept the praise willingly. People who don't think they are worthy of praise will do anything to detract from it. While there is a time to be modest, it often hurts us when others shed light on our accomplishments and we deflect it. Just like the ex-bf who stopped complimenting me, others will be less inclined to grant their compliments to you—and might start believing you when you say you don't deserve it.

Receiving helps restore balance. If you are giving, giving, giving and feeling resentful, yet are rejecting gifts that come your way—in the form of compliments, assistance, or actual gifts—you are effectively blocking yourself from receiving. You are telling people you don't want whatever it is they are giving. We can't complain we aren't getting enough support when we refuse it when it is offered.

How does it feel when you give a gift to someone and they reject it? Not good. How would you feel if a friend was struggling and needed your help? You would jump at the chance to help her! But if she felt she was being a burden or felt she could cope on her own, what would you tell her? That you would be more than happy to help—because you would be. You would be bewildered that she didn't accept your help when she needed it. Try to remember this the next time someone offers to help you—assume they are offering because they genuinely want to, not because they have to. You are doing them a favour by saying yes. It promotes bonding and intimacy with others.

Why is it so hard to receive?

Sometimes when we give, it is not from an earnest, heart-filled desire. Sometimes it is because we don't feel enough. So when we receive, we don't feel deserving of it. It feels foreign, and we don't accept it graciously (if at all). We might feel like we are conceited if we accept the compliment—this was conditioned in our grandmas' era as being humble, but what we are actually doing is deflecting, and not actually receiving. Giving means you're in charge; receiving leaves you vulnerable.

When we are at a place in our lives where we are taking care of our own needs, we naturally become happier people. We can relax because we are not dependent on others to meet our needs. We take things less personally, and we are more loving. Remember how good it feels to do something because you want to and not because you have to? It becomes an intentional act of love, and it is through this that we receive the most out of our giving. This is where giving is truly better than receiving—we just need to take care of ourselves first.

One way we can help balance the over-giving we are working on is to receive with gratitude.

How to Receive

Know that you are enough—you are worthy, just as you are. You are worthy of everything good that comes into your life, and you deserve good things.

Examine yourself as a giver—think about the times you give and ask yourself what motivates you. If it is out of a sense of obligation, you are probably not truly giving from you heart. Monitor when you feel the impulse to give to another, and ask yourself before you do if it's what you truly want to do. If there are strings attached, chances are it's not something you should do. Practice giving from the heart—expecting nothing in return—and see how different that feels from giving under a sense of obligation. Write a thank you note or send a quick text to someone you have been thinking about—it will probably make their day and helps you practice the flow of giving and receiving.

Examine when in your life you have been a remedial receiver—what did it feel like to receive in the moment? Did you shrug off a compliment or refuse help from someone, saying you were okay when in fact, you could have used the help? Think of times when you sabotaged the chance to receive, and make a promise to yourself to be more open to others' offers of compliments, gifts, or acts of kindness.

Allow the gift to be received—if it is a compliment, simply say, "Thank you." Don't argue or explain anything. Even if you don't believe the compliment is true, graciously accept it. If someone delivers a gift, thank them. If someone offers to help or extends an act of kindness, say yes. The more we accept these gifts into our lives, the easier it is and the more often they will come into our lives in the future.

Sit with the discomfort—when you are complimented, it can be easy to natter on to avoid the feeling that comes up. By saying thank you and nothing else, you can feel that feeling of discomfort that comes up. Just allow it to be there. By acknowledging that it is there, it will become less uncomfortable each time you do this, and pretty soon it will be natural to say thank you and actually *feel* the gratitude of gift you just received.

Resist the urge to reciprocate—when I received gifts or praise or whatever it was, I felt this impulse to give it right back. I felt so uncomfortable with just sitting with what I had just been given because I didn't feel worthy of receiving it. So I hastened to return the favour in whatever way that looked like. Friend brought me flowers? I'll bake her cookies! Co-worker tells me I did a good job? I immediately pass the attention on to her and what she did that day. In those moments, I wasn't truly giving with my heart, I was giving out of a need to feel worthy—and I didn't feel worthy of what I had just received until I gave them something back.

The world needs to flow, it balances itself with yin and yang. We give more easily when our cup is full. We are deserving of the care we give to others, in whatever form it takes.

1. Start small—accepting compliments is the easiest way to start receiving graciously. Saying a simple thank you without adding anything to it can be done with the smallest of kind actions.

2. The next time you are offered help in any way, say yes. Even if you don't technically need the help, accept the offer. Resist the urge to reciprocate in any way ("I'll have to buy you a drink to say thanks!"), and simply end the transaction by saying, "Thank you, I really appreciate your help."

3. Tell your loved ones you are practicing receiving, and ask them to help. "I need help practicing receiving graciously. Can you do something small for me without me paying you back so I can sit with how it feels?" If you are an HCW, this is probably something that will make you feel uncomfortable, but *trust me*—it might be the best exercise you do.

CHAPTER 10

Boundaries

"The only people who get upset at you setting boundaries are the ones who were benefitting from you having none." – Unknown

There has been a lot of talk around self-care these days. On top of having to work, juggle a family, try to exercise, eat right, and have a social life, we somehow have to find time for ourselves, too. Then we feel a responsibility to add *that* to our never-ending list. Just another thing to feel guilty about.

My good friend Star, an entrepreneur and mom with special-needs children, was speaking at a conference. After being told many times over to practice self-care, she exasperatedly stated to a room full of people, "I don't need a bubble bath ... I need a Valium."

For all the talk about self-care and "helpful suggestions" on activities of it, there isn't a lot of talk on how to actually do it. How are we supposed to find time to take care of ourselves when there are a million things to do, and so many people who rely on us? Single moms who work shift work, when is it possible to get time to yourselves?

The first step to self-care is self-awareness. Self-care activities are essential if we want to be healthy and happy, but if we feel guilty that we are not doing them, and doing them seems like a chore (e.g., squeezing in a massage appointment and then stressing the entire time about all of the things you need to do while you're on the table), they are no longer beneficial. We are human, life is crazy, and that probably isn't going to change.

What can help is deciding what is most important to you. Look at the values you identified in the earlier chapter. If there are a million things on your plate and you don't have time for all of it and you are barely keeping it together, try piecing together the things you are doing in life that align with your values. If you value family but are spending more time at work or with other commitments, then something doesn't add up—and it needs to change. If you value health but aren't taking proper care of yourself, then you will be feeling cognitive dissonance. That nagging feeling you have is telling you something isn't right. Shifting your priorities to what is actually important will help you have a greater sense of peace.

Once you have identified what is important and what is not, chances are you will have to start eliminating things from your life. Or, you will need to ask for help from others in order to make it work. Either way, having healthy boundaries is essential if you want to achieve a balanced lifestyle. If you only take away one chapter from this entire book, let it be this one. Setting boundaries is the single most important thing you can do to improve your life.

What are boundaries?

Merriam-Webster defines a boundary as "something that indicates or fixes a limit or extent." Boundaries define us. They tell us what we are and what we are not. They are like an imaginary line of what nurtures us versus what doesn't. They are the limits a person creates for themselves to identify safe and reasonable ways for others to behave towards them. They also describe how to respond to others when those lines are crossed.

What kinds of boundaries are there?

There are physical boundaries (e.g., the space you have between yourself and someone you are talking to—your "bubble"), mental boundaries (your thoughts, opinions, and beliefs), and emotional boundaries (your feelings, or who you are as an independent person).

You are setting boundaries all of the time during the day and don't even realize it. We try go to bed at a reasonable hour and eat healthy (choices), we study when we are preparing for an exam (goals), and we practice at our hobbies (skills). These are all positive ways we use boundaries on ourselves. If you thought you didn't know how to set a boundary, you are further ahead than you thought! You're already setting them.

The idea that people often associate with boundaries is when we are interacting with others. This can be challenging, as we cannot control how others think, feel, and behave. It is up to us to ensure that we are aware of our boundaries before setting them with others. But first we need to know what boundaries are, and what they are not.

Myths and Boundaries

"But empathy, minus boundaries, is not empathy. Compassion, minus boundaries, is not genuine. Vulnerability without boundaries is not vulnerability."
—Brené Brown

There are several myths associated with boundaries (adapted from *Boundaries* by Henry Cloud and John Townsend):[1]

Myth #1—Setting boundaries means I'm selfish.

Setting boundaries with others is actually a sign of mutual respect for the other person. By respecting your needs, you are honoring others because you are committed to being the very best version of you. The myth that setting boundaries with someone is being selfish couldn't be further from the truth. In fact, I would argue that the opposite is true. If you don't set healthy boundaries, it is often for self-serving reasons. Often, we take on too much because we want to make others happy, or we don't want to let them down. We don't like the uncomfortable feeling of telling someone no, so it is easier to just say yes in the moment and figure it out later. We are allowing our fear of being judged or the fear of feeling guilty come before everything else—which is self-serving. If you are too afraid to say no to others, you are not giving the people who matter most to you the best of yourself. Being discerning in who receives your time and energy will allow you to show up for those you have selected in the best way possible.

Myth #2—Setting boundaries hurts others.

Setting boundaries is not an attack on others, rather, it's a way of protecting our energy. Although it may not feel good at first, setting healthy boundaries with people will actually improve your relationships, as it will allow for equal balance. If you have been giving too much in a relationship, the other person is also not experiencing a healthy, balanced relationship, which will in effect hurt them in the long run. If they rely on you for more than they should, they are not growing as a person, and you are in fact doing them a disservice.

While it may be difficult for a loved one to hear that you are setting a boundary for yourself (and they might gripe or grumble), they need to respect the boundary you have set. If they don't (e.g., if they act hurt or angry), it is usually an attempt to get you to go back on your boundaries. This is when it matters most to keep them.

One common mistake people often make when they are learning to set boundaries is they set a "boundary" that controls others' behaviour. Boundaries are for you, not others. This can be tricky when the boundary involves others. "You need to call me more often" is not a boundary. Using "I" statements can be helpful when we are first learning.

Myth #3—Setting boundaries means I'm angry.

Anger is a symptom of not setting appropriate boundaries in the first place. People who have gone too long without setting appropriate boundaries become frustrated and resentful of others. They then have an outburst ("If you don't do this, I'm leaving!"). Boundaries that are set in an angry outburst are ultimatums, not boundaries. If proper boundaries had been set in the first place, this wouldn't be necessary. By knowing what your needs are and establishing them early on, this can be avoided.

Myth #4—When others set boundaries, they hurt me.

Having others set boundaries doesn't always feel nice, but if you have set healthy boundaries yourself with others, you know they come from a place of mutual respect. It's often not the boundary but the dependency on others that hurts us. Before I started working on my boundaries, I took it personally when people set them with me. Because I didn't have any, I didn't understand others who did. I've definitely been sad when a friend couldn't help me out due to other commitments. Now I recognize that it isn't personal, that my friend is prioritizing her needs and protecting her energy, and that I have the right to do the same.

Myth #5—Boundaries are forever, and they burn bridges.

Boundaries are more like gates than walls, they can open when you want them to, and can be flexible. My younger sister would often take advantage of me for rides and money—anyone else have a family member take advantage of your kind nature? This was not exclusively her fault—the responsibility for being respected by others lies solely with me. She didn't have the problem. She would ask, I would say yes. But I was feeling resentful that she was taking me for granted, so I was the one with the problem. While a nice character trait, it isn't her responsibility to ensure I am feeling appreciated for my favors, nor her duty to ensure that I am not feeling taken for granted.

I set a boundary with her that I wouldn't be giving her rides any longer. Did she like it? Nope. Did she complain? Not to my face. But did she respect it? Yes. Did it help her realize that she was taking me for granted? I hope so. And after a while, she became more independent and self-sufficient, which helped her growth. While not realizing it, I had been enabling her. After it was established that she could get herself around, I loosened the boundary and offered to give her a ride once and a while, and it is fine now.

If she had become angry and decided she didn't want to speak to me over this, it would be on her. Some of the boundaries we set may in fact cause people to be upset with us—for a little while, or longer. If someone "burns a bridge" with you over a boundary you have set, this is their decision and is not on you to own. By honoring your needs and putting yourself first, you are making steps towards real change. Unfortunately, some people will not like this, but their reaction to your boundary is not your responsibility, just as it is not their responsibility for them to ensure you are feeling respected. While unlikely to burn a bridge, if this is the end result, you might want to question whether this person was a healthy person to have in your life in the first place. Perhaps it will be doing you a favor not to have someone in your life who acts in this manner.

Myth #6—If I set a boundary with someone, they won't be able to handle it.

By assuming we know how someone is going to react to setting a boundary, we deny that person the ability to work with us. By avoiding telling them the truth, we are enabling a behavior we don't prefer. If we want authentic relationships, we need to be able to speak honestly.

How do I know if I have an issue with boundaries?

If you are feeling resentful of other people, this is the number-one indicator that you are in need of setting boundaries. This feeling, although unpleasant, is our internal response that something is off. Do your best not to shame yourself or ignore it if you are feeling resentful. Listen to it.

People with Healthy Boundaries	People with Unhealthy Boundaries
• Have high self-esteem and self-respect	• Do not know who they really are or what they really want
• Share information appropriately	• Either overshare or do not let people in at all
• Have a healthy sense of self-worth	• Base how they feel on how others treat them
• Have relationships where responsibility and power are shared	• Feel responsible for others' happiness
• Are assertive and can confidently and truthfully say yes or no	• Can't say no to others
• Are okay when others say no to them	• Get upset or become hurt when others tell them no
• Recognize that their boundaries are different from others	• Feel everyone should have the same boundaries as they do
• Take responsibility for themselves and their choices	• Allow others to make decisions for them

Unhealthy Beliefs that Lead to Unhealthy Boundaries

• I can never say "no" to others.	• I have an obligation to commit to work or my family.
• I can't trust anyone.	• I would feel guilty if I did something on my own and left someone out (e.g., family members).
• It is safer not to speak up.	• If I make myself invisible, I won't get hurt.
• I can never tell where to draw the line with others.	

Why do we allow others to intrude upon our boundaries?

Our awareness—usually, because we don't know it. We were never taught how to set healthy boundaries in school (quadratic equations were in the curriculum, though, as helpful as they were to us), therefore, some of us don't know what our boundaries are. I didn't know I had poor boundaries for a long time, but I knew I was feeling burnt out and resentful. Our feelings can be our guide when learning what boundaries to set for ourselves.

Our upbringing—was your mom a nurse? Or do you have a lot of health care workers in your family? Helping professions tend to run in the family, and with it comes learned behaviors. If you witnessed Mom coming home after work and cooking dinner, doing the laundry, and being responsible for all of the cleaning, you are likely not to think anything of it. Patterns of unhealthy behavior can be passed down, and if your parents had issues with setting healthy boundaries, you likely will, too.

Fear of rejection and, ultimately, abandonment—did you get into trouble when you were younger or lose someone important to you because you said no? This is actually pretty common. Your Inner Child remembers this and subconsciously learns not to repeat that behavior. She fears being rejected or abandoned and will go to great lengths not to feel that way again. We might consciously be aware that we are saying yes too much, but are subconsciously unable to say no in the moment.

Fear of confrontation—most of us would prefer to avoid confrontation, and it is easier (at the time) to say yes when asked. If we are working or living with people who get upset easily, we avoid having to deal with their emotions by appeasing them.

Fear of guilt—this is a biggie. Most of us are wired to fear feeling guilty. It is unpleasant and leads to feelings of not being good enough—either not nice enough or not caring enough or not thoughtful enough. Many of us HCWs have such an aversion to this feeling that we will do anything to avoid it. Being empathic, we hate to let others down because we feel their disappointment, too.

Unhealthy Boundary Setting

(adapted from *Boundaries* by Henry Cloud and John Townsend, and *Healing Your Lost Inner Child* by Robert Jackman)[2]

People with unhealthy boundaries fall into three categories:

1. *Compliant*—this looks like difficulty saying no. People who fall into this category fear rejection and can be overly dependent on others' opinions, becoming overly involved in their problems and accepting disrespect. They are likely to refuse help from others even when they need it.

2. *Rigid/Controlling*—this is where people can't hear no, and will do what they can to minimize hearing it, either through controlling others or by avoiding interactions. They can be aggressive (using intimidation), manipulative (using guilt or flattery), or deserters (ghosting, blocking people).

3. *Bubble*—this is where people have a seemingly strong exterior, but have nothing underneath it. They often get tired of keeping people out and will burst their own bubble, but with no boundaries to enforce, they are likely to overshare, and are not capable of saying no. Once they chase people away (often a test to see if people will stay), they will prove themselves right and go back into their bubble. The crusty person who has a gooey center can be described as having bubble boundaries.

I unfortunately fall into the last category. I can be strong when I need to be, but when I get close to people, the tough persona can evaporate, along with my self-respect. I would allow others to take advantage of me, the relationship would end, and I would go back into hiding. A doctor I worked with ironically used to call me "Bubble Girl" because I called him out on invading my space—he didn't know how right he was.

Sometimes we can fall into a few categories, depending on the situation. Some of us might be compliant with a family member but controlling at work (or vice versa). This is often done unconsciously in an attempt to balance our relationships—if we are feeling too lenient with our children, we can overcompensate by becoming controlling at work. What is important is realizing there is an imbalance, as having the awareness gives us the power to do something about it.

The issue with all of these is that the unhealthy boundary setter is too outward-focused, and not inward-focused. We focus our attention on what others might think, do, or say. We rely on others to get our needs met, and don't tune in to how we are feeling. This form of coping developed as children when we actually were reliant on others to have our needs met, and we haven't yet adapted to healthier ways to deal with our problems.

How do I set healthy boundaries for myself?

"Healthy boundaries are not created in a vacuum. They require healthy support in order to grow." – From "Boundaries"

Know that it is going to be work—setting healthy boundaries in a world where we are praised for working harder and being nicer is not easy. In fact, for many of us chronic people-pleasers, it may be the toughest thing we do. It takes courage to say to someone, "Hey, this isn't okay with me." It also takes a lot of inner work to figure out what actually is and isn't okay. Our superpower of empathy that allows us to tap into what others are feeling often prevents us from tuning into ourselves.

Know your values—knowing who you are and what is important to you are the two most important weapons you have in setting healthy boundaries. Having a strong sense of self helps you know what you will tolerate and what you won't. Having a strong sense of self is like an inner shield that takes in external stimuli and analyzes it before reacting, either to anger, criticism, or being asked to take on too much. It allows us to determine if the comment checks out.

To set healthy boundaries, you must know your own values and be able to clearly communicate them to others. It is important for you to determine what your boundaries are for YOU—what is right for someone else may not work for you. Knowing what nurtures you and protects you can help you convey to loved ones what your needs are. On the other hand, knowing what drains you or makes you feel used or resentful is a good indicator that you need to set a boundary.

Know to go slow—start small. Don't tackle big situations right away. We don't start a new workout routine lifting the twenty-pound weights when we've never lifted the five-pound ones. The same goes for boundary setting. It is unadvisable to tackle the people and issues that are the most emotionally charging right away. Start by saying no to attending events or volunteer work before moving on to the difficult co-worker.

Know that it is going to feel unnatural, and you are going to fail—it's okay not to do it perfectly at first. You didn't develop this overnight, so don't expect to heal it overnight. We are rarely good at something automatically. Following these steps will help strengthen your sense of inner self, and as you practice setting boundaries, it not only gets easier, but you will build a stronger sense of self-worth. Like with anything, it takes practice and determination.

We can beat ourselves up when we are just learning to set boundaries, say, "This isn't working," and give up. You didn't give up learning to drive just because you hit the curb when parallel parking, because you really wanted to have the freedom of driving. Setting boundaries is the same situation—having them really does set you free. It puts you in the driver's seat again, and lets your wounded Inner Child go back to being a passenger.

Know when you should and shouldn't set a boundary with someone—if you are dealing with someone who is physically dangerous or threatening to you, it may not be safe to attempt to set explicit boundaries with them. If you are in this situation, it can be helpful to work with a counselor, therapist or advocate to create a safety plan first.

Steps to Setting a Boundary

(adapted from *Fierce Conversations: Achieving Success at Work & in Life, One Conversation at a Time* by Susan Scott)[3]

1. *Identify the problem*—become clear where you have lost your sense of self and where your boundaries have been crossed. What triggered you to believe you need to set a boundary? Think of it in term of how X is affecting Y.
2. *Identify the need not met*—what was not fulfilled? Is it physiological (not enough sleep, missing meals), safety/security, belonging, esteem/respect?
3. *Name the emotion*—how is this making you feel?
4. *Act, don't react*—vent any strong emotion with someone you trust before having the boundary conversation.
5. *Speak in a firm but neutral tone*—this may feel uncomfortable at first, but the personal power you gain from this conversation will make it easier.
6. *Use simple and direct language*—often we are talking to someone who is in their Inner Child process. Speak to them as you would a child (but not in a patronizing way, this will upset them).
7. *Select a specific example*—keep it succinct. If you go on a long story, you will lose them, as they will be too busy making up a defense.
8. *Identify your contribution to this problem*—acknowledge your part in this, and what you will do to resolve your portion of it. It might be, "I waited too long to tell you how I felt," "I didn't speak up," etc. It acknowledges your accountability and will likely help lower the armor the other person is feeling the need to build.

9. *Tell them how you feel (if you feel safe to do so)*—letting the person know how this has affected you helps connect you both. It can be simply, "I feel hurt when you do x," or, "I feel like you don't value me."

10. *Don't apologize for your boundaries*—it gives the impression that you're not willing to enforce them and it makes you feel like you're doing something wrong by having them. There is no need to defend or explain your feelings, and any attempt to do so may be seen as a need to justify—you don't have to justify them. If questioned or faced with resistance, simply repeat your statement—they will get the hint.

11. *Back up the boundary with an action*—for example, "I have asked you for help around the house. If you continue to not help me, I will look for a cleaning service."

12. *Be prepared to carry out your stated action if the boundary is violated—*this is important**. If you do not follow through, the person you are conversing with may not take you seriously and will likely not respect your requests in the future. The most important step once you set a boundary is keeping it.

13. *Interaction*—give the other person a chance to tell you their perspective. They may be totally unaware how their actions are affecting you. Remember, we often have gone a long time without setting a boundary, and to tell someone you're suddenly not okay with something can be jarring for them. They also might want to lay blame or steer the topic away from the issue at hand. You are the one driving the conversation and may have to lead them back to the subject at hand.

14. *Start again*—assume that once the boundary has been set, you are starting fresh. You want them to acknowledge your new guidelines. Give the other person a chance to honor this. Don't bring up other issues or examples from the past. Expect to be respected from now on.

Situational Examples of Setting Healthy Boundaries

1. *Anger*—"I will not tolerate being yelled at. If you continue to yell, I will leave the room." "I don't tolerate this kind of behavior. If you need to cool down, excuse yourself."

2. *Delaying a response*—"I will have to check my schedule and get back to you. If you need an immediate answer, it will have to be a no."

3. *Criticism*—"It's not okay with me for you to make comments about my appearance. Please stop. If you don't, I will have to hang up."

4. *Extra commitments*—"Although I would like to help you, I can't commit to anything else right now. I have to put myself first."

5. *Money*—"I won't be lending you any more money. I care about you and you need to start taking responsibility for yourself."
6. *Agreements*—"I want to clarify this part of the contract." "Are we both on the same page when it comes to X?"
7. *Knowing who you are*—"No, that's not for me/my style/doesn't interest me." "I'm detail-oriented, can you give me more information before I decide?"
8. *Your values/commitments*—"Sorry, I need more time with my family this week."

Reactions to Us Setting Boundaries

People will have different reactions to us setting boundaries with them. While it doesn't feel nice to have a boundary set, if people want you in their lives, they will respect them. One thing you can do to ease the transition is tell people you are actively working on setting boundaries. This gives them time to process this information, and they will be less resistant to you when you need to set a boundary with them in future.

People with compliant boundary-setting often have people in their lives that benefit from this, to the point of taking advantage. One of the hardest things compliants have to do when they start setting healthy boundaries is end relationships that were one-sided. Once some people are not benefitting from the compliant, they either become resistant to the boundaries, or they disappear. This can be really painful for us to experience. Please know that you didn't do anything wrong by asserting yourself; if someone leaves because you are making positive changes, you probably are better off without them. Start surrounding yourself with people who have healthy boundaries, as they will not only be supportive of you, but they can mentor you as you learn to set healthier guidelines for yourself.

Other people generally fall into three categories when we start setting boundaries with them:

The Cheerleader—this person has your back. They respect you when you tell them no, they don't pressure you to say yes if they ask for something, and they encourage you to be honest. They probably won't even notice that you've started asserting yourself because you never needed to with them. They more than likely have healthy boundaries themselves. *These are your people.*

The Ponderer—this type of person will probably not be too thrilled that you are setting limits with them. Often, they are people close to us who have benefited from us doing more than our fair share. They are used to this, and telling them this is going to change doesn't always go over so well. These people may need time to adjust to the new situation (i.e., them doing more). This doesn't make them a bad person. They might grumble or protest, but if they want you in their life, they will adjust. Give this person space and honor the time they need. You are doing them a favor in cutting off the enabling, although they may not see it like that right away!

The Aggressor—this person puts up a fight when you tell them you are setting a boundary. They will argue, blame, make excuses, and do pretty much everything other than own up to their behavior. This person might try to gaslight you and make out that you're being irrational for setting the boundary. If you anticipate this reaction from someone, I don't recommend tackling this person first (or alone), even if they are the biggest source of your stress. This is like lifting a hundred-pound weight when you are just starting to explore boundary setting.

Unfortunately, many of us people-pleasers tend to attract this type of person to us, so there is a good chance we have at least one person like this in our lives. If it is a personal relationship, it might be worth asking if it is worth continuing to have a relationship with them if they have this reaction to us setting boundaries. If it is a colleague or a manager, and they don't respect the boundary you have set, there is recourse that can occur in a professional setting. Respect is not something that is earned, it is something that is expected.

Death of Your Persona

"I am not as sweet as I used to be, but I am far more loving." – Brené Brown

When you start setting healthy boundaries, similar to the stages of putting yourself first, there will be a grieving period. You might feel anger at others (and yourself) for putting up with so much. You might lose friendships. You will feel guilt.

Some colleagues might not like that you are not so "nice" anymore. Women are often praised for being "sweet" and derided for being "bossy" when they're actually being assertive. The most intense thing you might have to grieve is the loss of your "nice" persona, the one that was not allowing you to be true to yourself. This can be a very hard thing for us to let go of, as it has been who we are for most of our lives.

There is a difference between being nice and being kind. Remember, the "nice" person who takes too much on also doesn't have a lot of quality time with their loved ones, even if they are with them. The "nice" person is snappy, tired, and can be a nag. My guess is, if you are a nice person and are reading this book, some of these symptoms of being "nice" are showing up in your life.

A kind person is present with the people they are with. They are loving, make time for connection, and give out of a genuine want to give to others, not out of obligation (or guilt). They say no when they need to, and respect others for doing the same. When we put ourselves first, we become more kind—to ourselves, our Inner Child, our loved ones, our colleagues, and our patients. We respect our own time, and we respect the time of others. We live balanced lives, and we get more out of life for doing so. If you have a choice of being nice or being kind, choose kindness.

Benefits of Setting Healthy Boundaries

Boundary work is one of the hardest processes we go through. Part of the reason it is so difficult is that the people who usually support us in other areas of our lives tend to be the ones we are having boundary issues with. Working with a professional who can support you and remain unbiased is key to our success with setting boundaries.

As you set more boundaries for yourself, you will begin to notice:

• more energy, feeling less tired	• better quality and quantity of sleep
• more desire to eat better and exercise	• less anger and resentment
• feeling more empowered	• feeling calmer, more peaceful, safe to be yourself
• better relationships, more enriching relationships	• more confidence, increased self-esteem
• better communication	• more time for activities you want to do
• more trusting	• more giving out of a genuine desire to give
• more understanding of others	• less negative, able to see the bright side more often
• clarity about your goals and direction in life	• life seems less daunting
• more quality time with loved ones	• greater intimacy, more connection

As you go through this, be kind to yourself. If the goal for setting boundaries is to include more time for yourself, make sure you are doing things that nourish you. If that means a bubble bath (or a Valium, not judging!), then please indulge.

Boundary setting is the most important work we can do on ourselves. Congratulations for making it this far. Below are some scenarios that will help you as you begin to navigate this terrain.

Practicing Boundary Setting

For each situation below, practice what you would say to assertively set a new boundary or to enforce an existing one. Remember, treating yourself with respect will earn you more respect from others.

a. Your co-worker asks you to give a medication due for her patient while she is on her break. You are on your way to perform a dressing change for your patient that will take at least twenty minutes.

b. You miss transcribing an NPO (do not eat) order written for one of your patients, which causes the patient's procedure to be cancelled. The physician who ordered the exam finds you in the hallway and starts berating you in front of your colleagues.

c. Your friend shows up uninvited to your house after a long shift. She assumes you are okay to hang out, but you are exhausted.

d. Your mom phones to check in on how you are doing. She steers the conversation to your recent weight gain, and she asks you if you are doing anything about it.

e. You enter your patient's room to perform the morning assessment. She comments that she is glad to see you and be rid of that "immigrant" nurse, as she couldn't understand her. You feel uncomfortable with this statement.

f. You have a challenging day at work, and come home to your spouse. You want to vent about your day but notice he is barely listening.

g. Your friend has recently started jogging and is marvelling about how good she feels. She asks on several occasions if you would join her, even though you don't like running. You feel guilty, as you know it would mean spending quality time with her, and you have been wanting to get more exercise.

h. Your sister-in-law, a single mom, calls asking you to lend her money. She can't afford to pay her rent, and is worried she and her two young children will be evicted. This is not the first time she has asked you for money.

EXERCISES

1. Look back at the types of unhealthy boundaries. Identify if you are mostly compliant, rigid, or bubble boundary setting. Does this mostly pertain to work, family, partner, or friendships?

2. Think of someone in particular you are having boundary issues with. How could you start having healthier boundaries with this person? For rigid boundaries, it might mean opening up more, for compliant boundaries, it might mean saying no more often.

3.   What are some specific actions you can take right now with this person to have healthier boundaries?

4.   How do you think this person will react to these actions?

5.   How do you think your life would change if you had healthier boundaries with this person?

CHAPTER 11

Saying No

"Speak your mind, even if your voice shakes." – Maggie Kuhn

Your alarm goes off at 5:30 a.m.—you need to take the dog out for a walk before your morning shift. Your husband lies next to you, still sleeping soundly. He was up late working and disturbed you when he got into bed around midnight, yet your alarm didn't rustle him.

You yawn silently and rub your eyes as you walk out of your bedroom to greet your anxious four-legged friend. He was supposed to be the family dog—your children begged you for him—and the responsibilities were supposed to be shared, yet you find yourself doing most of the work. You don't mind, though, it gets you out in the fresh air for some exercise.

You return from the walk and start making the lunches—for you, your husband, and your kids. You ensure your children have their homework assignments completed and go and check their backpacks to make sure they are in there.

You make a list of reminders for your husband: "It's garbage day today! Make sure Allie has her lunch, she forgot it twice last week! Don't forget to lock the doggy-gate!" You are pretty sure he would remember, but just to be safe …

You head out for your twelve-hour shift. You are dreading going in. For the past three days, you've been given the same assignment, which includes a demanding paraplegic with C. Diff. This patient is a nightmare—demanding, verbally abusive, incontinent of loose stool constantly, and unable to turn or roll to help you in any way. Even when he is not incontinent, he is using his call bell multiple times an hour. You are in the room so much, and with extra time needed to don and doff PPE, you are not able to assess your other patients in a timely manner.

You know why you've been given that assignment—because everyone knows you won't complain about it. You make a pact with yourself to ask for another assignment if you have been given the same one again today … or, at least a lighter patient-load.

You get into work and see you indeed have the same assignment. Your face falls as you look at the rest of the staff names. No one on this shift would be willing to trade it. The charge nurse looks at you as you are studying the assignment sheet.

"Do you want to switch with someone, Keltie?" she asks kindly. "I wouldn't blame you. Bed Ten is a lot to handle, especially for more than one shift!"

"Oh, no, it's fine," you say with a weak laugh. "Everyone has to take their turn."

"Are you sure? I don't mind asking for you!" your charge nurse says with a kind smile.

You consider it briefly, but wouldn't want your charge nurse to go to the trouble of asking around for you—you know how some of your coworkers can be. "No, it's okay!"

You turn to get busy with your meds—you know you will be running for the majority of your shift. Sure enough, Bed Ten's call bell is ablaze. You tell yourself this is your last shift on this stretch, and that you just need to make it through today and you'll have four glorious days off!

Partway through the day, you are regretting not taking your charge nurse up on her offer. You are behind on your meds, and two of your other patients are having ten-out-of-ten pain. You look to see if you can ask someone for help. You spy two nurses in the hall, chatting. Asking either of these people is not high on your priority list—they are both less than helpful on most days. But your patients are in pain, and you are stuck in the isolation room.

You ask if one of them can give your other patients their pain meds. They roll their eyes at you. One of the nurses disappears into a patient's room, but the other sighs loudly and says she'll do it. You cringe at having to ask for help, but you can't do everything!

By the time your shift finishes, you are exhausted. You wearily drive home. You are looking forward to your days off immensely. There's a new book you bought weeks ago that you haven't had time to start, and you're eager to dive into it.

You get in the door and see supper isn't ready. Your husband and the kids are watching T.V. You had asked your husband the night before to make dinner, and he replied he would. Knowing he forgot, you curse yourself for not writing it down on the reminders list you set out for him that morning.

"Hank, honey, where's supper?" you ask, knowing the answer.

"Oh, sweetie, I'm so sorry, I forgot," your husband replies apologetically. You sigh, knowing that he has a lot on his plate right now at work.

"Okay, I guess we're having pizza!" you say, as you are neither cooking nor waiting for a meal to be made.

The kids cheer as you get on the phone to your regular pizza delivery—you order from them more often than you'd like.

"Mom, Mom, guess what?" your son Owen asks. You smile at him and try to listen to him as he recounts his day, but you are barely able to focus, you are so tired. "And you'll be at my soccer practice this week? You missed all last week because you were working, so you'll come this week, right?"

"Me, too, Mom? My dance classes?" Allie pipes up.

You sigh. You have a million and one errands to do on your days off. Your husband works Monday to Friday, so you do most of the errands on your days off because the stores are less busy during the day. You were looking forward to having some downtime, but it's true that you had missed many of your kids' activities due to work—you feel you should go as often as you can when you aren't working.

As you sit down to dinner, the fantasy of starting that new book starts to fade. When everyone has finished eating, they run back to the T.V. to finish the show they were watching. Another reason pizza is a good option? No clearing up. You wrap up the leftover pizza as your family relaxes in the next room.

"I'm heading up for a bath!" you call out. You feel guilty that you haven't spent much time with your family, but you are bagged. A bath and then bed is all you can think about. You'll have more time (and energy) with them on your days off.

You don't even look at your phone, which has several messages from family members and friends. Most of them haven't heard from you in a while. While you'd love to chat with them, you can't even muster up the energy for spending time with your own family, let alone extended family and friends. You think about some of the friendships you have drifted from since you started having a family, and wistfully wonder how those people are doing. You run into each other now and then, and of course always say you should meet up—but it never happens. This is life now, and it's crazy hectic for everyone. This is normal.

But should it be? You muse about that as you head to bed. You look over at the clock – nine p.m. This is a pretty average bedtime for you. Some days it's hard to stay awake past eight. As you turn over to go to sleep, you start mentally going through the list of all of the things you need to do in the morning. Despite being exhausted, you start tossing and turning. You have difficulty sleeping on many nights, and it looks like tonight will be another. You reach for your nightstand drawer and take a sleeping tablet. Hoping to get a few good hours in, you succumb to a fitful sleep.

Does this sound familiar at all?

Saying no—Why is it so hard?

No is one of the shortest words in the dictionary—and one of the most difficult to utter. Growing up in Canada, I was conditioned to be polite. We Canadians are proud of our reputation for being nice, almost to a fault. We don't want to be labeled as difficult or as someone who rocks the boat, so we will do almost anything to appear docile. This culture is so inherent in us that we often sacrifice our own happiness for others—which may make us "polite," but it doesn't make us kind. We may smile to your face, but rest assured, if we don't like something, we are complaining to someone else about it—which makes us passive-aggressive.

Females have it even worse. In her book *The Assertiveness Guide for Women*, Julie de Azevedo Hanks recounts how women were dependent on men for centuries as our providers, and it makes sense that we kept them happy because it got our needs met.[1] We've inherited this. Fear of saying no is natural to us, especially to people in power. Self-sacrificing is still rewarded in our society. Instead of being respected for being assertive as our male counterparts often are, we have a tendency to be branded aggressive if we don't agree with something or speak up for ourselves. While the #MeToo movement has shed light on areas where there were tragic examples of women not being able to speak up for themselves, we still have a long road ahead of us. Women still have to work against reputations their male counterparts don't have to deal with. "Ballbuster," "bitchy," or "bossy" are all labels applied to women, not men, and often are a result of a woman who refuses to be the nice girl.

While we don't all aspire to be the next Arlene Dickinson, we should feel comfortable saying no when it's what we truly want. As health care providers, our superpower of empathy allows us to put ourselves in others' shoes, and we often feel for people in our lives who may be struggling. The colleague who has a code brown to clean up, the friend who is without childcare, the charity struggling to feed the homeless. We truly feel the pain of these people, and desire to do something to help.

We fear disappointing others, we fear appearing selfish, we fear feeling guilty, we fear no one else will do it, we fear we will be a burden on others. There are a multitude of reasons why we fear saying no. So we say yes.

And this is where we get into trouble. We say yes to everyone else, but we are, in effect, saying no to ourselves. If you have a hard time saying no, congratulations, you're already doing it—to yourself. Over-cluttering our schedule with things we don't really want to do isn't good for our family, isn't good for our careers, and isn't good for our soul.

When we have put ourselves first and attended to our needs, we can actually say yes out of a genuine desire to help from our hearts. Salmon et al. define this as "compassion satisfaction," or the gratification we get when we give from our hearts. [2] This is the feeling most of us HCWs went into our field of work to experience, not the compassion fatigue most of us are experiencing now.

Fear

As kids, we stretched ourselves every day. We didn't think about falling down when we were learning to walk, we fell down and kept going. As we get older and have more experience, we become more averse to things that make us uncomfortable. We've been burned in the past, and we as humans are naturally inclined to step away from our fears. While it may have served us from an evolutionary standpoint, it also makes us stagnant. Saying no invokes a fear in us that people won't like us, that we won't have support, or that we will be punished or reprimanded. Fear is one of the strongest emotions we endure, but if our fears are preventing us from leading the lives we want to be leading (or are causing us to become sick or burnt out), then the fear of living our lives for others becomes greater than a fear of not being popular. If life is becoming unsustainable for you, it might be a nudge that things aren't working.

When is the last time you did something that scared you? Fear is where the most growth happens. It doesn't have to mean quitting our jobs and joining the circus (it totally can, though). It can be a simple as joining a new gym.

Steps to assisting us in getting over our fears:

1. *If you have a spiritual practice, use it*—even if it's just getting out in nature.
2. *Journal*—this gets us in touch with the deepest parts of ourselves.
3. *Inner Child dialogue*—conversations with our Inner Child help draw out our true feelings; creative practices help draw us out of our heads where the fear builds.
4. *Focus on your strengths*—this helps remind us that we have them. We can do hard things.
5. *Get more training/education*—if your fear of leaving a bad situation involves not enough skills (e.g., leaving a job you have been in for a long time and you don't feel you are experienced enough for something else), find ways to improve your skillset.
6. *Practice*—makes perfect. Doing things to get you out of your comfort zone will condition you to do the bigger things that you are working towards. This can be as simple as taking a new fitness class, or learning to cook a new dish.
7. *Support*—we need comfort with facing our fears, and knowing others have our backs really helps.
8. *Mentors*—look to people who have done what you're about to do, as they can often give you advice and insight that you might not get from researching on your own.
9. *Remind yourself of when you did something hard*—you can do it again. Ask loved ones to remind you of times you overcame something scary, as sometimes we forget our own achievements.

Be Honest with Yourself—and Others

*"The truth is like poetry. And most people f*cking hate poetry."*
– Adam McKay

Saying no is a very important part of setting healthy boundaries. Often if we had said no in the first place, we wouldn't need to set boundaries with someone who has been violating them. For example, say you agreed to volunteer for your child's hockey bottle drive. You didn't really want to, but you felt obligated to do your part, and maybe the parent who asked you was a bit pushy, so you didn't want to say no at the time. Then, she begins asking you to organize other fundraising activities, carpooling, and logistics aspects of the team. Now you feel like you are committed, and don't know how to get out of it. If you had been honest with her that you didn't want to do it in the beginning, this may not have progressed to her asking more of you than your fair share.

Saying no in the beginning can also prevent hurt feelings. One of my coworkers once went out on a few dates with someone she met at work. She didn't really want to, but she said yes to avoid hurting his feelings. After a few dates, she knew she wasn't interested in him and broke it off. He was hurt when she explained that she hadn't really been into him and asked her angrily why she went out with him in the first place, to which she didn't have a great reply. Being afraid of saying no to avoid hurting someone's feelings can hurt them more in the long run than if we had been honest in the beginning.

The Art of Saying No

Saying no is a skill that takes practice, and, like anything else, gets easier the more you do it. Here are some tips on starting:

Check in with yourself—before committing to something, do a mental check—do you actually want to do it? If you said yes, would it be out of an actual desire to help, or out of obligation? Remember, put yourself first. Have you met all of your physical and psychological needs? Would saying yes to the request cause you to jeopardize those needs? If this is outside of work, you definitely have a minute or two to respond to whatever is being asked of you—usually that's all you need. The "let me check my schedule" tactic will grant you time if you need more. If you're at work and it's an imminent task, it's a bit trickier, but it can still be done courteously: "Let me finish what I am doing and I will come back to you."

Be gracious—thank the other person for thinking of you. Take it as a compliment that the other person trusts you enough to do something for them, as they obviously think you are capable of whatever it is they are asking for.

Explain, if necessary, but briefly—the more often you say no without an explanation, the easier it gets. You don't owe anyone a response as to why you can't say yes, and the more you try to explain, the more it just feels like an excuse. You are not obligated to do anything, and you are also not obligated to explain why. A simple, "It's going to have to be a no from me," or "I can't make it this time around—have fun!" is all you have to say.

Depending on the nature of your relationship, you may want to give a reason. If you do feel you would like to explain, keep it brief. "My family time comes first," or "I have another commitment that day," works well—even if that commitment is time to yourself. YOU are the most important person in your life—you definitely outrank your friends, colleagues, and extended family. Care for yourself first, and don't feel the need to explain why. If you are concise and honest, others will (usually) understand.

Propose something else—to soften the blow of a no, offering another option will ensure the other person knows you care about them, and gets you off the "guilt" hook. The alternative you offer should most importantly be something you are willing to do, something that is less time-consuming, and doesn't cost anything.

For example, if you are at work and a colleague has asked you to do something for her that will take too much of your time, tell her no but offer to do something small instead. It could look like offering to answer a call bell instead of doing a dressing change. If you are being asked to volunteer at your child's soccer games, offer to donate bottles for the bottle drive instead.

Handle objections kindly—sometimes, a simple no won't do. Some people may be used to hearing no, and will have tactics to address it. Instead of getting offended or upset, simply repeat your statement, as many times as necessary. If the other party becomes offended or upset, this is usually done as a way to manipulate you. Don't fall for it. If this is someone close to you who does it on a regular basis, you may want to reconsider if you want this person in your life.

Here's a sample script you can use if you are replying in a written response:

Hey, Angela,

Thank you so much for thinking of me for this opportunity! I am so proud that you are committing to it and I'm flattered that you asked for my contribution.

I have to say no, as I already have too much on my plate right now, and I need to stay sane!

I would love to support you in a different way. I could do (offer something less time-consuming). Would that be helpful?

Thank you so much for being such a great friend and colleague. Good luck with this opportunity, I know you will do a great job!

Sincerely,

Kristin

Some other useful phrases:

"I would love to, but … "

"I get that you're in a bind, but … "

"I don't have the capacity right now."

"I can't do x, but I can do y."

"I'll let you know if anything changes."

Asking for Our Needs to be Met

In addition to being able to say no, we often have difficulty asking for our needs to be met. Not wanting to be a bother or a burden to others, we go without meeting our own needs and can burn out in the process.

As health care providers, we often don't ask for help because *we* are the helpers. Asking for help with a patient is very different than asking for help for ourselves. Sometimes having our needs met looks like saying no to others; sometime it is asking for others to help us in some way. Asking yourself how you are feeling and what you need are two great questions in order to get your needs met.

When we interact with others, asking for our needs to be met not only helps satisfy our needs, but it also gives others permission to have their needs be met as well. This teaches people in the long run how you typically want others to support you.

What is the Desire?

Sometimes, when we are asking for our needs to be met, we have gone so long feeling resentful that we come across as exasperated or nagging. We have done it all for everyone for so long that we are burnt out, and our request comes out as more of a complaint.

In her book *Unbound*, Kasia Urbaniak invites us to shift our perspective. Instead of focusing on what we are fighting against (e.g., doing all the work), she asks us to focus on what we are fighting for (e.g., a team-playing household).[3] A complaint of our loved ones not helping around the house is really a desire to have the work doled out evenly, a wish to be closer with our loved ones and have more quality time together, a yearning for cohesiveness and respect.

What would you ask for if there were no consequences? Sometimes, we can be surprised by what happens when we ask for our needs to be met. In *Unbound*, Kasia recounts how she and her partner were having difficulties spending quality time together.[4] Her partner was going overseas and requested they spend the afternoon going to the movies. Kasia, being brutally honest with him, said she not only didn't want to go to the movies, but she gave the ballsy ask of inviting him to help her with her work. To her amazement, this invite was met not only with eagerness, but her partner actually gave up his humanitarian work overseas to help her create her own vision, as it was the purpose he was looking for. This never would have happened if Kasia hadn't been honest with herself and what her needs were, nor if she hadn't had the courage to ask a seemingly impossible ask.

We have been conditioned as good people, many of us girls, not to take up space, not to ask for more than what is our "fair share," and look where it has gotten us. Begging for the bare minimum in our workplaces. Nagging our spouses to empty the dishwasher. Pleading with our kids to clean up after themselves. It is time we had the courage to go after what we really want in life. We may not always get it, but there is a 100-percent guarantee that we won't if we don't start asking for it.

The Door Slam

Sometimes people who have difficulty expressing their needs suffer from what is termed "the door slam." The door slam occurs when someone has allowed someone in their life to take advantage of their generous nature for too long. The pressure builds and builds as the person becomes more and more resentful of others asking them for help. We become so angry that we finally say enough is enough, and we blow up at the person, or we cut them out of our lives. The other person, blindsided by this, has no idea what happened and is left in the dark.

The reason the other person is confused is because we have not communicated to them how we are really feeling. We keep saying yes because we don't want to disappoint the other person, but secretly we are seething. Instead of being open and honest with the other person, we continue to allow them to take advantage. The other person does not see an issue with this. Perhaps they are knowingly taking advantage of us, or perhaps they are simply trying to get their needs met.

The door slam is your Inner Child effectively having a temper tantrum. She has put up with too much, and is unable to deal with it anymore, and this is the most effective way she knows how to stop it. My Mum told me when I was upset with her when I was younger, I used to close my eyes and turn my back on her. I thought that by not seeing her, the problem would go away. The door slam is the adult version of closing our eyes and turning our back on a problem we aren't consciously able to deal with, and this is how our subconscious helps us deal with it. The real issue is that we are uncomfortable confronting the person, and instead we look for more comfortable ways to function—by avoiding it.

Sometimes the door slam is necessary. Sometimes people are knowingly taking advantage of us, and it is best to not have them in our lives. Yet without working with the person we are having boundary issues with, we will never know if they are someone who is unhealthy for us, or just someone who is adept at asking for what they want. In her book *The Assertiveness Guide for Women*, Julie de Azevedo Hanks reminds us that other people do not have any power over you.[5] You are an adult, and you get to decide if you want to say yes to their request or not. Avoiding them or blocking communication with them without having actually told them the issue is not only unfair, it is unkind.

It might feel empowering at the time to cut someone out of your life who has been taking advantage of you knowingly. In fact, it might be the empowering move you need to start asserting yourself better. But it should be used as an exception, not a rule. Most people are reasonable when you tell them you are overstretched. They might not like it, they might grumble, but in the end, you have the power to choose how you are running your life. Period.

Getting Your Needs Met

Sometimes we need specific things from people in the moment. Ever had a friend bombard you with advice when you just needed them to listen? We have all been on both sides of this. Others can't read our minds, and while most people are just trying to be helpful, we can become frustrated when others misinterpret what we actually need in the moment. This is why we have to ask. It will create more cohesion in your relationships, and it will allow you to become more assured in knowing what you need at the time and actually asking for it.

Here are some sample scripts for situational needs:

When you need listening, not advice—"Thank you so much for the advice. I know I will figure it out eventually, but right now I just need someone to talk it through with."

When you need acceptance, not being preached at—"I know I screwed up, and I'll fix it, but right now I just need someone to listen to me and accept me. Can you do that?"

When you need validation instead of being cheered up—"You are so good at looking at the bright side, thank you. I think I just need to honor that I'm feeling upset."

When you need to just talk, and not listen—"Hey, I normally would love to hear about your day, but right now I just need to let it out. Can you do that for me?"

When you need praise, not one-upping—"Thank you for sharing that, but can I just finish sharing my accomplishment so we can celebrate it together?"

When you need action, not just words—"I really appreciate your support! It's really hard for me to ask for help, but I think I need more than just words. Are you open to discussing other ways you could support me?"

As we are wired to help, sometimes we can be the person who is offering advice to our friends and not letting them just vent if it's needed. When we are conscious of what we need in the moment, we can begin to ask for that from people. Do we need to just be accepted? Are we feeling low and in need of cheering up? Or is the problem we are facing something that we might need advice for from others? When we begin a conversation, be clear about our intention from it. Asking yourself what you need can help figure this intention out, and how we can gain it from others.

EXERCISES

1. Journal about a problem you are facing. How are you feeling in the moment about it? Imagine yourself when you were younger and you were facing a similar issue. What would you have told yourself if you were your own parent? Would you try to give her advice? Or would you just listen and hear her out? Tapping into this space will help you figure out what you truly need in the moment.

2. Think about something you are afraid of saying no to. Write out all of the things that you're afraid might happen. "If I tell my Mom no to visiting, I am afraid she will be lonely," "I'm afraid if I say no to my co-worker, she will report me." Write down all of the fears bottled up, including worst-case scenarios. Then, look over all of what you've written. Chances are, you'll feel better just getting it down on paper. Study the fears that you have written. How likely are these fears to come true? Are they actually legit? Separate what is legitimate from what is not, and come up with some solutions that you can do to nullify those fears (e.g., if you are worried your elderly mom might hurt herself when she is home alone, you could arrange for a community volunteer to visit once a week).

3. Take yourself out of the "good girl" role for a minute. What would you ask for if you knew you would get it? Don't hold back—living on a luxury yacht, travelling the world, egging your ex's house... If you acted on some of your deepest desires, what would it look like? Picture yourself getting it—what would you do? How does it feel in

your body? How would your life change? When I did this exercise, it actually started the ball rolling on some of the major changes I have made in my life—for the better. Allow yourself to daydream and see what your imagination comes up with.

4. Have an intentional conversation with a trusted friend. If you know you are going to be discussing an issue you've been having, stop and think: What is it that you are looking for from your friend when you discuss the issue? Are you looking for advice? Do you need a shoulder to cry on? Would it be helpful for you both to brainstorm ideas on how to solve the issue? Often when we are facing a problem, we know deep down what we need to do, we just might not be ready to do it. That is okay, and it is what friends are for—to support you. Identify what it is you need from that friend and tell her, so when you bring the topic up, it will help her be more conscious of how she can best support you, too.

5. Practice saying no. If this seems daunting, start by saying it once a week, then once a day. Let your friends and family know that you are doing this—it's not cheating! By letting them in on the exercise you are doing, you give them the opportunity to be supportive of your goals and will be less likely to be rejected when you are first starting out. This is a crucial time, as you are more likely to succeed if you have support. Even if it is simply saying "no" to passing the salt, your body has the same gut reaction as saying no to something more important. It gets our feet wet and allows us to practice overcoming that fear we feel in our bodies.

CHAPTER 12

Burnout

"Burnout is what happens when you try to avoid being human for too long."
– Michael Gungor

Burnout is something I am unfortunately well-acquainted with. During my parents' illnesses and passings, I was working full-time, traveling between hospitals from ill patients to ill parents. I knew burnout from a personal perspective, having been a caregiver for most of my life with my parents' substance abuse and illnesses.

At work, I have felt the symptoms of burnout periodically throughout my career. Growing tired of the politics, the rushing to get too much work done with not enough resources, the constant overtime and call-backs. I was challenged to set boundaries in order to have some semblance of a healthy work-life balance.

Unfortunately, the pandemic has only created more intense burnout for all of us. My most recent position is a prime example of this—as a vascular access nurse, they disbanded the IV team in the hospital I work in, and I am currently expected to do the work that five nurses used to do by myself. While the pandemic is hitting us, most HCWs are going to work with less staff on the units, as many of us have burnt ourselves out. This only expedites our own burnout, as doing the same amount of work with less bodies becomes an impossible task to sustain.

At first, I tried to keep up with all of the work that five nurses used to do. We were still getting upwards of forty calls a day. This, while inserting outpatient PICC lines (fancy IVs), and having ten to fifteen inpatient PICC requests at a time. We were also expected to go to the lab to access ports, perform all of the T.B. screening for the hospital, and respond to Medical Assistance In Dying (MAiD) procedures. When I realized I couldn't physically do this, I tried phoning the units to tell them I couldn't come and suggested they find another resource.

This, as you can imagine, was met with a less-than-warm reception. I encountered aggression, demanding I come up there and fix the situation. I experienced threats to escalate to upper management. I had to endure pleading, stories of how the patient wouldn't get the blood they needed because they had no access, that the patient would miss their dose of antibiotics and they were septic, or their CT scan which would diagnose a pulmonary embolism was cancelled because the patient had no IV. The weight of this decision to cut the IV team was now placed solely on my shoulders—there was only one person scheduled per day, and I was expected to do it all.

The more I couldn't respond, the more the units called. The floor nurses, understandably frustrated that, on top of being chronically short and in the middle of a pandemic, they were now expected to add more to their plate. They would call multiple times, escalating to their nursing managers or even physicians. I tried being diplomatic with each call, explaining that I wasn't ignoring them, and that by calling more, it was just another message for me to listen to. Some staff were understanding, some less so. The more I tried to explain, the more abuse I received. It got to the point where I was afraid to even answer the phone. I would go home and lay in bed at night, wondering about the patients I didn't get to, if they got their blood products, if the nurse changed the overdue PICC dressing, or if they were now being poked for the tenth time. And it took its toll.

One day I snapped. I had been up to the same unit five times that day for IV starts. When I got up there to help with the fifth they had called about, the nurse asked me to do a sixth patient.

I lost it.

"*What* is going on here?" I snarled at her.

She gave me a dirty look and muttered, "Don't worry about it," and walked away.

I knew I had been out of line. I went over to her to apologize. I started to give excuses, but she wasn't having any of it. I finally just said, "You know what? I snapped. I can't keep up with everything, some of the nurses who call are rude, and I just lost it. I'm sorry," I finished defeatedly, tears in my eyes.

Her eyes welled up as well, and she said, "I know, I've heard them, they're horrible to you." We both just sat there and cried. Neither of us were enemies, we both were doing the best with what we had, and we both wanted the best for the patients. The pandemic, the already low resources, and now the cuts had taken its toll on both of us, and we felt angry and powerless.

I started the IVs, went down to my office to change, and I walked out of the hospital, not knowing if I was coming back. The next day I called my manager to tell him I was going on stress leave.

The first week, all I could do was stare at the wall. I felt like a fuse had short-circuited in my brain. I couldn't watch TV or even listen to music, as the images and noises were too overwhelming for me. I had been burned out before, but this was unlike anything I had ever experienced.

I'd been given this lesson over and over, and I. Still. Wasn't. Listening.

My self-sacrificing, despite having all the tools and knowledge on the importance of self-care and putting myself first, *still* hadn't sunk in. I was actually a good chunk into writing this book, teaching others, while I was not following my own guidance. Well, I finally got the message—only, I suffered much longer and harder than I had to. I am now walking the walk, and I implore you to heed my words and not fall into the same trap that I did.

The End of the Road

As I write this, we are in a critical health care crisis—like anyone in health care could have predicted. My story is not unique—in fact, in some ways, I am sure I am very fortunate. The emergency rooms are backed up like never before, the floors are critically short, and the ICUs are downright dangerous.

The fact that new nursing grads are leaving the profession within the first five years at an alarming rate tells us there is something wrong. No, they are not weak. No, they are not lazy. They have experienced what nursing life is like, and before they get too committed to it, they quit. We can learn a lot from people coming in to our departments, young or old, as they have fresh eyes to witness what the culture is actually like. Unfortunately, the culture is often the same, unit to unit.

In a cross-sectional study that reviewed ninety-one peer reviewed articles, six predictors for staff burnout were identified:[1]

High workload—obviously.

Value incongruence—not being able to practice our values and embody what is important to us, e.g., work-life balance, not being able to take care of our patients in a safe or nurturing manner, etc.

Low control over the job—mandatory OT, our suggestions and concerns not being heard.

Low decision latitude—not being part of the decision-making process (we all know the frustration of higher-ups making calls that don't affect them, nor knowing how it will affect others), low autonomy.

Poor social climate/social support—toxic work culture, no one to turn to for help or to make change.

Low rewards—why am I doing this? When we get to this point at a job that used to be rewarding, and we now don't even know why we are showing up, something is very wrong.

Other factors identified were low staffing levels, low schedule flexibility, time pressure, high psychological demands, and poor leadership.

Definition of Burnout

Miller-Keane's Encyclopedia and Dictionary of Medicine, Nursing, and Allied Health defines burnout as "emotional and physical exhaustion resulting from a combination of exposure to environmental and internal stressors and inadequate coping and adaptive skills. In addition to signs of exhaustion, the person with burnout exhibits an increasingly negative attitude toward his or her job, low self-esteem, and personal devaluation."[2]

People who are suffering from burnout in the workplace will allow their entire lives to unravel, and they might not even notice their world is falling apart. Their health will suffer, their relationships will suffer, but they will still come to work every day and give themselves up to it, even as they become less and less well.

Know the Signs

According to Dall'Ora et al., the outcomes of burnout include reduced job performance, poor quality of care, poor patient safety, adverse events, patient negative experience, medication errors, infections, and patient falls.[3] Much of the literature identified outcomes of burnout that affected the work setting; less involved actually investigating the effects on the people suffering from it.

One of the precursors to burnout is compassion fatigue. Compassion fatigue (sometimes referred to as secondary trauma) can be conceptualized as the emotional, moral and physical distress which occurs as a consequence of caring and bearing witness to the suffering of others. It manifests itself through a gradual erosion of empathy, optimism and compassion. It differs from burnout in that it is often more acute and refers to professions that provide direct patient care. Compassion fatigue can have repercussions on HCWs' professional lives, and consequently, progress into burnout. When we have reached our limit with being compassionate for others, we go numb. We then are unable to connect with the feelings and needs of others.

Signs of compassion fatigue:[4]

Withdrawing—disengaging with social aspects of your life, not seeing your friends or extended family members, not replying to texts/calls. Being with people becomes a chore. It becomes difficult to express yourself. You would rather be alone. This is a sign that you are struggling, and it might be related to your job.

It is quite common for HCWs to have friends who are also in health care, as not many other people truly understand what we go through. But talking shop all of the time is unhealthy, too. We need people in our lives to talk about things outside of our colostomy comparison notes.

Poor judgment calls—this can look like being irrational, or impulsive behavior—it can be with our diet, our money, or our relationships. Our poor fatigued brains are fried from working on overdrive all of the time, and we start acting out in ways we wouldn't normally. This is not our fault. There is no shame in acting out of character when we are fatigued—this is our Inner Child shouting from the rooftops because we have been ignoring her. Wolfing down junk food, being careless with our finances, and picking fights with our spouses are all coping mechanisms. We are using these as outlets to cope with the overwhelm as best as we can. We aren't always conscious that this is why we are acting out; this is our Inner Child trying to get our attention. It is a cry for help, hoping that someone, anyone, will notice. But our bodies and our loved ones can only help us carry the load for so long before they start to get tired, too. We need to go within and start really looking at ourselves.

Procrastination—have you ever been late for work, an important event, or just didn't do something until the last minute and had no good reason for it? It could be poor planning, but it could also be self-sabotaging. When we are overwhelmed and unable to process information, our brains stop being able to make decisions from a grounded place, and we don't prioritize properly. And when we have a million things on the go at work and home, it may just be too much to handle, and this is our way of coping—by not showing up at all.

Substance abuse—wine o'clock, anyone? We all joke about using alcohol (or cannabis, where it's legal), or caffeine, to survive a hard day. This is conditioning. It has become socially acceptable to drink to "take the edge off," or caffeine to "power through." It's not okay that we need something outside of ourselves to get through life. If I have to rely on something external to cope, it can easily turn into a dependence, which can turn into addiction.

Confession: I loved reading our college journal that came out—not for the interesting articles or new technologies, but the disciplinary page. This journal would come out monthly, and one page was dedicated to all of the disciplinary actions taken against nurses. Paragraphs entailing the naughty things nurses did (usually pilfering narcotics, but sometimes for inappropriate comments and other unprofessional behavior) and how they were punished for them, was published for everyone in the profession to see. I revelled in reading other nurses' reasons for being reprimanded (not something I am proud about today – the empathy was definitely lacking here). But it was alarming how many of them had pilfered narcotics; I would estimate it was usually half of them in any given month. And no one is asking why so many nurses are addicted to narcotics—was it because they sustained injuries at work, and this was the only way they could function? Or is it something bigger? My evolution from glee to sadness for these nameless registration numbers listed has caused me to really look at why this is happening. With so many nurses (and I'm sure other HCWs who don't necessarily have a regulatory body that prints it in their journals for all to see—shaming us is all it really accomplishes) being affected by this, there's obviously an underlying problem that isn't being addressed.

Numbing out only perpetuates a real problem, and for some, it becomes such a habit that they have another problem on their hands. While there's nothing wrong with enjoying the occasional beverage or edible, when we use it to cope instead of as an experience on its own, there is a problem. Clever marketing for #MoscatoMondays has made alcohol socially acceptable to abuse. We are dulling down our emotions that are there for a reason—to deal with, not stuff down.

Calling in sick—yep. We have been doing this at an alarmingly high rate—we either are getting sick more often, or are unable to mentally handle going in (which means you're sick, btw, no need to feel guilty with this). Our jobs are causing us to be sick—and if we are sick, how are we supposed to take care of the sick?

If we don't recognize these symptoms and implement change, they can lead to full-on burnout. Signs of burnout:

Exhaustion—physically and emotionally. You are spent. This one may seem obvious, but if you are doing all of the right things—eating right, drinking enough water, getting enough sleep—and are still exhausted at the end of the day, it may be something at your job that is affecting you. Stress eats up a ton of energy, and we only have so much to spare, as we are giving constantly. If we are taking care of our physical health properly and still feeling exhausted, there may be something else going on.

Not taking care of yourself—that being said, when we are not taking care of ourselves, burnout could be to blame. Ever not bothered washing your face before bed because you were just so exhausted? Or not put any effort into your appearance when you used to love dressing up? It could be either because you have left no time for yourself, or you couldn't be bothered to. It may start out as missing a few exercise classes or social events, but could lead to daily activities becoming more and more challenging for lack of energy.

Lack of motivation—you feel unmotivated to do much of anything outside of work. Going out, doing hobbies that you used to love, keeping your home clean. Do you see how much of this is the same as depression? Which came first? The depression or the burnout?

Apathy—this is a biggie. After dealing with frustration, anger, and sadness, we are often unable to sustain these feelings long-term. Without hope that things will change, or becoming exhausted or defeated from trying, we slip into acceptance that this is just the way it is. We don't try, we don't hope, we just exist. We survive our daily work life, getting involved as little as possible. We do our jobs and go home. We are resigned to the fact that this is how it always will be, and we don't deserve anything better. We may snipe and complain to others, but we are unable to change our perspective, nor are we willing to help those who want to make changes.

How many colleagues do you work with who are here? How long have they lived in that energy? It is scary how many of us over time would rather stay where we are, miserable, for fear of change than actually try to make a better life for ourselves. Some don't have the awareness that they are here, some don't have the energy to change it.

Some HCWs recognize they need a change, and luckily, there is never a shortage of areas that need care. Tired of emerg? Try a nursing home. Don't like the intensity of an ICU? Try peds. Or home care. Or call centers. Or working privately with a family. But even after we make this change, we find the same issues in other departments, and we believe the problem exists everywhere. Some make a career change, but some, resigned to that fact that this is just life in health care—settle back and suck it up.

Apathy is like a poison that seeps into a department: The more people that are affected by it, the more it spreads to others like a plague.

If you have been here like I have, the most important thing you can know is that there is always hope. If you are feeling defeated or bitter that things won't change, be the change you want to see in the world. It starts with you, and I mean that with every fibre of my being. It is amazing how much one person's positive energy can shift an entire room, much like someone's bad mood can ruin it.

It starts by looking within yourself. It doesn't mean you have to stay somewhere that you are unhappy, but shifting your perspective from apathy to hope will give you the push you need to either accept where you are working and be happier in that environment, or give you the push to start looking elsewhere. It can be scary to contemplate change for those of us who have been in the same area for a long time, but sometimes it is necessary.

Cognitive problems—increased stress hormones can cause difficulty concentrating, brain fog, and impaired memory. This often mimics depression, and in fact, it's difficult to tell which came first. But it is also easier to treat depression than stress—you don't have to quit your job, you just need to swallow a Zoloft. I wonder how many people prescribed antidepressants would still need them if they removed themselves from their unhealthy work environments, or were given proper tools on how to cope with them.

Chronic illness—this can be due to many things, not just work. But with chronic migraines, gut issues, and diabetes on the rise, one starts to wonder how much of our profession is contributing to the illnesses we have. I had chronic neck and back pain that I thought was due to multiple car accidents, yet when I spent a vacation away from work, I barely noticed the pain. My physiotherapist would remark, "You love your job, right?" as I went in for an IMS treatment for the umpteenth time. I did, but I had to face facts that it was affecting my health.

Taking work home—as HCWs, we often see tragedy around us, and it's easy for us to take it home and sit with it long after we've left the hospital. This is normal to us. It might not happen every night, but every once and a while a patient might come along that leaves an impression on us. This is healthy; it means we are human. But when poor working conditions, disrespectful staff, or administration that are deaf to our concerns starts creeping into our home life, something is wrong.

You feel guilty for relaxing—ever felt guilty when you sit down to chart while others are busy around you? Actually?!? Because we are in a profession that is notorious for workers being overworked, we feel we have to live up to that reputation. We actually feel guilty when we are not busy.

Our management and supervisors contribute to this, as their presence instills in us a need to always be doing something. I distinctly remember running around all morning without a break, and the characteristic click-click of administrative shoes came upon me just as I was sitting down for a second to rest—I jumped to my feet, embarrassed that I had been "caught" sitting. It's ridiculous.

It isn't normal to be rush-rush all of the time, yet we as humans adapt quickly to the environment we are in. This doesn't mean it's right. In fact, it's so unhealthy that we eventually burn out—and then we have a bigger problem on our hands.

This can be transferred in the home as well. Go-go-go with our kids to their sports activities, cleaning, cooking, helping with homework, we are constantly in motion. We have created just as much chaos in the home as we have at work, and we don't know how to relax. Or we feel guilty when we try. Society has rewarded us for being "productive," so much so that when we try to rest, we think about all of the things we could be doing instead. We might not be conscious of it, but we are not used to sitting, and we often don't actually know how to be still. It takes a lot to get over that initial hump of discomfort when we feel guilty for relaxing—but it is necessary for us if we want to live a long and healthy life.

When I eventually did deal with my stress, years of built-up anxiety came rebounding back, far more intensely than if I had dealt with it in the moment. Going on stress leave was hard—harder than actually going through what I went through. I was thinking all sorts of things. What would people think of me, would they lose respect? Would my manager be supportive, would my colleagues suffer in my absence? None of which had anything to do with me or the issue, and that was another sign to me that I needed to stop and focus on my mental health. On my first day of stress leave, I felt I needed to be doing something in my house—clearing clutter, wiping baseboards, all of the things I had never had time for. This was transferring one place of distraction for another. I needed to be still and sit with my feelings. And you know what? A lot came up. It was amazing what I had been avoiding by always doing something. Once I sat still (it was super uncomfortable at first), I got quiet enough for long enough to hear the voice that I had been ignoring for so long, the one that told me I needed to take care of me. And thankfully, I listened.

Our jobs have always been prone to burnout. Our workload has increased significantly over the past decade. The population is aging, getting sicker, and more acute. There have been significant cuts to the health care system. Combine this with the fact that we work long hours, shift work, and a boatload of overtime, and it is no wonder that we are burning out. Many HCWs are not able to cope with being full-time, and many leave the profession in the first five years. We are at a higher risk of depression, anxiety, and more likely to commit suicide than the general population.[5]

There is a ton of literature around stress and burnout among nurses and allied health. Yet, despite it being studied so extensively, we have little to show for what is actually being done about it. I can give stats on the rates of burnout, stress, depression, PTSD. I can give you tips about how to handle it. Yet, without feeling empowered to do something about it, nothing will change.

The motivation behind the extensive research from an employer standpoint has little to do with our well-being and more to do with the associated costs and patient safety—makes us feel real special, right? Until we actually start caring for one another and everyone's well-being, not just the cost of absenteeism or the risk to patient safety, there will be no real, lasting change. No one is coming to save us—we need to put ourselves first. Our outward focus on the system, the suffering, the lack, is causing us to focus on the negative. We are not going to fix the system overnight. What we can do overnight is make the decision to put our needs above all others.

Many of us have been made to feel like we don't have the power to make significant change. One person can't make a difference. I am here to tell you this isn't true. I did make significant, lasting change in my department. And I did it mostly on my own. Now, I don't recommend that you do it my way, because I did burn out from it. The more people who realize that they do not have to take the constant cuts to health care, the poor working conditions, the abusive treatment, the more change can occur. By shifting your perspective on yourself—what you are worthy of—you will wake up and recognize that this isn't okay. And the more people who recognize this, the more we can do collectively. Strength in numbers. Put your foot down and refuse to settle for unsafe working conditions.

Helpful Hints for Burnout

Moral resilience is defined as "the courage and confidence to confront distressful and uncertain situations by following and trusting values and beliefs."[6] Building moral resilience helps us see the situation for what it is, recognizing what is out of our control, and being able to focus on what is in our control. Accepting what is, is the first step to achieving moral resilience.

Know the signs—they can be different for everyone. Pay attention to your body. Have you been getting sick a lot lately? Are you more tired than usual? Are you having difficulty sleeping when you usually have no issues? Your body can tell you a lot if you slow down and listen to it. Anything that deviates from the norm is probably something that needs to be looked at. Do your body a favour and pay attention to what it is trying to tell you.

Suffering from injuries—repetitive motion that causes shoulder injuries, plantar fasciitis, carpal tunnel—all of these are indicators that our jobs are too hard on our bodies. This is an early sign that we often ignore that something is wrong. Your body is trying to give you signs that you are overworked—listen to it. It may seem normal because many of us suffer from these physical ailments. Just because many of us have these issues doesn't mean that it's right, it's a sign that we are overworked, and something needs to give—hopefully it isn't your spine.

If you have succumbed to an injury, this is your body's way of telling you to *slow down*. Sometimes, it does so in mysterious ways. My friend Kristin had uttered one day that she just needed a break from work—and later that day, she broke her leg.

Don't be in a rush to go back to your life; maybe your life is the reason you got injured in the first place. If you cannot work—DON'T. Don't worry about what your manager will say or how your coworkers are coping, this is time you need to rest. If your unit can't function without you, that means your unit has a problem, not you.

Many of us get impatient when we have injuries that prevent us from doing all of the tasks we have set out to do. Take this time to reflect. You can't do anything about it anyway, you may as well use this time to figure out what is actually important in your life. Instead of being irritated, be grateful that your body has given you this time to slow down. It is sending you a message, and it's up to you to listen. If you try to hasten your recovery so you can get back to doing all of the things, you are not getting the message.

Have the courage to admit you need help—the hardest thing I had to do was admit that I needed help. I had always been the "strong" one, and I had taken that role too seriously. I am sure, as a HCW, that you can relate to this misnomer. Part of me didn't think that I needed it. I was going to work, I was functioning. Stress leave was supposed to be for people who couldn't get out of bed, right? But it wasn't apparent to me how badly I needed this until I actually went off and had time to be still.

It was a huge hit to my ego to take the stress leave. I felt like a failure, I felt like I was giving up, and that people would look at me differently. Truth be told, I did encounter people who treated me with kid gloves when I returned from stress leave, but the people closest to me (the people that actually mattered) were relieved that I was finally putting my needs first.

Take relaxation seriously—like I said, when I first went on leave, I wanted to clean, de-clutter, do all of the things I didn't have time for when I was working. Yet I realized this was just transferring one task for another—I was still keeping myself busy.

Are you the type that goes on "vacation," has to have a ton of activities planned, and are so busy during your vacation that you come home more tired than when you left? Hint: YOU ARE DOING THE SAME THING. I know, I had a lot of OT that I filled with busy trips sightseeing. I took a lot of envy-inducing pictures, but I wasn't truly relaxing.

If you find you have a hard time sitting still, and you also have a tendency to burn out, ask yourself why you can't sit still. What about it is uncomfortable? The go-go-go mentality can be an addiction in itself, and the only way to break that cycle is to experience stillness. Sometimes we need a little boredom in our lives to be fully present.

Rich non-work life—simply put, it's not healthy to be at work all of the time. I found that work caused me to be too tired to do much else, and I didn't have any hobbies or much of a social life outside of my colleagues. My life was not as rich as I would have liked. I didn't do anything creative. I couldn't even tell you I had creativity in me, when the truth is, everybody does. We're just so focused on work and family and paying bills that many of us haven't tapped into that creative side of ourselves. Once I went casual in my position, I realized how much of the world opened up to me—there was so much more out there! And I stopped caring so much about contributing to my pension and started caring more about actually living the life I had in front of me, now, here. My parents both passed away young – there is no guarantee that I will make it to retirement. It was a gift that my parents both gave me to live life to the fullest I could, every day.

Focus on the positive—I know, I know, it sounds cliché and cheesy. But it really makes a difference. Coming from someone who was a Negative Nancy most of her life (and I still revert back into it when I don't catch myself), I can tell you that this is a hard habit to break. Being pessimistic is a sign of early trauma. If I expect the worst outcome, I can't be disappointed, and therefore I can't get hurt. Looking at the world negatively causes us to seek out deception and abuse of power, and it keeps us in victim mode. We start seeing it in everything we do. Where we put our focus is what we experience. If we are too focused on the negative, that will be all that we see. By focusing on what we do have, we can become less pessimistic. Even if you don't believe that having a positive attitude will make a difference to your department, it will make a difference in your life—and that's really all that matters.

**A note on toxic positivity*—there is a difference between being positive and being toxically so. Being positive does not mean ignoring the issues or pretending they are not there. "Good vibes only" does not allow for empathy for those who are struggling. Coming from an unhealed place, false positivity can cause just as much damage as negativity. The way we navigate this is by accepting what is—not denying it or stuffing it down. We can admit that things are tough when they are—but this does not mean we have to get bogged down in it. We can instead focus on our power and what we can do, and slowly, little by little, our perspective shifts.

Find better ways to decompress—at the end of a long day, many of us are tempted to reach for a glass of pinot, a bowl of chips, or the remote. In moderation, none of these are a problem, but when we start using them regularly to numb out from stressful jobs, they can become a crutch and even lead to a serious addiction. Instead, go for a run or a walk, play with your pets, journal, do yoga, meditate, spend time with children — yours or someone else's. Find a different outlet for dealing with stress, one that isn't harmful to your health, and one that keeps you consciously in your life—not numbing out of it. Use this as a time to explore your creative side. Finding a hobby that relaxes you, such as painting or music, will help you come down after a long day. You don't have to be good at it, it just has to feel good when you do it.

Know when it's you, and when it's them—if we are taking care of ourselves the best we can, and we are still having issues at work, chances are it is the working conditions (duh). When we are in a recession, employers often cut costs by limiting resources. We are expected to do more with less. And while we may be able to "handle" it for a short time, we are actually shooting ourselves in the foot by working to impossible standards. Making things work in the interim doesn't pay off, because the employer does not plan for this to be temporary. When we work harder, it proves to management that we can function with less. Often how hard we work and how exhausted we feel isn't because of us, it is because of the working conditions imposed on us. And unless we are willing to put our foot down and say we are not tolerating it any longer, it will continue to plague us.

After a critical event, ask for debriefing at work—we HCWs are exposed to really difficult things at our jobs. Even if it doesn't feel challenging at the time (you might still be in shock), if a critical event happens where you work, you are entitled to a debrief with the people involved, including upper management. It helps give closure and provides an opportunity to hear others' perspectives of the event, which can assist in healing. If it isn't available, reach out to a therapist or to your employee assistance program.

After the death of a patient in our department, I needed a debrief with the staff involved. It seemed a moot point, as I had already discussed it with my manager and a few colleagues, but it made a difference to have an official debrief with the people involved. If you have a critical event on your unit and feel you need to discuss it, ask for an official debrief, even if it isn't offered. You can get closure from this that will help you move on, even if it doesn't feel like it at the time.

Advocate for a change in workload and more control over your schedule—small changes to your work can have huge payoffs in your health—mentally, physically, and emotionally. If you are concerned about talking to your manager, just be honest. Tell her that you are feeling apathetic and want to explore options for improving morale, and see what you can come up with. Knowing that you are being heard is sometimes all you need to feel better in your position. Improving your morale can have a ripple effect for the morale amongst your coworkers. It can be as little as having a radio in the med room that makes a big difference to your day.

Have the courage to discuss the real issues with your manager—in her book *Fierce Conversations,* Susan Scott discusses how not talking about the real issue is what is contributing to much of our work stress, and keeps us miserable.[7] Many times, we sugar-coat, minimize, or skirt the real issues. Getting down to the meat of the matter is scary, but it often resolves issues that keep coming up in different forms. If you could tell your manager exactly how it is, what would you say? Having the courage to discuss the real problems on the unit, whether it be a difficult staff member, the low morale, or how you are struggling to come into work, can help you resolve the problem quicker than beating around the bush about it. If your manager is competent, she will have to take what you say seriously, even if she wasn't aware of the problem. Speaking up, though scary, gets us closer to our healing and living a happier life. If it is taken positively, you are on the road to making change. If it is not handled well, then you have some insight into whether or not it is worth it to stay somewhere that your honest thoughts and feelings aren't respected.

Take some time off—whether you have ample banked overtime or sick leave, or you need to go off on disability, nothing is more important than your health. You may not be fully supported in this by management (be prepared for this), but catering to the needs of others to the point of exhaustion among health care workers needs to stop. We are in the health care profession, and we are not taking care of our own health. I've witnessed enough of my colleagues suffering serious illness from ignoring their own bodies. I've lost a few to terminal illness, a few to suicide. It's time to put our own well-being first, even if that means displeasing others. You are the most important person to you. You are no good to anyone if you are neglecting your health, and your body will surely tell you this eventually. No one who has your best interest at heart is going to give you shit for taking the time you need to, so fuck anybody who does. Health care workers have been seeing a spike in suicide rates for a long time, and I'm sure they are sky-rocketing now with the pandemic. This is no joke—it's time to put ourselves first.

Unfortunately, my most recent burnout was not handled as positively as I had hoped. Being on medical unemployment insurance with only a percentage of my income was more stressful than being at work. As I was filing a work safety claim, I was required to make a statement of all of the issues I had to deal with, causing me to relive the harassment, bullying, and overwhelm all over again. With multiple doctor visits, dealing with the union, OH&S, and the work safety department, as well as navigating government forms and contacts, it was all too much for someone who was on a stress leave. I will NEVER go through this again. It's not worth it. I let it get away from me, trying to do more than what one human should have to. Don't repeat the same mistakes I made—if you are feeling overwhelmed, or even have an inkling you are burnt out—DO something about it, before it gets to this stage.

Know when enough is enough—be proactive with your health, get the support you need, and work with your employer. If your employer is not willing to work with you on making necessary changes to the department, ask yourself if it is worth sacrificing your health over. It may be necessary to move on.

The Bottom Line with Burnout

If you are experiencing burnout, this is where you need to practice your super-power of empathy the most. If you imagined that a close friend was going through what you were going through, what would you tell her? Would you tell her to suck it up? To stick it out? To just deal with it? Of course not! So why do we tell ourselves this? The empathy that we have for other people needs to be calibrated to include ourselves.

We are so hard on ourselves, and we don't often seek the support we need. If you knew a friend was having a difficult time, would you want her to be dealing with it on her own or would you want her to ask for help? And would you feel that friend was being a burden to your life? Again, of course not, but this is often the reason we feel hesitant to reach out. We often don't treat ourselves with the same respect and kindness that we give to others. Our Inner Child is desperately wanting us to treat her the way we are treating others.

If you are in burnout or have dealt with it, I am so sorry. I hope you have the support you need. It is my wish that this book, in addition to getting proper care from a professional, will give you tools to help prevent this from happening to you again. When I was first debating whether or not I should go on stress leave, I allowed myself to focus on others instead of my own needs—even when contemplating a stress leave. I felt like, because everyone else was dealing with it and *seemed* fine, that I didn't have a right to do this. I wasn't special; we all were experiencing the same issues. Who was I to take stress leave?

My Inner Child was listening. If I told myself I didn't matter, that meant that she didn't matter. If I could ignore my own needs, I could ignore her. While I don't have children, I know how it felt when I was ignored as a child, or deemed unimportant. The Inner Child persona is real, and she hears us. And for those of you who do have children, by ignoring yourself for everyone else, you are teaching them that this is okay. They will grow up to either expect others to over-give or become the person who does. We need to break the cycle of unhealthy parenting, and it starts with parenting ourselves.

If you think you might be suffering from burnout now, I urge you to seek support. We all deserve to be living happy, healthy lives—it is our birthright. Don't settle for less than you deserve. We all deserve to be treated with kindness and respect. We all deserve to be healthy, happy, and joyful. Make yourself the priority. Make the necessary changes that you are worthy of. Instead of worrying about how others will cope without you, start thinking about how happy they will be for you when you actually start feeling better, like your old self.

If you are a health care worker, know how special you are. You are so amazing, and you have no idea how powerful you are. You have no idea what your empathy can do for others. You don't have to suffer with feeling powerless. You are worthy of better working conditions. You are worthy of having your voice be heard. You are worthy. Do not underestimate your ability to make change—one person can make a difference. You need to be determined, you need to be active in the change you want to make, and you need to ask for help.

You deserve to feel better. The world is a better place with you in it. We need you, and we need you to start making yourself a priority.

EXERCISES

1. Imagine you are the parent of you. Or, if that is too difficult, imagine that your daughter or son is in the same predicament you are in at work. What would you say to her? What advice would you give to her? How would you nurture her, how would you help her? Say it out loud, roleplay, or write your Inner Child/daughter/son a letter expressing how you feel when you see her ignoring her needs.

2. Gift yourself some time to sit still, even just a minute. Gradually increase the amount of time that you sit still in silence—without your phone, or TV, or other distractions. Even if you say you don't have time, you have five minutes. This will help you get into the groove of relaxing and undo the need to be constantly doing something. Just be.

CHAPTER 13

Perfectionism

"The curious paradox is when I accept myself just as I am, then I change."
– Carl Rogers

Ask yourself a question—if you had a task that you gave yourself permission to do imperfectly (a dressing change that was done sterilely but messily, cleaning the kitchen but leaving a few dishes in the sink), how would you feel? Would that sit well with you? Would you still do whatever task or accomplishment you want to achieve, knowing that it wouldn't be done exceptionally well? Or would it annoy you, knowing that you wouldn't be satisfied with "just okay"?

Have you ever stopped yourself from doing something that you had a mild interest in (e.g., a hobby—painting, or learning a musical instrument) because you didn't feel like you're talented enough, even though you had the desire to try?

Have you ever procrastinated on something for so long because the conditions weren't optimal—you didn't have enough information and needed to "research more," or waited for the "right time"? Have you ever started something, realized you weren't kicking ass at it right away, then gave up because you didn't want to fail (and perhaps tricked yourself into saying "It's not for me," or "I don't like this," or "I'm not naturally gifted at this, therefore it wasn't meant to be")?

Guilty. On all of the above counts. The universe actually played a cruel joke on me when I was writing this chapter. I had edited all of the chapters, including this one, to my liking. As I was reading through my work, I discovered that my editing of this section hadn't saved. I had to do it again. The irony of the chapter entitled "Perfectionism" being done improperly is not lost on me. Touché, Universe, touché.

What Perfectionism Actually Is

Adapted from the "Perfectionism in Perspective" module from the Australia Psychology Department, the definition of perfectionism is "the relentless striving for extremely high standards (for yourself and/or others) that are personally demanding, in the context of the individual."[1] It is when we base our self-worth off of how much we *do*, and not who we *are*. This then leads to experiencing negative

---

consequences of setting such demanding standards, yet continuing to pursue them despite the high cost of doing so.

There is a big difference between the setting of healthy goals for ourselves and the harmful striving for perfection. Setting goals helps us to achieve things in life. Having our sights set on something we desire and then taking necessary action to make it happen is a key component of feeling fulfilled. However, when these goals are either unachievable or only achievable at great cost, it becomes overwhelming. Continual overexertion of our time, energy, and finances can lead to perfectionism.

Perfectionism is much more than simply doing something "perfectly." People who suffer from perfectionism aren't able to handle constructive feedback because they associate themselves with what they do instead of who they are. This means if they fail, THEY are a failure. They equate their achievements to their own sense of self-worth. This is obviously hazardous for our ability to function in society, as making mistakes and failure is a part of being human.

I used to wear my perfectionism as a badge. I thought it was a good thing to strive for perfection, and I wasn't alone. I would hear others claim with a haughty air, "Oh, well, I'm a perfectionist, so ..." thus justifying their over-attention to detail, the long hours spent bent over a creative project, the reason they just couldn't relax. While it was exhausting just to listen to all of the tasks the self-declared perfectionists had set for themselves, I witnessed them also complaining about all of the things they needed to do, how their spouses were no help because they couldn't do a task properly, and how they had to do it all because only they could do it right. They clearly weren't happy with their situation, yet they continued to flaunt that perfectionist pin.

Beliefs associated with perfectionism:

- I have to do things right the first time

- I have to do everything well

- If I can't do something perfectly, then there is no point in even trying

- If I make a mistake, it means I am bad

- If I do everything perfectly, others can't criticize me

- I constantly judge my achievements and rarely give myself credit when I do well because there's always something that could be improved upon

- I become hyper-focused on getting one task done perfectly that I don't have time to complete the rest of my work

I allowed perfectionism to keep me in a prison for most of my life, starting from when I was a child. When I got a test back and received ninety-eight percent on it, I didn't need my parents to ask where the other two percent went, I was already searching for it myself. My perfectionism was costing me my happiness from an early age. While most kids would be overjoyed by the marks I was achieving, I was constantly trying to strive for the best results. And if it didn't beat my grade's smartest kid, it wasn't good enough.

These perfectionistic beliefs continued into adulthood. When I set a goal and happened to achieve it according to my standards, I couldn't pat myself on the back or revel in my accomplishments—I was already setting my sights on the next thing. For me, the need to achieve was in all areas of my life—career, friendships, family.

I couldn't handle making mistakes. If I made a med error at work, I would be upset about it for days. I would repeatedly bring it up to colleagues who had long forgotten about it, and they would try to persuade me to do the same. If I cheated on my healthy eating diet or skipped a run, I was "off the bandwagon" and figured I screwed up, so I may as well just keep chowing down.

My ego (my Inner Child) could barely function when I messed up. I was compassionate with others who made errors, yet I beat myself up when it was my turn to screw up. I thought if I could do everything perfectly, I wouldn't be prey to criticism from others—which was the true underlying issue. My sense of self-worth was based on what I could achieve.

Underneath, I was a fragile little girl who hadn't been given enough support to develop a healthy sense of self. I was so afraid of being wrong, of making a mistake, of being seen as incompetent. I went to every length possible to be right. If I read enough books or memorized the policies, people wouldn't be able to call me out. If I checked everything twice at work, I wouldn't mess up and no one could hurt me for making an error. I didn't allow myself to be human.

And I did mess up—a lot. Being "perfect" all of the time became exhausting—and I became fatigued and unable to focus on the tasks at hand because I had this underlying conflict within myself running all of the time. If my mind was like electricity in my home, I was like someone running the air conditioner while having all of the windows left open. My perfectionism was sucking up all of the energy and causing the air conditioner to run on full blast in an attempt to keep the temperature regular. I was leaking energy all of the time trying to be perfect—and it was draining me of my ability to do my job properly. In fact, it was probably causing me to perform *worse* because I was so focused on not making a mistake with a task that I tended to miss other things.

It also sucked away all of my happiness. I wasn't able to enjoy my relationships, being on constant watch for any imperfections I might be showing to my friends and family. If I always acted perfect instead of just being myself (irritable, sad, angry feelings and all), then they wouldn't be able to criticize. I would be able to argue my way out of any conflict because I had performed "perfectly" (even when the suppressed anger bubbled up and spilled over and I shamed myself even more).

My fragile Inner Child couldn't handle being wrong, as this meant that she wasn't loveable. And unfortunately, she had a lot of data to support this notion. Some of the unhealthy relationships and people she had around her growing up blamed her when she wasn't perfect, and her self-fulfilling prophecy of being unlovable unless she was flawless was enacted when she messed up and was abandoned for it.

Working in health care, there is pressure to get everything done, and we work extremely hard to do so. Setting unreasonable amounts of work on us can lead us to perfectionistic qualities, as we feel the need to do every task, with good reason: If we miss doing a task, patients suffer. So we endeavour as much as we can to get all of the work done in a day. This can be seen as perfectionistic to have all of the tasks done in order to tick all the boxes off in a day. Our culture has created this tendency in many of us.

Areas of perfectionism affect different aspects of our lives:

- *Decision-making*—taking a long time to decide or ruminating over making the wrong choice

- *Overcompensating*—being overly detailed or justifying your responses to others

- *Not knowing when to stop*—arguing a point over and over, pursuing a task and not giving up even when it is clear you should stop

- *Controlling* —needing to know what is going to happen at all times, influencing others to maintain control

- *Validation-seeking*—needing constant reassurance from others

- *Excessive organizing*—making lists, being rigid in cleanliness, checking over your work multiple times

- *Avoidance*—being afraid of failing or not doing something well and therefore not trying

- *Procrastination*—putting things off because the time isn't right or you won't be able to do it perfectly, or fear of failure

- *Failure to delegate*—not allowing others to help because they won't do it properly

- *Attempts to change other people*—correcting grammar or offering unsolicited advice in order to "educate"

Perfectionism can live in certain areas of our lives and not necessarily others. You may be bending over backwards to be the perfect Mom, but be more realistic and down to earth at work. You may be an easygoing spouse and parent, but extremely rigid in your career, hyper-focusing on little details that don't really matter in the big picture.

Left unchecked, perfectionistic tendencies can lead to a diagnosis of clinical perfectionism. Clinical perfectionism is linked to anxiety, depression, obsessive-compulsive disorder, and eating disorders.[2]

Why do we become perfectionists?

If any of this is sounding familiar, it's not your fault. Growing up in the conditions that most of us did, it isn't any wonder why we have this little part of us that feels the need to prove ourselves as adults. The conditioning of not being good enough has been instilled in anyone who owned a TV, or had parents, or is human, essentially.

Society is often to blame for creating perfectionistic personalities. We are rewarded and given positive reinforcement when we get good marks, when we "behave," or when we achieve. This starts when we are young and our teachers and parents praise us for being "good." We get awards for being on the honor roll, or for winning at sports. Other areas society rewards us for is cleanliness, being attractive, or being promoted at work for our achievements. Our child self, only seeing things in black and white, may misconstrue the adults' pleasure of getting good grades and generalize it as, "People are only proud of me when I succeed." This is reinforced further when we are punished for our mistakes, and instead of believing we *did* something bad, we simplify in our young minds that we *are* bad. Unless we listened to Fred Rogers nonstop, the positive messages in our lives were probably outweighed by the negative ones.

We also learn through our parents. If our parents had perfectionistic tendencies, they would (often unknowingly) pass it on to us. If our parents worked very hard or long hours, it might be deemed as normal—thus, we believe anything less than this is being lazy or unmotivated. If our childhood home had to be spotless, we are likely to be unable to tolerate clutter or mess in our own homes. The helicopter parenting expected of parents today probably began in our parents' generation.

Acknowledging how we got here, knowing that it isn't our fault, and admitting that we have an issue with perfectionism (read: not good enough) is the first step to doing something about it.

How Perfectionism Affects Us

It affects the standards we set for ourselves—those of us who struggle with perfectionism set extremely high standards for ourselves and others, and it is impossible to achieve them 100 percent of the time. When we do not meet these standards, we tend to believe we didn't work hard enough. "I should have …" is a common phrase that perfectionists utter when we feel remorse over not doing something perfectly. Sometimes we will go to great lengths to achieve these goals at great personal cost—sacrificing sleep, finances, or time with loved ones.

It affects our beliefs—we humans tend to pay attention to things that validate what we believe. If we have perfectionistic tendencies, the belief that "we must not make a mistake or we will be punished" will have us looking out for mistakes or errors and correcting them. We will overlook or minimize all of our achievements and all of the good things that we do, and only focus on what we did wrong. This can also affect our relationships, as we can become nitpicky or negative by only seeing faults in others.

It affects our self-worth—perfectionism causes us to be extremely self-critical. We blame ourselves for not meeting unrealistic goals, and it causes us to feel like we are not worthy. This can lead to guilt, stress, anxiety, and depression.

It affects how we see the world—black-and-white thinking is quite common in perfectionism. How a ten-year-old sees the world is how perfectionists have a tendency to see it. You are right or wrong, good or bad, a success or a failure—there is no in-between. The kitchen must be spotless or it's not clean. The dressing must be neat and tidy or it's not done properly. This all-or-nothing thinking causes us to not be able to see the grey zones. The us-versus-them mentality discussed in a previous chapter can be traced back to black-and-white thinking ("If you're not with me, you're against me").

It affects what we believe might happen in the future—when we are afflicted with perfectionism, we tend to jump to conclusions about what might happen if we don't perform perfectly ("If I mess up, they will laugh at me/reprimand me"). We only see what could go wrong and don't think about anything else. This causes us to work even harder not to mess up.

Perfectionist Armor

Perfectionism, far from shielding us from harm, only shields us from getting in touch with ourselves. It's scary to let people see the less desirable parts of ourselves when we have been taught for so long that we should be ashamed of them. When we wear the armor of perfectionism, what we show to the world is something that doesn't allow anything in. While it may protect us from pain or getting upset in front of people, it also prevents the good from getting in, too. Ever have a compliment just bounce off? Like, you hear it, but you don't let it in? The armor of perfectionism that we have built piece by piece has done its job. It doesn't let anything in, including the good. Including the compliments. Including the love and affection of others.

This also includes your own love and affection for yourself. Sure, you can list off all of the accomplishments you have achieved over the years, can probably acknowledge that you have done a lot, can smile politely when others praise you for how far you have come. And if you are anything like me, you can even fool yourself into believing that you are proud of your accomplishments.

But do you actually feel it? Are you feeling it in your heart or your head? If you have a tendency to move on to the next goal often, always looking for the next achievement without being fully able to appreciate where you are at, then you are likely suffering from perfectionism. If you were to stop and listen to your inner voice, you might hear the critic that says that you should be doing more. That you shouldn't have made that med error and should do more to prevent it. And if you allow her to lead you, she will have you focus on the next big project you should be setting your sights on. Because if you are always focusing on the next big thing, you can't hear the air conditioner working on overdrive just to maintain a comfortable temperature. She is being critical because she is afraid that if people see her not achieving, she will be criticized. She's essentially beating them to it by criticizing herself. The heartbreaking truth of the matter is that perfectionists don't believe that they are truly good enough, as is, just because.

My perfectionism didn't just affect me, it affected others. When I wasn't fixing myself, I was fixing the "wrong" things that were around me. Working in a hospital is like a buffet for someone who needs to fix things. I saw so many issues that the uncomfortable feeling of not having something to control was quickly extinguished. There were so many obstacles to sink my teeth into, I was spoiled for choice. First it was the ultrasound department, where the nurses were working in suboptimal rooms despite having larger rooms as an option. Then it was the call schedule, not yet in existence and marked with inconsistency in how it was divided. Then it was attaining another nurse in the department.

While the issues I settled on were genuine problems and not simply make-work projects, and I was sincerely passionate about making the department a better place to work for myself and my colleagues, the motivation underneath it had transformed from a desire to improve things into something I needed in order to focus on something other than myself. My perspective that zeroed in on the negative aspects of the department was so ingrained in me, I could only see what was wrong. When I heard colleagues echoing these issues, my bias was confirmed. I was on a mission, and they were happy to receive the spoils of my toils.

The Dark Side of Perfectionism

Perfectionism isn't a badge to be worn. It's more like a tattoo of pain, misery, and self-loathing. It was a heavy, ugly, dense energy in my stomach that meant I had to do everything right, everything perfectly, so I didn't prove to my subconscious what I truly believed underneath it all: that I wasn't good enough. That my self-worth is derived from my actions, my accomplishments, my good deeds, and not simply because I am a human being who has a right to be here. I had to constantly be earning my keep.

Every human being on this planet is entitled to a healthy sense of self-worth, whether a man or woman, black or white, cop or criminal. Whether we have made mistakes (really bad ones) or not, we are still entitled to our self-worth. That does not mean we should not be held accountable for our actions, or not feel sorrow or pain when we make a mistake. But it also does not mean we should feel ashamed of who we are.

This is very much a Western societal issue. Many people who live in a traditional Eastern culture do not suffer from issues with self-esteem. The Dalai Lama, when questioned about issues around self-esteem, had to have it explained to him what it was—he had never encountered the concept of low self-esteem before. It is taught in our society to not feel good enough (mostly as a way to sell us something that will fix that). Feral children who have been rescued and have somehow survived, while they have many other psychosocial issues, do not display this aspect in their behavior. They can be barking like a dog and not have an ounce of shame—they missed this important lesson that Western society drills into us. Our attempt to be perfect is often a script written into our behavior from an early age.

The more exploring I did with my therapist, the more I realized how insidious it was. It colored every aspect of my life—my career, my relationships, and my health. If I did my job perfectly, nobody could critique me. If I was the perfect girlfriend/friend/daughter, I would be loved and protected. If I ate "perfectly" and worked out "perfectly," I would look a certain way (because it was rarely about my actual health, it was how I looked on the outside). My fragile ego couldn't stand being wrong or being rejected, so I did everything in my power to avoid these situations—which translated to doing everything "right" all of the time.

This is perfectionism. This is what being a perfectionist really is. This is how it plays out.

It was like wearing shit-colored glasses, and everywhere I looked there was a code brown. It tainted everything I touched. It didn't matter how many certificates I received, or miles I ran, or foods I eliminated, I always needed to be doing more. I was hypercritical of everything, yet it all stemmed from me being hypercritical of myself. The armor I wore to protect myself from criticism was turning on me. It worked so well at keeping criticism out that it kept everything out. I couldn't take a compliment if I tried. No matter how much praise or reassurance or love I received from others, it didn't get in. Nothing could. I was always on the hunt for the thing to make me feel better. Maybe it would be a new exercise class, or a book, or a course. But nothing did—until I started the Inner Child work and really began digging into my perfectionism and the root of it all.

For those of you who relate to this account, I am so sorry you have had to endure this. For those of you who don't, but maybe have a severely pessimistic or a highly critical coworker, know that this probably stems from a similar issue. With our empathy laser beams, we can see that the negativity and criticism our coworkers emit are simply projections of how they feel about themselves. While it isn't easy to deal with, know that they are suffering more than they are letting on.

It was the little girl who first learned she wasn't good enough. It was the little girl who had to be quiet, had to be independent, had to be *just so.* Children are just as smart as adults, soaking everything up like a sponge, they just don't have as much information yet as adults do. But they learn, very quickly. All of the experiences we have as children shape who we become as adults, whether we are consciously aware of these behaviors or not. Time doesn't heal all wounds, we just get better at ignoring them. When we start diving into the reasons why we don't feel good enough and start actually talking about it, it feels as fresh today as it did twenty years ago. To a small part of us, this happened yesterday. This is why it feels so real to us when we do discover old wounds that we had compartmentalized and forgotten. To our Inner Child, everything is still very real, raw, and undigested. Any behavior that triggers us as an adult is the Inner Child trying to get our attention. "Hey, this is still a thing, look at it, please!" She is waiting for us to finally listen to her and heal something we neglected to notice before. With perfectionism, it is not being good enough.

To us, we might logically be baffled as to why certain events have contributed to how we behave as adults. Not all childhood wounds have to involve trauma. For instance, it was pointed out to me that my first memory may have contributed to feeling unheard. I was sliding down the stairs and was told to be quiet so I didn't wake my Granny who was sleeping in the next room. This was significant as I was being silenced from the get-go—that my voice didn't matter, and I was "bad" for doing something that all kids do—playing. You didn't have to have had a difficult childhood for events to make an impact. As a child, you were always learning and absorbing, and you did whatever you could to stay safe and happy. And if you were scolded for something innocuous—being too loud or breaking a plate—you as a child would collect that data and store it for next time. As our parents are human, they were not perfect—and we learned to react to them, however their parenting styles developed. If we were continually scolded for the same thing over and over again, we would learn not to do it to avoid punishment. For me, the silencing trend was continual and varied—I learned that I didn't get a voice.

Shame

"If you put shame in a Petri dish, it needs three ingredients to grow exponentially: secrecy, silence, and judgment." – Brené Brown

Shame is something everyone experiences. Sometimes, after doing the amount of work I have done on myself, I will feel shame for not knowing something I "should" know. When I remember that everyone experiences shame (and I am not immune to it, no matter how much knowledge I have on the subject), I relax and let myself feel it. The best way to overcome shame is to bring it out into the light. Have you ever hid something from others for fear of being judged, only to hear someone courageous share their story of a similar plight, and it suddenly didn't seem like a big deal? That it was not as ugly as it looked before, whether it be something grave we experienced in our past, or a less serious bad habit (a TikTok addiction, for example?) Bringing our "shame" out into the light effectively kills any power it might have over us. We simply need to have the courage to share.

Shame is often the emotion we repress the most. Shame is extra weight that we carry with us, dragging us down and keeping us from living our best lives. If you were to see yourself on a path trying to reach a destination (a goal, for example), shame is like a big black cloud. We lose sight of the destination, get lost in the fog, and use our precious energy trying to escape from it. We usually do make it out, but we have wasted too much of our time and energy trying to escape it. Often the things we are ashamed of were never ours to begin with, but what society has told us we should be ashamed of. Our bodies, our skin color, our sexual orientation, our bank accounts. Our childhood selves were bombarded with information that proved that we weren't good enough, and so we spend most of our lives trying to fit into a box to be accepted, meanwhile denying who we truly are.

For me, my body causes me a great deal of shame for not being perfect. It has caused me to miss out on activities that I would enjoy because I wasn't the right size. If I didn't have shame about my body, I would be on the beach and not caring about covering up, I wouldn't put off dating until I was the right size, and my eating habits would change. Shame has caused me to miss out on opportunities, and even though I still reach my goals, it feels heavier when I do than if I wasn't carrying the shame.

How to Shed the Armor

So what can we do about perfectionism? First of all, throw away the badge of honor, whatever form your perfectionism takes—it isn't something to be proud of.

This is a big thing to unpack. It can color every aspect of our lives, from our career to our relationships to our health. This is not something to take on by yourself. Working with a therapist is essential to being given enough support. Even when you begin to work on this, you will be actively dealing with your perfectionism in your therapy work. My therapist sent me many modules to work on (some of which I have referenced here), and I had them all completed by our next session—I kind of missed the point!

If you are anything like me, this will be something that you work on for the rest of your life. Be kind with yourself. Like characteristics of your personality, there are aspects of perfectionism that you won't be able to change. You have been critical of yourself for a long time – this isn't going to go away overnight. Your Inner Child has been overly critical because she felt it was the best way to keep you safe from harm. You know better now. It's time for change.

You can try having a conversation with your Inner Child about why she is feeling shame. Or, you can imagine it being a loved one who is feeling it. I personally love Elizabeth Gilbert's method for self-parenting: She writes a letter to Love, pouring her heart out to Love as a compassionate witness, asking Love what She would do, and Love writes back to her. It is a sweet way to get in touch with the tender parts of ourselves. I have been told many times, by different people, how hard I am on myself, and I never see it. When I stop and check in with myself, I uncover the part of me that feels shame and is afraid to come out. I grant it compassion, and accept it for what it is.

Knowing that this part of ourselves is present doesn't mean we can't work on making our lives better. Like an introvert who plans their social events around their energy, we can make changes to our lives to help us with our perfectionistic tendencies. Being a perfectionist, you're going to want to tackle all areas at once, but resist the urge to overachieve here—that's part of the work.

Changing Our Thoughts

Our minds chatter incessantly all day long. Like taking a train every day, the first time you hear the announcements of where to get off, you hear them very clearly. After you've been riding for a while, you don't even register them anymore, but they are there. We go on autopilot with our thoughts. If we have heard many times that we are not worthy, or good enough, through conditioning (parents, teachers, friends, TV, colleagues), our thoughts will reflect this whether we notice them or not. Changing our thoughts is important for our beliefs, our feelings, and our behaviors. Being conscious of them is one way we can begin to reverse our negative thought patterns.

One way to do this is through meditation, where we "watch" our thoughts. We don't attach to them or let them affect us—we treat them like they are passing clouds.

We can also check in with ourselves throughout the day. If we are thinking pessimistic thoughts, we can consciously choose to course correct to more positive ones. Even if we simply notice our thoughts more often than we usually do, we can begin to notice patterns. When we notice patterns, it gives us data that can support change (e.g., if we notice more negative thoughts when we are around certain people, we can choose whether we want to address this with them or perhaps not be around these people as often).

Changing Our Beliefs

Once we are more conscious of our thoughts, we can challenge them through identifying our beliefs around them. The best way to do this is through self-reflection. In *Loving What Is,* Byron Katie quotes four questions she has christened "The Work" for identifying negative thoughts that affect our beliefs:[3]

1. *Is it true?*

2. *Can you absolutely know it's true?*

3. *What happens when I believe this thought?*

4. *Who would I be without this thought?*

For example, let's say I left dishes in the sink. I identify that it annoys me. *Why* does it annoy me? Here are some thoughts that run through my head:

"You're lazy." "Only a slob lives like this." "Trailer park." (Sometimes I only can catch snippets of words, but as you can see here, I know what I can infer from the words "trailer park.")

So now I do "The Work":

1. Is it true?

    Am I a slob for leaving dishes in the sink? No.

2. Can you absolutely know it's true?

    I would say no, leaving dishes in the sink once does not make me a slob.

3. What happens when I believe this thought?

I feel sad, dirty, gross, unworthy, that I need to overcompensate by being excessively clean to prove the thought wrong.

4. Who would I be without this thought?

I would be able to relax, allow others to come over without having to madly scrub the baseboards, allow them to see the real me—who leaves dishes in the sink sometimes.

Do you see how a few dishes can play havoc because of a thought? This is the work that shifts those beliefs.

Changing Our Behavior

While doing this self-reflection is helpful, it is not going to shift long-stemming perfectionist behavior overnight. It might be affecting multiple areas of your life. Our all-or-nothing thinking probably wants it all to go away, just like that—and that isn't realistic. By breaking our actions down slowly, piece by piece, we can begin to change some of the unhealthy behaviors we have adapted. Working with a therapist concurrently while altering some of our behaviors can bring support as well as enlightenment as to why we developed some of the behaviors in the first place.

Here is an exercise I worked on with my therapist. I decided to work on delegating, as I needed help. I noticed that I was afraid to be rejected and I didn't like that others might not do the tasks the way I would prefer.

Taken from *Perfectionism in Perspective*:

1. Think about the areas of your life that are affected by perfectionism. It may be work, home, relationships, diet/exercise, hobbies, etc.

Delegating at work.

2. List the actual behaviors that you are doing (e.g., excessive list-making, cleanliness, working too many shifts, having to do tasks perfectly, not delegating to others, procrastinating, etc.)

Doing all of the tasks, not accepting help from others even when I need it, being afraid to ask others for help because I know they are also busy.

3. List all of the positive outcomes/rewards you get for having these high standards (e.g., people praise me, I get a lot done, it feels satisfying to complete a task perfectly, etc.)

I feel like a rock star for getting it all done, I feel satisfied that the work I've completed is done the way I like it, I feel happy that I am able to help others.

4. List all of the negative consequences of having these high standards (e.g., missing time with family, losing sleep, etc.)

I am exhausted at the end of the day, I don't want to be around loved ones because I need to decompress, I'm not doing other activities that I'm interested in, I notice I want to eat junk food to make myself feel better, I feel resentful of others even though I am not asking for my needs to be met, and I feel they should just "know."

5. List the potential long-term costs for continuing to have these high standards. What might happen if you continue down this path? (e.g., health suffers, lose important relationships, etc.)

    My health is suffering (eating poorly, not exercising, being too hard on my body), I'm not having quality time with loved ones and my relationships are drifting away, my mental health is suffering.

6. What might happen if you were able to overcome some of these tendencies?

    I would have more energy and feel more satisfied every day, I would get to see loved ones more, have deeper connections with them, I would have more time and energy for hobbies.

7. Pick one area that you want to work on—JUST ONE. For example, it might be working too much. Select a goal specific to that area that might help you. For example, it might be "picking up less shifts" or "delegating to others." Break this down and make it measurable. For example, it might be, "I will only pick up one extra shift this month instead of the usual two or three," or "I will delegate tasks at work three times this week."

    I will delegate at work one time each shift for one week.

8. Think about what might prevent you from breaking these habits (e.g., "My manager might pressure me," or "My family won't help out"). Do what you can to mitigate this, and get creative with solutions. For example, you can tell your manager ahead of time that you won't be picking up this month so he/she is less likely to ask you on the spot, or you can tell your family if they won't help out around the house that you will hire a cleaning service (and it can come out of their allowance). Anticipating what might stop you can help make things easier.

    I might feel guilty for asking others to help when they already have so much on their plate, I might feel fear of being told no or getting flak from others, I might be annoyed when the tasks I've asked others to do don't get done the way I'd like them to, or when. I can remedy this by telling people I need to work on delegating more, and ask for their help. I can be specific in my requests so that the tasks are done in a way that I am satisfied with.

9. What can you do to reward yourself when you have met this goal? Remember, the goal is to do something less perfectly—if you don't do it perfectly, that is the point! Sit with the discomfort of not doing something perfectly, and give yourself positive reinforcement.

    I will get a pedicure if I meet the goal at the end of the week.

Tips and Tricks for the Recovering Perfectionist

1. Remember that life isn't black and white. You are not going to do this perfectly, and that is the point! Life is messy.

2. This is going to feel uncomfortable. In order to overcome perfectionism, you are going to have to do things in ways you aren't used to, and leave things not done, not clean, and not in a shiny bow. What that might look like is a large load of laundry, tasks being done by others that may not have your high standards, or not getting everything done at work. THIS IS OKAY. Just because you don't do the dishes one day does *not* mean you are going to turn into a slob (which is probably what the inner critic is accusing you of)! And if your house is messy for a while, so be it. It might be a phase you need to go through in order to accept your imperfections a little better.

    The same goes for tasks at work. We try so hard to get everything done that this goal is more important than our own welfare. If we are skipping meals and holding our bladders to ensure our patients are getting their meds on time, we are not putting ourselves first. It becomes about the task and not about what is actually important—our own health. Get used to living with imperfection. Trees don't grow perfectly straight, but we don't criticize them, we admire them for their uniqueness. Be a tree.

3. You might be tempted to go back to your old habits. It is normal to feel anxious or uncomfortable during these times. It is especially hard to deal with when others are not getting their needs met anymore because we have started to prioritize ourselves. In the home environment, this might be okay, but it is hard to say no to our patients who need us. The system is broken, and the only reason it is still running is because we are enslaving ourselves to make it work. While we know we need to put ourselves first, it is still very uncomfortable to do this in the work setting. This is why working with a therapist is imperative to overcoming some of these unhealthy coping mechanisms. Remember the costs in the long term of going back to these habits – it might mean *you* become the patient. It will help you when you are feeling the need to use them again.

4. Changing these habits (like any habit) requires a commitment of time and effort. If you are in an exceptionally stressful situation or period in your life, now might not be the time to pursue this. Make sure you have the support, time, and dedication that you will need. But make sure this is the truth, and not just an excuse to procrastinate. If you are unsure if perfectionism is a problem for you, ask people you know and trust if they think it might be affecting you.

5. Give yourself permission to make mistakes. This might seem scary at first, as we have been conditioned to avoid any situation where we might make an error. Like becoming accustomed to anything new, getting used to making mistakes can be hard. One way you can practice this is by learning a new skill. Try taking an art class or learning a new sport. I signed up for a dance class, and the ladies in the group and I just laughed as we messed up the steps. The instructor was reminding us that her other students, who were children, were able to memorize the dance quicker than we did—I retorted they don't have useless information like quadratic equations knocking around, and we all laughed at this. When you sign up for a new skill, it is expected that you will mess up, and by being the newbie, you will be supported by others when you do. This can do wonders for your self-esteem, and helps you relax in other areas of your life and not be so rigid.

6. Don't take yourself too seriously. Life gets heavy sometimes, and we all have things we are working on. Make sure that you are doing things that you enjoy that help you feel lighter. Watching comedy movies, being out with friends, or spending time with pets or children can help with this a lot!

7. Reward yourself often. Setting up little treats can bring positive reinforcement to change. The way it worked on us when we were young still works today! Give yourself the compliments and praise that you have denied yourself so long, and do it especially when you don't do it perfectly.

EXERCISES

1. In what ways do you find yourself having perfectionistic tendencies? Do you procrastinate, or make excessive lists, or fail to delegate?

2. Do these tendencies tend to show themselves more at work or at home? With tasks or relationships?

3. Do the exercise listed above, selecting ONE area you would like to work on. Tell people you are doing this, as it will give you more support and help you stay on track with it.

4. Once you have a measurable goal, what will you do to reward yourself? Remember this reward when you are having a hard time sticking to it.

CHAPTER 14

The Drama Triangle

"What is drama but life with the dull bits cut out." – Alfred Hitchcock

You are an OR nurse in a busy inner-city hospital. You go out to speak with your patient before his procedure. He is tired, weak, and hasn't had much sleep. He is having doubts about his surgery and wants to speak with the surgeon. You go to speak with the surgeon, who is abrupt and only half paying attention. He exasperatedly states he doesn't have time to speak with the patient, that he already spoke with him extensively when he obtained consent from him to operate, and that the patient is being ridiculous, as it is a routine procedure.

You, feeling you should advocate for the patient, proclaim that it's normal for the patient to be nervous and that he has a right to express his feelings. The surgeon, surprised and annoyed at your reaction, becomes angry, exclaiming that he has done a ton of these procedures and he is well aware of what is normal for patients to be feeling. He retorts that he will speak with the patient when he has a free moment.

You, feeling a bit annoyed but satisfied that you have done right by the patient, go out to tell the patient that the surgeon will speak with him when he is free.

"When he's free?! It might not seem like a big deal to a hotshot surgeon, but this is a big deal for me! Why didn't you say something to him? Oh, but, you're just a nurse, you obviously have no power around here. I guess I'll have to wait for the big cheese to come out when he feels like it."

Seething, you go back to the OR where they are preparing the room. How dare that patient speak to you like that? "Just a nurse"?! What a jerk! And after you were advocating for him! Of course, you couldn't tell him that the surgeon didn't want to speak with him, as this would make him look unprofessional. But then it starts sinking in how little power you do have in this situation. You're not a doctor, you don't get the respect that physicians get, no matter how much education or knowledge you have, or how many times you've saved the patients from a physician's error. Feeling powerless and deflated, you lament how rude the patient was to Cally, one of your coworkers. She rolls her eyes as she hears the "just a nurse" phrase, having heard it many times. Feeling slightly better but still irritated at the powerlessness you feel, you go back to check on the patient consent situation.

You see the patient and the surgeon having a conversation. The patient, who had just been badmouthing the surgeon, is laughing and joking with him, apparently all being forgiven. You silently seethe some more. The surgeon comes back to the procedure room.

"So the patient is okay with going ahead with the procedure?" you ask coolly.

"Yeah," the surgeon replies, still smiling from his interaction with the patient. "He just wanted some reassurance, that's all. It's a big deal for these patients, however routine it seems to us."

You stare at him, using all of your willpower not to smack him. "That's exactly what I told you before you went out there!" you cry exasperatedly.

He looks at you, wide-eyed. "Alright, I hear you," he says, in an attempt to calm you.

But there's no reasoning with you now. All of the little digs that you didn't respond to before come boiling up to the surface. "No, you don't hear me at all! I tried to explain to you that the patient has a right to be scared, and you snapped at me!"

He tries to interrupt. "No, I'm sick of this!" you cut him off. "You treat us like garbage around here, and then go out and suck up to the patient that you were just dissing before you went out there!"

The surgeon eyes you, stone-faced. "You better calm yourself before the procedure, or you can find someone else to scrub. I'm not going to work with you like this," and he storms off.

You, not calm by any stretch but refusing to prove the surgeon right, go into the theater regardless. You are still worked up, but you can't back down now. You scrub the procedure together, the air in the room frosty. You, flustered by your anger, make a few mistakes, the surgeon says nothing, and your coworkers quietly try to do their jobs without upsetting either of you.

Afterward, you realize you should have let someone else scrub the procedure, as you could have made a serious error and you were putting the patient in jeopardy. You bitterly justify your behavior, blaming the surgeon and the patient for riling you up. Neither of them respects you or appreciates all that you do for them. You sigh, knowing that you have to get up and do it all over again tomorrow.

Questions

1. Can you identify the roles being played out on the Drama Triangle?

2. What do you notice about the role of the nurse as she goes through the procedure?

3. What do you think may have contributed to the situation as it played out?

4. What do you think could have helped the situation?

The Drama Triangle

The Drama Triangle is a model developed by Stephan Karpman in 1968 to describe intense, unhealthy relationship transactions that can occur between people in conflict.[1]

It does not pertain to healthy disagreements or arguments, only destructive behavior that is damaging to its participants.

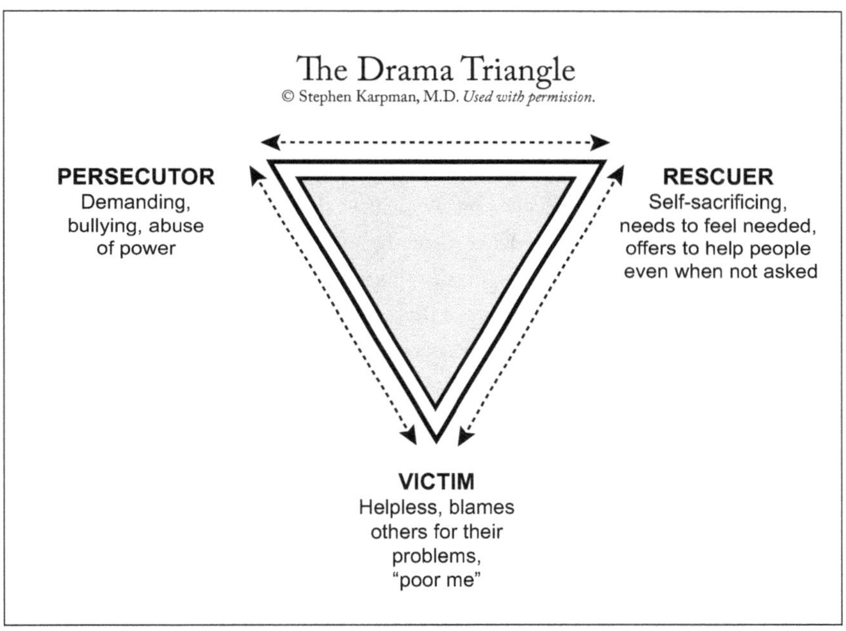

The Three Roles in the Triangle[2]

The Persecutor: Aggressive, controlling, blaming, the persecutor always has to be right. They perceive themselves as someone who has to stand up to the abuse others are inflicting upon them (essentially self-identifying as a victim). They need someone to blame (the victim), which keeps them from accepting responsibility for their actions.

The Victim: "Poor me!", indecisive, ashamed, can become hopeless, depressed and passive-aggressive. They need someone to validate their powerlessness and will seek out a persecutor to do so. They also allow a rescuer to come in and save them, thus maintaining their helplessness.

The Rescuer: Jumps in to help the victim who is being persecuted, enables and causes dependency in the victim, smothers them, feels guilty if they don't help.

The rescuer may sacrifice to the point of harming themselves, causing them to feel resentful. The rescuer needs a victim to serve to keep them from focusing on their own problems.

More About the Drama Triangle

The Drama Triangle is fluid—we can enter the triangle with one role in a situation and switch partway through. When I first learned of this model, I was certain I was a Rescuer—wanting to help out the department, feeling the good feelings it brought when I "helped." The more I became familiar with this model, however, the more I realized I didn't just play the one role. I could be a Victim, too, especially when it came to feeling unappreciated at work after "rescuing" others. And (gasp!), I also occasionally became the Persecutor. I really didn't want to admit to being anything other than a Rescuer, though, and thought it was interesting that I unconsciously skimmed over the other roles when I was learning about them.

That being said, people on the Drama Triangle do have a tendency to play a recurring role, be it the Rescuer, Persecutor, or Victim. This tendency is usually learned behaviors from childhood—for example, the children of neglectful/abusive parents tend to become rescuers because it helped serve their need for attention. It also can be learned from parents' behaviors—for example, mothers who are Rescuers can pass this on to their children, who witness their mothers' over-giving and deem it as normal. This also may contribute to the high incidence of helping professions running in families. All of the roles on the triangle are coping mechanisms – we often use what we learned when we were younger, and keep playing the roles out because we don't know how else to get our needs met. And, as anyone who has been sucked into the drama knows, these behaviours can and do get results – so we keep using them.

As health care professionals, we have a tendency to enter the Triangle as Rescuers. We have a natural tendency to want to help—this is good! What we have to watch out for is it growing into a need to be needed—this is especially true if we grew up with unhealthy families, endured trauma, or suffer from low self-esteem.

All roles on the Drama Triangle have a theme: they distract us from the actual issues we are suffering from. By focusing our attention on The Drama, we don't have to accept responsibility for our own actions and beliefs, and it keeps us stuck.

The Empowerment Triangle

In 2009, David Emerald released a book titled, *The Power of TED* (*The Empowerment Dynamic).*

This built on Karpman's work and put a positive spin on the roles. Instead of identifying the roles as weaknesses, the Empowerment Triangle identifies the role as strengths and how we can use these to improve situations we might come across.[3]

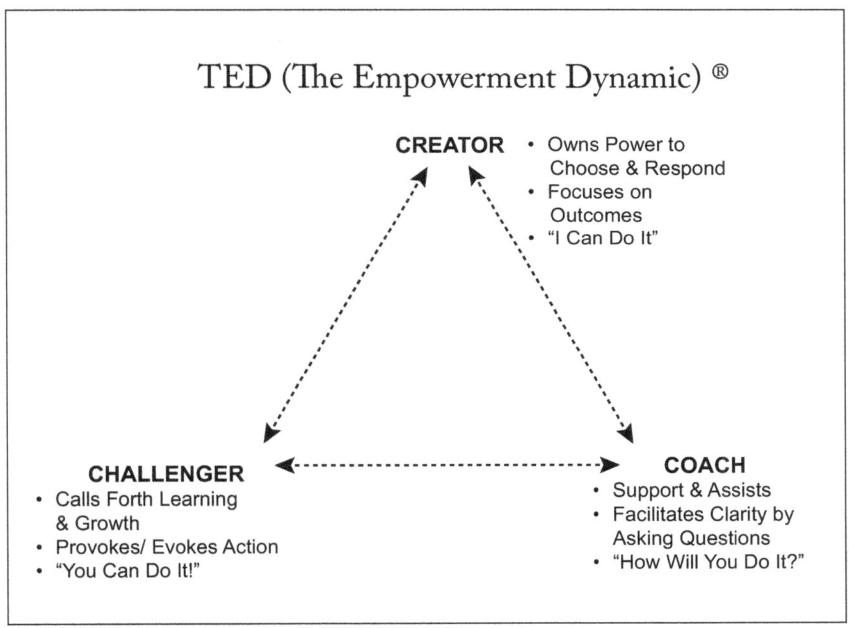

The Empowerment Triangle® by David Emerald. Used with permission.

We all have a role we tend to play most on the Drama Triangle. Instead of viewing it as an affliction, we can change our perspective about it and view it as a strength.

The Persecutor becomes the Challenger—The Challenger uses his/her assertive behavior to challenge and encourage others to grow, set goals, and inspire positive action without punishing/controlling others. They ask themselves, "How can I motivate?"

The Victim becomes the Creator—Instead of focusing on the problem, The Creator evaluates their situation from an objective position (without attaching shame or powerlessness) and asks of themselves, "What do I want?" They then create a new reality for themselves by focusing on solutions and recognizing that they always have a choice.

The Rescuer becomes the Coach—By using his/her natural affinity to care for others, the Coach helps people empower themselves to make positive changes in their lives without promoting dependency on the Coach. They ask themselves, "How can I empower?"

The Health Care Worker as The Coach

As HCWs, we have a tendency to enter the Drama Triangle as Rescuers, where our "Victims" (usually our patients) are enabled by us to keep them being victims. Obviously, some patients are completely reliant on us for total care. But our natural question, "How can I help?" tends to involve "What can I do for them?" instead of "What can I do to help them help themselves?" Think about it: When was the last time you transferred a patient who has partial mobility because it was just faster? Or looked up medications for them because they weren't aware of what they are taking?

With technology, we now have access to our patients' medication list, their health history, and we can do more procedures for them than ever before. While medical science is expanding, it is causing an unhealthy disempowering effect on our patients. With so much medical knowledge on our part, patients are overwhelmed with everything. From specialists to medications to procedures, they are no longer in charge of their health, and they are becoming reliant on us to make decisions for them. Our society is sicker, more helpless, and more reliant on the health care system than ever before. We are always trying to help our patients and brainstorm ways of making their lives better … but when do we ever empower them to make their own lives better? Educate them to do as much for themselves as they can?

As HCWs, we can go from Rescuer to Coach by changing our perspective on the power our patients have. They may require our support, but our best healing can be done by empowering them to help themselves. Asking patients what their preference is, encouraging them to carry a list of medications (and knowing why they are on each medication), and ensuring they know THEY are in control of their body and have a right to make an informed decision (even if it doesn't align with our views) are all ways of empowering patients and helping them truly heal.

Steps to Getting Off the Triangle

1. *Recognize you are on it*—When you recognize you are on the Drama Triangle, congrats—awareness is the first step to making change! Don't be too hard on yourself, as this is a lifelong learned behavior. We all get sucked into the drama

from time to time. When you recognize yourself on the triangle, simply observe yourself and your actions.

2. ***Identify what event caused you to enter the Triangle***—What triggered you? By keeping track of events, you are more likely to identify what often gets you sucked into the triangle and, therefore, will make you less likely to enter it again. For example, is it abuse of power? Not being heard? Being labelled?

3. ***Walk away***—The Drama Triangle is a play that needs people to enact the roles in order to continue. No actors = no drama. If a Persecutor is trying to blame you (make you a Victim), you have the power to walk away from the situation. If a Rescuer is attempting to pull you in to support their cause, you can politely decline. Or, if a Victim is shaming herself and looking for someone to come to her rescue, you don't need to enable her.

4. ***Transform your role into the Empowerment Triangle***—If a physician is trying to blame you for making a mistake (Persecuting), you can be your own Creator and realize you have a choice to stand up for yourself. For the patient who doesn't know what medications he is on (Victim), you can Coach him by encouraging him to carry a list and to go over it with his family doctor so he is more in charge of his own care.

EXERCISES

1. What role do you identify with most on the Drama Triangle?

2. How do you think your childhood and family dynamics contribute to the role you identify with? Where do you see your parents/siblings fitting in on this Triangle?

3. Where can you see your relationships playing out this triangle now? At work? At home?

4. Keep track of times where you enter the Drama Triangle, what role you were playing, and what triggered you. Notice what role you play most—it might not be what you think! For example, you might be a Rescuer at work but a Victim at home.

5. Once you have identified which role you most often play, practice playing the Empowered version of the role (e.g., if you identify as the Victim, envision acting out as the Creator). How does the shift in perspective make you feel?

6. Once you get better at identifying and getting off the Drama Triangle, notice how it affects your relationships—have they improved? How so?

CHAPTER 15

Interpersonal Conflict

"A negative emotional wake is not caused exclusively by thoughtless or unkind comments; it is created at times by a lack of appreciative comments."
— Susan Scott, Fierce Conversations[1]

Health care workers have a myriad of interdisciplinary relationships they deal with on a daily basis. Nurse-patient, patient-doctor, staff-manager, unit-unit, the list goes on.

Our scope specific to our roles encompasses many tasks when dealing with patient care, and may overlap with other modalities. Navigating this on a regular basis requires us to know our roles and the roles of our health care team. Sometimes this can be confusing and becomes a cause for interpersonal conflict.

As health care positions shift and change, our responsibilities are ever expanding. Because all of our roles are becoming increasingly busier regardless of whether we are a paramedic, a pharmacist, or a social worker, we are having to be creative in making it work. Many of us who function as a team are beginning to overlap our roles in order to get the work done. Working in radiology, I was so grateful to have amazing technologists that were able to look up bloodwork, perform the safety checks prior to the procedure, and even help with code browns, despite none of it being in their job description. They knew nurses were busy, and they were willing to help out where they could. While this worked for us, it shouldn't have to be this way. People in many roles are stepping up in order to help, but they may not have the expertise or proper training in whatever aspect they are assisting in. If you've ever been a nurse waiting on a respiratory therapist when your tracheostomy patient is having issues and you are fumbling your way through varying equipment that you aren't familiar with, you know how unsafe this can be.

Where we need a paradigm shift is in the working conditions set for us. What we have come to accept as normal are actually impossible standards that are being put upon us. No human being should be coping with the current work conditions of a busy hospital (or busy clinic, or home care caseloads, etc.) that our aging, acutely ill population is causing. We have more complicated patients, and we are expected to do more complicated care with less. This shift is affecting all modalities in the hospital, from our physicians with more complex cases, to our RTs who have a higher patient load, to our managers who have to somehow balance decreasing staff ratios with a workforce who are already operating with limited resources. It is a slippery slope we are all feeling.

It is therefore unsurprising that issues with interpersonal conflict would be an escalating issue among HCWs–we are all feeling the pressure. And sometimes the colleagues we rely on can also be the people who irritate us, who won't cooperate, and generally add more stress to our days.

While these people can be vexing, they are also here with the same goal in mind—to ensure the patient receives good quality care. Sometimes it doesn't feel like a manager has the patient's best interests at heart when she is focused on the budget, or a doctor who misses writing orders may seem like they are being sloppy. In these times, it is important to remember that we are all human, and we all make mistakes. In times of imperfect human behavior, try to remember this when it causes you more time or effort spent. Remember, empathy is our superpower, something not everyone has the power to exercise. While this does not excuse inappropriate behavior, having empathy for our colleagues in the back of our minds will help us as we navigate interpersonal conflicts.

Patients

While our priority is patient care and we may have less interpersonal conflict with patients than we do with our colleagues, it can still be a challenging dynamic. Angry, demanding, or condescending patients can be a challenge to navigate, and one that we often don't receive a lot of management support from as there is fear of retaliation from patient relations.

First and foremost, recognizing that the patients' behaviors are fueled by feeling vulnerable and out of control can help us interact with them more effectively. They are feeling scared, uncertain of their future, and may have a myriad of other issues going on that we know nothing about. As HCWs we often receive the brunt of their frustrations, as we are an outlet for their aggravation. Also, in female-dominated professions, we garner less respect than what we are worthy of receiving. This is a trend that needs to stop. While we can have empathy for people who are going through health issues, we are not responsible for taking on their issues. Accepting verbal abuse in lucid patients is something we have tolerated for many generations—the right to refuse care has been a hotly debated topic for our governing professional bodies.

You do have the right to demand respect from a belligerent patient. You do not have to tolerate abuse, and you have the right to exercise that. Our empathy can also seem like a weakness, but often a patient who is angry just wants to be heard.

By asking the patient questions, you can gauge whether or not this strategy will be effective in deescalating a difficult situation.

If they do not respond favourably and remain angry, setting a boundary may be necessary. Simply stating, "I understand you are frustrated, and we are doing our best, but I will not tolerate you speaking to me in that tone. If you continue to speak to me in this way, I will take this to my superior, which may delay your care." This is usually enough to snap the patient out of whatever behavior they are assuming. If it doesn't, then it is important that you follow through on this boundary—then wash your hands of it. It is not your responsibility to tolerate abuse, and you do not have to carry it alone. It is natural that patients become upset, and with our health care system suffering, I only foresee this becoming a more common occurrence. Being armed with this strategy, you can know that you always have a game plan in how to deal with this quickly and effectively. Remember, you are the one in control of how you want to be treated, and you have every right to express this. Respect is not a privilege, it is an expectation, regardless of what role someone is in. The more we create a culture of demanding respect, the more it will become common nature.

Some of the roles we interact with on a daily basis don't always receive the credit they deserve, often because the roles they are in demand more professionalism, which sometimes looks like being standoffish or aloof. I assure you, the people in these roles are human, and often tasked with being seen as superhuman.

Physicians

Physicians work an insane amount of hours—they are on call more, sacrifice more time with their families, have an increased amount of pressure on them to "fix" the patient—and fewer people to turn to for support. They are told from the beginning that this career choice is a vocation, a calling, that they are in a position of prestige, and they should be grateful to be in it. They are financially well compensated for doing so, thereby negating the sympathy they so often are in need of, whether they realize it or not. Every hardship that occurs, from the pressure of getting into medical school to the exams to becoming a resident, reveals this career is considered a vocation for a reason—there is little time for anything else. Their residency, where they go from a medical student to an ordering physician overnight and are expected to know everything, is basically an initiation to pile more pressure on to them. The breadth of knowledge their field necessitates leaves little else for them in their busy lives. They need to live and breathe science and textbooks, and are taught little else. In his review of "Love, Medicine, and Miracles," A.B.R. Thomson, a gastroenterologist at the University of Alberta, where I studied and worked, questioned back in 1989 whether physicians are "medical mechanics or caregivers."[2]

They endure the same difficult patients, the same deaths, the same stresses as we do, and all with a stoic, strong expression, having been taught to be less personal and more professional to garner respect. They are not taught much about the power of empathy or bedside manner or alternative healing. They are not taught to trust their intuition. Everything about their education is mechanical, scientific—and we expect them to be human? They go through medical school with the goal of making it through—and though some realize halfway in that it isn't for them, they've already invested so much time, money, and effort that it would take a brave person to walk away from this dream.

The next time a physician snaps at you, use your superpower of empathy. Did he sleep at all last night? Is she missing her daughter's recital right now? Did a patient he treated yesterday have complications? This does not mean you have to accept the behavior; having empathy will soften the need to retaliate and prevent escalation.

They have an immense amount of pressure on them to "fix" the patient. As people are sicker and more complex than ever before, they are fighting a losing battle—and they know it. They feel just as frustrated as we do that patients are not receiving the care they should.

Some doctors are arrogant: fact. Yet we know underneath most arrogant people lies a feeling of inadequacy. Medicine is still very much a hierarchal, masculine structure. It is outdated, chauvinistic, and based on elitism and prestige, even more so now with the cost of schooling: Only the very rich or the very dedicated can afford to go to school for that length of time. And in order to survive this environment, you are more likely to join them than beat them. With most physicians being male (although a trend that is shifting), and most other HCWs being female, we know what often occurs as a result. Unfortunately, with all of their time dedicated to schooling, it doesn't leave a lot of time to work on themselves. Many physicians with attitude problems would never know or ever seek help, as they are in good company. Unless their behavior has been mandated to change (usually in the form of anger management), it is unlikely they will do so. Part of the problem is that perhaps not all of them see health care workers as colleagues—which we are. Helping shift this perspective by saying the word out loud will help shape how they view other members of the health care team. We all have the same goal of helping heal the patient, and therefore are on the same team, even if it doesn't feel like it sometimes.

While we need to remain empathetic to their plight—the long hours, the social awkwardness of some MDs—it is also our responsibility to call them out when they are behaving inappropriately. This can seem intimidating, and it is. Yet the more people who stand up to bullying doctors, the better the work environment will be. Sometimes it doesn't seem worth it, and it is easier to remain quiet when you have had an altercation. Allowing someone to talk to you that way once will just ensure that they will try it again. Setting a boundary early on is the best thing you can do. Often doctors may seem intimidating, but I promise you most of them are decent people, and most of them will respond favorably if you assert yourself. This may not change their behavior entirely, but it will change their behavior with YOU. And your colleagues will notice this.

If an MD does not respond well to you asserting yourself (as long as you are doing it in a respectful way), you might have a difficult person on your hands—see the following chapter for more guidance around this.

Physicians carry a heavy load, and they are mostly unsupported in carrying it. They are often expected to be superhuman, never calling in sick, or being able to show vulnerability. Nurses and allied health workers have a lot more support rallying around them, and they are fairly capable at seeking it out when they need to—doctors, not so much. We have the power of being empathetic when they may not be feeling that way towards themselves. It might be difficult for them to admit they are struggling, especially to their physician counterparts. Yet just showing them the kindness that you would with anyone—how is your day, how are you coping—may give someone the opening they desperately need.

Managers

"People don't quit a job, they quit a boss."

A recent study showed 39 percent of Canadians who were surveyed left their jobs due to a bad manager.[3]

Managers in health care have a stressful role of balancing the budget while trying to maintain a healthy working environment. As soon as they step into this role, they go out of scope, possibly losing skills they had gone to school to learn, as well giving up security. They therefore are not safe from layoffs if management is eliminated. They also are not always the same modality as the people they are managing (e.g., a social worker in charge of an ICU), which can be even more challenging as they have to navigate a unit that they are not as familiar with. They won't know the roles and duties, or the contract of their employees, or education of the majority of the people running it. They have many things they need to juggle, attend constant meetings where very little gets accomplished, and deal with frequent complaints/issues from staff who have not been able to deal with issues on their own. They take on poor staff ratios, sick calls, increased patient acuity, beds shortages, etc. Chances are, if you are dealing with issues on your unit, management is also dealing with these issues, too.

Again, empathy is our superpower. I have struggled with issues with management myself. I went to my managers with many concerns that I felt were important, and I wasn't always met with (what I felt) was adequate concern or response. I felt like I was in a war with management, as we were making them aware of the issues but nothing was happening—I felt like it was falling on deaf ears. And with some of my colleagues either too afraid or too apathetic to second my concerns, I was mostly on my own, which meant that poor working conditions continued. In the beginning, I felt like my manager didn't listen or care about what I had to say. Having a bit of an authority complex to start with on my part, this was not a good working relationship.

What changed this for me and our relationship was having empathy for her. I implored her to help with morale in our department, to show appreciation for her staff, to recognize the hard work we were doing. I was trying to help her see that her showing genuine appreciation for us would help. It eventually dawned on me that she was probably just as starved for this recognition as we were.

Be the change you want to see in the world.

I wanted her to appreciate me and my colleagues, so I started showing what I wanted to see in others first. I wanted to feel appreciated, so I strived to show it first—with my colleagues, and my manager. I asked her questions, I took interest in her life, her other duties, I told her I could see how difficult her job must be. And it helped. It helped our relationship, and it helped her see what I had been saying. Sometimes actions speak louder than words.

I know it can be difficult to see eye to eye with your manager, but I'm telling you—if I can do it, anyone can! Using the empathy we have for our patients can be challenging to use with our superiors, but it can make a huge difference.

Go to your manager with problems early. You are less likely to have emotions get in the way, and your manager will be more likely to view it as a concern instead of a complaint. There may be nothing done about the situation at this time, but it allows this to be on her radar should something more serious come up. Ask questions related to your problem when you first go to her with concerns as well. She will be less likely to think you are questioning her ability to lead instead of the issue at hand. Sometimes, we expect our managers to be our eyes and ears in the department, but they aren't privy to everything. Even if the issue may have been brought to her attention by someone else, you going in to vouch that it is a valid concern increases the likelihood that she will look into it, as there is now more than one person bringing it to her attention.

Sometimes your immediate manager may be sympathetic to the concerns you voice to her, but her hands may be tied with her managers. If there is an issue you feel strongly about and it is affecting multiple people, I highly recommend that you seek your colleagues out for their support. If multiple people are being affected by a situation, she can't reasonably ignore it if you come together as a unit to address the issue. This may be difficult to convince others, but again, it comes down to asking "What gets everyone's needs met?" and asking yourself what your needs are.

If you need help from your colleagues, ask for it. We run the units we work on, not anyone else. We are powerful, and together we are even more so. Ask yourself what you are willing to tolerate, and what you are not. If your colleagues are in agreement with you, going to your manager as a unit demonstrates how important the issue is. It is also to your benefit to come up with some possible solutions to the problem. While this may not be your responsibility, showing that you have given thought to the situation and are willing to explore options with your manager will help you become a collaborator in the issue and not just at the mercy of whatever she decides.

Sometimes, unfortunately, we end up with a dud. If your manager is consistently unprofessional, ineffective, or absent, you do have the right to seek outside counsel. This may be something that you need to think long and hard about, as there is no going back once you have done this, and it may permanently affect your relationship. That being said, sometimes the benefits outweigh the risks, and if you feel it is worth pursuing, you have the power to do so. Don't ever feel that you don't have the right or are powerless to create change. If you are unionized, going to a union representative would be helpful (but I recommend speaking directly with your manager before doing this, as it can put her on the defensive if she hasn't been approached first). HR and your professional governing body can also be points of contact.

It's easy to see management as the enemy, and when they are aware of the problems on the unit and are not doing anything constructive, it can be very frustrating. Focusing on yourself and your own needs can be the best form of action you can take, and not getting pulled into the Drama Triangle can give you the peace you need to get through difficult times.

Miscellaneous Modalities

This interpersonal aspect can be many and varied, depending on your location. In a hospital, it can mean respiratory, physio, or occupational therapists, technologists in the diagnostic imaging department, dieticians, social workers, psychologists, health care aides, food services, housekeeping, porters, HR, unit clerks, lab techs.

Outside of the hospital, there may be less of these specific roles, and we may actually take on some of these roles as there are less bodies to do them. All of these positions play an important function in patient care. If the porters are short-staffed, it means our patients are delayed in receiving necessary procedures. If housekeeping is delayed, it means a patient who is waiting on a bed in the hospital stays in a busy emergency longer, not receiving adequate care. The pandemic has highlighted this; everyone has a role, and every role is important.

Sometimes it is easy to forget how important these roles are when we are busy taking vitals, performing life-saving tasks on a regular basis. I definitely have been guilty of this, having taken out my frustrations on other modalities ("lab specimen hemolyzed" are words that give me insta-anger). Again, having empathy for busy RTs who float within the entire hospital, or a PT whose report a patient's discharge is relying on, or a porter who does not have time to wait for you to transfer your patient onto a stretcher can mean a better working relationship. This comes in handy when you are the one who the other modality is waiting on. Recognizing that we deserve respect also means that we are expected to give it, regardless of title or education of our interdisciplinary colleagues.

This is especially important to recognize, as other modalities may be dealing with their own stressors. As there are sicker patients and reduced staff ratios, the PT/OT/RTs workload is extremely high. They are expected to know and remember many patients throughout the hospital, not just one unit. Roles that require less education, such as health care aides (HCAs), often face discriminatory behavior from patients (and unfortunately staff) who deem them less important than other modalities. As I was an HCA while going through nursing, I experienced this firsthand more often than I should have. While someone being defensive of this is not "our problem," it is important to recognize discrimination, as it has most assuredly happened to them at some point. Recognizing my privilege, how lucky I am to have the skillset, education, and compensation that I do helps me when I come across someone who is experiencing this in their workday.

Also, it may be helpful for your unit to have a meeting discussing the different points of view from different modalities, getting them all together to allow each other to see each other's viewpoints. Having the big picture through multiple eyes can help with coming up with solutions.

When I worked in the DI department, we would have to coordinate pediatric cases with the unit, anesthesia, parents, radiologists, and the nursing team, and it could be extremely challenging to plan. Often anesthesia would be running behind, and the patient would be fasting for a long period of time, the parents might not be able to be at the bedside, or we wouldn't have a room or a doctor to do the procedure. There were so many people and factors involved, it would benefit us to meet with anesthesia and the unit managers to try to come up with solutions, not just try to figure it out ourselves, as we only were one piece of the puzzle. If your unit is consistently having issues with other modalities, a meeting with representatives of all parties affected would be beneficial to suggest.

Nurse-Nurse, PT-PT, Tech-Tech, etc.

This is the most common type of interpersonal conflict, and despite being members of the same profession, there is much complexity within our own career field. Health care workers are primarily female, which has its own cause for strife. Women are more likely to overthink, to be sensitive to interpersonal dynamics, and to feel defensive within our profession, as we constantly have to prove our worth. According to Kasia Urbaniak in *Unbound*, much of that is due to our good-girl conditioning.[4] While males are conditioned to be action-oriented, we received reward/positive attention for being "good," and any time we step outside of that persona we feel shame or unworthiness. That being said, there are issues within the spectrum of a specific modality that can cause conflict, ranging from generational differences to differing levels/focus of education, and different areas (e.g., emergency, ICU, home care, etc.) being the main reasons of conflict within the profession itself.

Older Generation versus Younger Generation

This is the most common and the most studied form of interpersonal conflict within many professions, especially nursing. The construct of "nurses who eat their young" has existed in this career for years. Despite it being studied extensively, it is still happening. I remember learning about how to deal with this in university, thinking, *Why are they teaching this to us when they should be teaching it to the people who are doing it? It won't happen to me!*

It's true that they can offer education seminars about the effect of older nurses treating newer grads with disrespect, but the people who are doing the bullying are not likely to be the ones attending a seminar on it. Therefore, it obviously seemed prudent to the Faculty of Nursing to teach nursing students how to deal with it instead of actually preventing it from occurring. There will always be generational differences in the workforce, so this situation isn't going away. And while we believe that most of the conflict is instigated by older nurses, bullying behavior can occur regardless of age or experience.[5]

Again, the answer starts with empathy. As a new grad, I had the knowledge fresh in my mind—I knew my anatomy, I knew my pharmacology, and I was privileged to have learned things in school that my more experienced colleagues never had the opportunity to learn, with so many changes having been made to nursing education over the years. I also had a fresh set of eyes, and had my health, my energy, and my motivation to help (and also the motivation to work, as I had been a broke student for four years). I couldn't understand why some of my colleagues seemed so bitter, with little compassion. I started my career in the NICU, and some of the comments made by my colleagues astounded me—judging drug-addicted mothers, questioning why we were putting so much into saving twenty-two-week gestation babies who would just grow up to be a drain on the system, sniping at each other over silly things like not making enough feeds for the shift. We were adults, right? We had a prestigious career that we were lucky enough to get to go to every day. I didn't get it.

Until I did.

Working long hours of shift work, working every other weekend, working short nearly every day, not being able to go to evening activities with my schedule, missing family and friend get-togethers, being denied vacation, seeing the same situations crop up over and over again, more and more acuity and illness, I began to feel the fatigue.

These issues transferred into my next job in diagnostic imaging, which I had applied to as a way of having more of a life, with it being mostly daytime hours. But that meant being on call and being woken up in the middle of the night by a pager. We would come in on a call back after doing a full day's work for a dialysis patient who had skipped their run and was now in a crisis. Or a patient who had been in emerg all day and wasn't seen until they became septic, and it was now a middle-of-the-night emergency. We aren't allowed to discriminate or complain about what justifies being called in, even though we are human and can see the issues clear as day. So after only a few years into my career, I understood where the older generation was coming from, and why some of them seemed so bitter.

I also recognize that much of the older generation dealt with being discriminated against for being women in health care far more severely than my generation. While it is still very much an issue, nursing twenty, thirty years ago wasn't seen as a "profession," and some of that generation bears the brunt of maltreatment over their entire career.

We have also taken on too much, for too long. Not being given the tools or feeling like we have the right to say no in my generation, I know that this must be a long-stemming issue. If I burned out in my thirties over the workload and stress, I know nurses who are older than me have endured much of it themselves, and either feel trapped or helpless to change, or don't recognize that they are burned out. While their self-reflection is not my responsibility, I strive to understand just how hard they had it.

It can also be intimidating when younger staff have more extensive knowledge bases or skillsets. A nurse who has worked in long-term care is not going to have the same experience that a nurse in emerg does, and while we shouldn't compare the two, it often happens. Couple this with a nurse being younger and having more acute care experience, and this can cause a nurse with more longevity to feel vulnerable about her expertise. I have definitely felt this myself. Having been out of ICU for most of my career, new hires who have ICU/ER experience can cause me to feel out of my depth when discussing patient care. My memory of what I learned in school is dwindling, and I don't have the motivation to study what I learned in university like I used to.

In my thirties now, I am in the middle of the new grads and the older generation, and I can appreciate both elements of where each group is coming from. An element that Millennials/Gen Z get tarred with is being lazy or entitled. While there may be some individuals who embody this, I think it's an unfair representation of the younger generation. I think they see how hard it is to work in the environment that health care workers have been living in with fresh eyes, and they have decided they don't want it to be that way for the rest of their lives.

As our workload has slowly increased, we don't necessarily see how much we are putting up with until someone comes in and is aghast at the situation. It has become so normalized that we don't recognize the extent of the problem. And I think the younger generation coming in does see it. With our union rules granting vacation time in order of seniority, it often means having to work twenty years in order to get time off in the summer. This hardly seems worth it. No wonder most new grads would prefer to work part-time. Can we blame them?

We were raised by a generation of people who told us that if we worked really hard, we would get ahead. But as we are witnessing our parents' and grandparents' generation working harder, becoming more ill, and dying before they can actually enjoy the fruits of their labors, we are adjusting our priorities. And working ourselves to the bone isn't one of them. I am happy to live with less if it means having a better quality of life, even if it means I have to stay in the workforce longer. What is the point of working that hard for your pension if you are crippled by the time you earn it? My parents both passed in their fifties, so I might not make it to my pension. Thus, I've decided I want to get the most of my life now. Sadly, several of my colleagues also became ill/passed away before they retired. Life has no guarantees.

Yet the older generation has worked this hard for years. And can we blame them if they are disgruntled that younger people coming in don't want to work as hard as they did—and in some cases, get away with it?

The problem is not ourselves, the problem is the culture of the society we live in that rewards hard-working behavior—verbally, that is. Our sense of working hard gives us a sense of self-worth, yet no one is there to pick up the pieces when we are too battered and broken to continue.

So instead of preying on each other, we can empathize with where each group is coming from and start to make a commitment to change. Let's not eat our young or vilify our elders, but unite in fixing a system that is pitting us against each other. Just because this is the way it has always been does not mean this is the way it has to stay.

LPN versus RN

This is a problem that I have to admit: My privilege as an RN was showing. Until recently, I didn't think there was a discrimination problem with licensed practical nurses and registered nurses working together in my unit. I worked with some amazing LPNs, and value them very much. In the fifteen years I have been practicing, the LPN scope of practice has accelerated so much I can barely keep up. This led to a scarcity mentality when our jobs came on the line. Everyone was out for themselves, and we RNs were definitely feeling vulnerable. White RN pins started showing up on my colleagues' scrub tops, declaring to everyone what level of education they had, which was basically a slap in the face to my LPN colleagues. Questions of "Can an LPN do that?" started cropping up in an environment that never used to question it.

I will be honest, I used to think LPNs who complained that RNs treated them differently were just being defensive. The two years difference in education and focus on different skills in a clinical setting didn't make a huge difference in our department. I felt that they may have been suffering from self-worth issues, like some RNs who feel inadequate around physicians. Until I saw the discrimination firsthand, I didn't believe it was true.

I had to recognize that as an RN, I had privilege within my own profession (some nurses even discuss degree-holding versus non-degree-holding amongst RNs). Because I set more store by a nurse's character and experience, I didn't think much of it. I didn't have a problem with LPNs, so I didn't pay too much attention to it—which is the definition of privilege. While LPNs and RNs may have different education focus and length, we do have much that unites us. Experience and character affect our capabilities much more than education does, and this is the case for any profession. We are much more similar than we are different. Focusing on what unites us instead of what makes us different is something we can do with any group of people, whether it be race, religion, or educational background.

Privilege

Coming from an Irish upbringing, it would infuriate me when I spoke to an English person about the suffering of Irish people during its troubled periods. Especially as Northern Ireland is part of Great Britain, it would anger me to no end how ignorant most English people were about things that happened in their own country. Then the news of what happened in residential schools to indigenous children came out. This happened in Canada, and I never once was taught anything about it. How the indigenous must feel was similar to how I felt about Irish trauma. And I realized that privilege lies everywhere we look.

In her book *Caste: The Origins of Our Discontent*, Isabel Wilkerson discusses the history of separatism and how it has affected generations of people, passing on low self-worth like DNA.[6] By dehumanizing a particular group, whether it be by race or religion or gender, we allow that group to become the scapegoat for whatever ire we are experiencing.

In the book, she describes an experiment done on school-aged children by a teacher named Jane Elliott. The teacher separated blue-eyed children from brown-eyed children, and gave the blue-eyed children special privileges and denied the brown-eyed children ordinary privileges. After a day of this, she switched the groups and gave brown-eyed children special privileges. She stated, "I watched my students become what I told them they were." After only a day, she noted the "privileged" children treating the "underprivileged" children poorly, and the "underprivileged" actually started to take on low self-worth attributes. This happened after only a day; imagine a lifetime of being treated poorly. Some of us in health care are those people. Though it may not be for our eye color, it might be due to our race, or gender, or socioeconomic status. And it affects how we see the world, and how we are treated.

While I am a female and encounter sexism in my job, I am also white, educated, and have my health. I may be discriminated against for some things, and hold privilege in others. Now that I am aware of it, I can be more understanding to the discrimination some of my colleagues go through.

Us versus Them

The common theme underlying all of these interpersonal confrontations is an "us versus them" mentality. In the book by the same name, Ian Bremmer discusses confirmation bias.[7] "Tell me which party you vote for and I will tell you which newspaper you read, which channels you watch, what websites you like, etc." As social media changes its algorithms to show us more of what we like and none of what we don't, we become more and more polarized. If you watch Fox News, you are a Trump supporter. And we all know how Trump divided a nation. Only, he didn't invent the us-versus-them mentality, he just knows it exists and used it to his advantage.

Bremmer writes, "If your goal is to boost your popularity by pitting people against each other, it's a smart political tactic. If your goal is to promote a stronger, healthier, more prosperous society, then this tactic is a dangerous one. It produces anger over unity."

People vote in extremist leaders because they are scared. The people who vote for them aren't bad people—that is something we come to believe due to conditioning. It is possible to be a caring person and also be concerned about the economy. While politicians know how to use the system, it isn't in their interest to unite people—that responsibility falls on us.

Think about it: If we were united, in our work, our families, our communities, we would have less to be afraid of. I remember seeing a news story of an elderly gentleman who had health issues. He was fearful he wouldn't be able to pay his rent, shovel the walk, get groceries, afford medicine. The whole neighborhood stepped up and helped him out in his time of need. If you knew you had a community who would help you when you needed it, you wouldn't be as afraid of all the things that could go wrong—you know you would be okay. And with that mentality, you would make better decisions, decisions best for everyone, including yourself. We wouldn't be as reliant as we are on the government to fix things—and in that, they wouldn't have as much power over us.

There is a man by the name of Daryl Davis whose story I will never forget. He is a black man who sought out the leader of the KKK in order to understand him. He averred that hate and fear develop from a lack of understanding. Through conversation and a genuine desire to understand each other, the two formed a bond. While they didn't agree with each other, they respected each other. Eventually, because of this relationship, the KKK leader left the KKK. Mr. Davis attests the ability to understand one another is something we all are capable of. If you haven't watched his TED Talk, I highly recommend it, as it is one of the most powerful things I have seen.[8]

There is a difference between discernment and judgment. With discernment, we can see a contrasting viewpoint for what it is and choose to see it differently – not invalidating it, allowing it to exist. Judgment is where we bestow our opinions as superior – this alienates people with opposing viewpoints, and only adds more fuel to a damaging fire. Every viewpoint is valid from that person's perspective – even the KKK. And when we don't judge these viewpoints, even the ones we deem wrong, we don't give energy to them. We can even, as with Daryl Davis' case, invite curiosity in as to how the opposing viewpoints came to be.

It is so easy to blame the other unit, or the manager, or the government. If we view all staff members we come into contact with as part of our health care community, we can begin to have an easier time investigating instead of blaming. We can gain more from being open to others' perspectives, and perhaps learn something that we didn't see before. If we don't address the issues that come up with the people involved, we all can't learn. We are a team of professionals who are here to help our patients. We are all on the same team, and we are all in it together. We are in a health care crisis, and it is imperative that we stop looking at others to blame, and start uniting. We don't have to all think exactly the same in order to be united – our differing perspectives are valuable. But we do need to look at each other as being on the same team. Don't hate war, love peace.

EXERCISES

1. Think of an area where you feel discrimination. It may be in your work, among family or friends, or in society in general. What do you believe the person/people who are discriminating against you feel about you, or how do they misunderstand you? What is one small way you could change this?

2. Think of a person or group that you have a genuine strong dislike of. Explore what you think you know about this person or group. Is there a possibility that you don't have all the facts? Take a step forward in trying to understand this person/group. Use your power of empathy to put yourself in their shoes. How do you think they became the person/people they are today?

3. Find a media source that differs from your point of view. It can be the news, a documentary, etc. Go in with curiosity instead of looking at where you disagree with the information given. Do your best to see the situation from the differing perspective, and focus on what you agree on, not what you disagree on. What did you learn?

CHAPTER 16

Bullying

"Some people try to be tall by cutting off the heads of others."
— *Paramahansa Yogananda*

As a child and teenager, I was bullied by girls in my grade. Having moved to a new school at the age of seven, I wasn't accepted by the girls in my new class. They taunted me, deliberately left me out of playing with them, and even physically ganged up on me.

This trend continued in my teens. At thirteen, I was ostracized by the girls I had previously been friends with. They not only called me names and spread false rumors about me, but they sabotaged any chance I had of obtaining new friends by telling lies about me to anyone I got close with.

I thought that once you grew up and became an adult, this behavior would stop. That adults were too mature to do this sort of thing to other people. That it was only something that happened as a child or teenager.

I was wrong.

While the bullying tactics may not be as childish or obvious with adults, it is unfortunately just as present in the workplace as it is in the playground. I thought I had put that aspect of my life behind me. Unfortunately, I have very recent experience with it—again.

I recently moved to a new city, and I had unlucky timing in being hired to an area that was in the process of laying nurses off. The staff facing layoffs were confronted with the task of training me, their replacement, while still embroiled in a bitter dispute about how the situation was handled by senior management. The air was heavy with resentment every time I walked in. I knew it was a shitty situation for them to be in, and I did my best to be kind. My superpower of empathy enabled me to put myself in their shoes, and know how terrible it was, some of them close but not quite able to retire. The process took months, and I was exposed to this environment every day, while trying to learn how they operated compared to where I was trained.

One nurse in particular seemed to have it out for me. She made snide remarks, forced me to re-scrub three times in one sitting, claiming I had done it wrong, despite it being a skill I had been doing for most of my career. She nit-picked, fussed, and scrutinized every action I made. At one point, she even yelled at me.

I had allowed her to treat me this way. It started out slowly, little comments here and there. But as I remained silent, she ramped up her abusive behavior, obviously seeing it as a sign of weakness. I gritted my teeth and decided it wasn't worth speaking up about—she was bitter and resentful with many people, not just myself, so I knew it was her problem. And I knew she would soon be gone. I just wanted to get through it and make it to where I could be on my own.

My "superpower" of empathy had been my blind spot. I had tolerated abuse for weeks due to feeling more badly for someone that was in a shitty situation than I did about myself. Unfortunately, it did lasting damage. Long after she was gone, I could still hear her voice criticizing me while opening up a sterile tray. Despite this being a skill I had been doing for as long as she had, her criticism caused me to question my own competency. I started second-guessing everything. I became paralyzed and started to feel the need to double-check things I *knew* how to do. My self-esteem had taken such a hit that it began affecting me outside of work. It came to a point where I could barely get out of bed. It wasn't until I was paired with other staff members who told me I was doing just fine that it dawned on me what had happened.

This is how abuse happens. This is how people lose their sense of self-worth, their confidence to perform in their jobs, and their ability to maintain a healthy disposition. Having done so much work around this, I questioned how I could let it happen to me again. I realized that my ability to empathize with my tormentor's plight caused me to be blinded to the fact that she was inflicting her anger back on to me. I put myself in her shoes, but while I recognized that I would also feel horrible in her situation, I neglected to appreciate that I wouldn't take it out on anybody else. She gleaned (correctly, I have to admit) that I would be an easy target to take out her frustrations on, as she knew she would never have to work with me again.

Research on Bullying in the Workplace

The American Nurses Association's definition of bullying is "repeated, unwanted harmful actions intended to humiliate, offend, and cause distress in the recipient."[1] There is a ton of research out there on bullying in the workplace, specifically in nursing. In fact, it is almost laughable how much research exists on this subject. I can give you stats, details—you can have all the data and info you want on it—it's out there. But the fact remains that it has always plagued the nursing profession (as well as other health care professions). Despite our supposedly caring nature, and despite many studies and a lot of funding to combat it, bullying still remains a prevalent issue among the caring professions.

Bullying in health care starts early: seventy-eight percent of students experienced bullying in nursing school.[2] It only continues as we enter the workforce and have to deal with our intense environment. Intimidation is more likely to occur in workplaces with high-stress settings.[3] Our heavy workloads, high patient acuity, and lack of autonomy all contribute to the bullying epidemic occurring in health care. Up to thirty-four percent of nurses leave or consider leaving the profession as a result of bullying.[4]

What Bullying Looks Like in Health Care

As health care workers are female dominated, much of the bullying that exists in health care is covert. Covert bullying looks like:

• belittling or demeaning	• gossiping
• withholding crucial information	• refusing to help
• spreading rumors	• name-calling
• favoritism	• giving difficult assignments
• hostility or silent treatment	• leaving people out

Bullying Affects Our Health

Bullying in the workplace poses a significant threat to health care workers, and it also affects our patients.[5] It is having a serious impact on our health and well-being. Nurse bullying has been linked to psychosomatic symptoms such as "headaches and frequent illness, depression and anxiety, reduced productivity, absenteeism and fear of going to work, impaired relationships, poor quality of life, and suicide."[6]

Left untreated, these symptoms can become more serious: bullying can lead to symptoms of PTSD.[7] Long after the traumatic event occurs, we can have physiological symptoms that affect our nervous system, including increased stress hormone secretion, modifying how our brains filter information, and remaining in a continuous hypervigilant state. One book that explores this in depth that I recommend is *The Body Keeps the Score* by Bessel van der Kolk. When psychological trauma occurs, areas of the brain such as the prefrontal cortex and the limbic system are affected, reducing the brain's ability to come back to balance. This can look like severe symptoms of depression and anxiety, as well as re-experiencing the trauma, having flashbacks, and avoiding people and places.

Why Bullying Flourishes

Bullies were often bullied themselves. They are more likely to have a history of trauma, suffer from low self-esteem, and feel out of control. Bullies often lack self-confidence and may see certain colleagues as threats.[9] Since many of us have experienced bullying as children at some point, it is reasonable to expect that some of us will end up bullying others as adults, and health care is a perfect storm of stress and lack of control that may trigger bullying behavior. Also, since many of us in health care are nurturing and kind, we may attract bullies as they deem us easy targets.

The quality of leadership affects the degree that bullying exists. Managers who use intimidation will enable their staff to do the same. Also, since much of the bullying strategies in health care are covert, it can be difficult to discipline. Often, staff who are bullied report that it is more a feeling of hostility they get—most gossiping occurs behind their backs. A manager may be aware of bullying conduct, but without concrete behaviors that can be measured (i.e., no proof), it may be challenging for her to address it.

The main reason why bullying is so rampant in health care, however, is due to toxic systems. When we are forced to operate under critical conditions, it puts unsustainable pressure on frontline workers. We can only tolerate so much before we break. In order to survive, many of us employ strategies of defense, and that can look like bullying others to get our needs met. While much of the literature surrounding bullying in health care acknowledges that toxic systems create toxic workers, the solutions still put the onus on the people to adjust their behavior, instead of fixing the system that is creating it.

Practicing Our Superpower

When we feel bullied by another, we tend to feel defensive and see the other person as the problem. While the person who is doing the bullying is of course accountable, we need to shift perspectives. Changing the culture from defensive to collaborative modifies how we approach bullying in the workplace. The offense needs to be directed at someone else, namely the organization. Practice your superpower—having empathy for the person who you are being targeted by may seem difficult. What is the point?

Having empathy for someone doesn't mean you have to be besties, and you definitely don't have to be nice to them if you don't want to. But taking a moment to understand why they may be acting this way will help you release any resentment you may be carrying for this person (which is affecting you, not them). Ask yourself: Would you want to be this person? If the answer is a *hell, no*, then it might be easier to not allow this person to get to you. And it will also help you be less reactive when you have to engage with them. Showing strong emotion around this person is granting them the exact reaction they are hoping for—that they are getting to you. That they have power over you. By being empathetic to their situation, you take out the emotional charge that is firing you up, and you are more neutral around them. This will help you calmly interact with them the next time you have to, and will also help you converse more clearly with them—when you are standing up to them, especially.

Picture the bully as a small child. What do you see when you picture them? Are they still angry? Or are they lonely, frightened? That being said, remember that your Inner Child does not deserve to be treated with abuse. You can be respectful while maintaining your integrity, something I neglected to do. The next time you interact with the bully, try to picture their Inner Child inside of them. Doing this exercise for the nurse who bullied me didn't make me want to be around her at all, but it did take out the emotionality of it, and I could speak to her from a more collected place.

The Paradigm Shift

Much of bullying exists due to the toxic environment we are in. While we definitely should not be tolerating bullying behaviors, our focus needs to shift. Bullies are often simply people who are overwhelmed and not coping with the stress of our unhealthy working environments. Using our superpower of empathy can help us see these people as victims instead of threats. This is much easier when we have put our own needs first. When this occurs, we are less likely to be defensive or in victim-mode. This decreases the emotions that can build up when a bully targets us, as we can see the situation more clearly for what it is: someone who is stressed and not adjusting to it in a healthy way. Bullies feel like they need to control. Once they realize they are unable to control us, they will often move on.

When we start putting our needs first, the system needs to adjust to us no longer putting up with toxic workplaces. Bullying is not the only toxic behavior that exists in health care. Because many health care systems are toxic, many toxic behaviors thrive. When we put our needs first, we become more grounded and clearer in our communication and decision-making. It creates an inability for these toxic behaviors to exist. Therefore, persistent situations like bullying would taper off, as we would no longer feel triggered every time we walk in the door.

Here are some other things that you can do:[10]

1. *Accept there is a bullying issue*—since much of bullying is covert, we don't often acknowledge it is present. Bullying thrives in secrecy, so getting it out in the open takes away its power. Management won't be able to support the unit if they aren't aware that there is an issue.

2. *Do what is possible to mitigate stressors*—bullies are unable to cope with stress well, so minimizing factors that cause them to be triggered will help ease tension (easier said than done, of course).

3. *Ensure respectful workplace practices are being followed, and bring it to management's attention when they are not.*—most workplaces have these practices posted or documented.

4. *Call it out when you see it*—when you or someone else is being bullied, speak up. Name the behavior (e.g., gossiping, name-calling, favoritism, etc.). Do so in a non-accusatory manner, but be firm. Sometimes it is so ingrained in culture that people don't realize they're doing it. If you don't feel comfortable speaking up to someone who is gossiping, walk away—they will get the message not to do it in front of you again.

5. *Follow policy in reporting bullying behavior*—involve all parties that need to be included (e.g., management, HR, etc.), and ensure the process is taken seriously by said parties. As stated above, it can be detrimental to our health to endure this behavior. Management needs to treat it as the serious issue that it is. If the bully in question is your manager, seek outside workplace support, such as a union rep or HR, and request a second person when you discuss issues with her.

6. *Seek support of a loved one or therapist*—if you are being bullied and have followed the above, it will still be a difficult experience. Make sure you have support of loved ones, or better yet, an impartial professional such as a counselor who can help you as you navigate your next steps. You may not wish to continue working in the same area, and a professional can help you work out your thoughts and feelings so you make an informed choice.

Have You Ever Been The Bully?

Take a moment to reflect on this for a moment. Have you ever bullied someone else, either as a child or as an adult? If so, how did it feel to bully someone else? What else was going on in your life that may have caused you to seek power over another person?

I enjoyed witty banter with one of the doctors I worked with. He would say a teasing remark, and I'd give it right back to him. For the most part, we enjoyed this and it allowed us to have some light-hearted fun in a busy, sometimes stressful work environment.

One day, however, I went too far. One of my coworkers had brought in an old-fashioned inflatable clown, the kind that you punch down and it comes right back up again (it was a great stress reliever!). I had thought it funny to put this particular doctor's face on the clown and joke that we were using him as a punching bag.

He walked in, saw his face on the clown, and went bright red. He immediately tore it off, sputtering something about bullying and walked away. The rest of us just looked at each other and laughed, insisting he couldn't take a joke. I laughed it off, too, but it stayed with me that night.

I realized that, despite his sometimes-mocking nature, he was still susceptible to hurt feelings, and I had obviously done just that. I thought about all the times I had "teased" him, and I realized that I was bullying him.

This was surprising to me. Having been bullied so extensively, I never would have thought I would be capable of bullying anyone else. But after this occasion, I had to admit that I had been bullying the doctor that I worked with. It didn't immediately dawn on me because he wasn't the typical person you picture when you imagine someone being bullied. I wasn't being funny—I was just being mean. I never would have realized this if he hadn't shown how upset he was about it. From that point on, I was more careful about what I teased him about. I loved our banter, and I wanted it to continue, so I was more mindful about what I said after that.

When I picture bullying in my head, I imagine a shy, reserved, sweet person being taken advantage of by someone who is loud, angry, and intimidating. Yet in health care, with more bullying being covert, we know this isn't always the case. If you've ever gossiped about someone (let's be real, we all have), then you have effectively taken part in an act of bullying.

What to do if you realize you've bullied another person:

1. *Accept it*—we're human, we all make mistakes. None of us wants to think of ourselves as a bully, and having the awareness that some of our actions might have hurt someone else will give us the power to own it and not do it again. But first, we need to admit to ourselves when we have done it in the first place to prevent it from becoming a habitual behavior.

2. **Have compassion with yourself**—if you've been the victim of bullying in the past, this may have caused you to go on the offense before you can be bullied again (a symptom of PTSD). Since most bullies were bullied themselves at

some point, it is important to have the same compassion for yourself as you would for someone else. It is a form of survival that you are using to keep yourself safe. It was a survival tactic, but it is one you don't need now.

3. ***Reflect on why you feel the need to assert control over someone***—is there something going on in your life that is contributing to you behaving in this way? It may not seem related, but if you are stressed in other areas of your life, you may be taking it out on others. What do you need right now?

4. ***Ask for help***—if you notice you are having a hard time, it is not only the right thing, but the strong thing to seek outside assistance. For many of us, we are going through the most difficult time in our lives—no one is okay. And that's okay. Getting the help we need will help us get on the road to feeling better.

5. ***Use your judgement***—what is the best way to rectify this situation? Sometimes apologizing may be the best route. However, once you have asserted that you won't behave in this manner again, sometimes the best thing to do is to just move on. Bringing it up to the person might embarrass them. However, it might be just what they need to bury the hatchet with you. Be honest with yourself. Would avoiding apologizing be simply a way out of accepting responsibility for how you've behaved?

Bullying in health care has been a long-standing issue. We are doing the best we can with the limited resources we have. By using our superpower of empathy and really putting ourselves in the other's shoes, we will not only be less likely to be bullied, but also less likely to be the bullies ourselves. We work in higher-stress occupations than most. There will always be conflict, and there will always be difficult people. But when we put our needs first, we feel more empowered, more in control, and more grounded. We can handle situations that arise from a more realistic perspective and will be less likely to feel the need to defend ourselves.

EXERCISES

1. Think of a time you were bullied. This can be as a child, or in your current work situation. What do you think was the underlying cause for this person to bully you? (Hint: it has nothing to do with you, and everything to do with them). What needs do you think weren't getting met?

2. Is there a time that you were a bully? There is no shame in admitting this; we are the product of an unhealthy culture. How did you bully (gossiping, leaving someone out, hostility/silent treatment)? What needs did you have at the time that were going unmet? Can you forgive yourself for this?

CHAPTER 17

Dealing with Difficult People

"Be hard on the problem, soft on the person." – Henry Cloud

I have worked closely with radiologists for over a decade. A lot hinges on them; their ability to detect subtleties in a scan can change the trajectory of a patient's life. They are an extremely important piece of the health care puzzle, and with technology advancing as much as it has done, they are more and more at the forefront of guiding our health care decisions. I have great respect for what they do, and I would trust many of them with my life.

I also jokingly refer to them as the "Dungeons and Dragons" of doctors.

If medicine was high school, surgeons would be the jocks, dermatologists the preps, and radiologists would be the ones in the basement gaming. They sit in the dark and look at computer screens all day. Some of them chose this specialty for the money, some for the hours, and more than a few for the ability to introvert.

I worked most closely with interventional radiologists, who have to "people" more than most rads. They discuss and perform procedures on patients, requiring them to have some semblance of bedside manner. They rely heavily on the team involved in the procedure, including technologists, scrubbing nurses, and circulating nurses. This requires them to communicate clearly what they need, and trust the team to carry out their requests effectively. With some of the procedures being high-risk, tensions can run high.

Sometimes the stress spills over from the person in charge on to the people in the room. As many of us work in high-stress, acute areas, we can all be guilty of this sometimes. But when the stress is taken out on others frequently, it could be labeled as a pattern. It could be labeled as a difficult behavior. After attending Stacey Holloway's seminar entitled "How to Deal with Difficult People," I walked away with much more insight—into myself and into others. While I realized that in fact, difficult people are everywhere, underneath it all, everyone is experiencing the same thing. We all want to feel safe, we all want to feel loved, and we all want to be able to do our jobs and have meaningful lives. We all experience difficult emotions—it's what we do with it that matters.

Check Yourself First

Sometimes we have to ask ourselves if we are having our needs met. If the answer is no, we are more likely to be irritated by others. Have you been fed, watered, and burped? Have you had enough sleep? Is there a situation outside of work that is causing you stress? Sometimes we are simply just hangry, and when we have attended to our needs, we don't find the situation as upsetting as before. In health care, we often skip breaks because we are too busy. This can negatively affect our mood, and as our blood sugar drops, we become more sensitive and/or irritable. Unfortunately, we have often ignored our body cues so often, for so long, that we don't even have the physiological signs of hunger until it is way overdue. I noticed in myself that I could go hours without even feeling hungry, but I was definitely hangry. I had to admit that something that seemed like a big deal before I went for break was less world-ending once I had my snacky-snack.

Are you being triggered? What I would define as difficult may not be what you would define as difficult. If you have a history of maltreatment, you may be more sensitive to certain behaviors. It may be someone who is angry, or it may be someone who is overly sarcastic/condescending. For me, I find people who are anxious and rushing to get the work done very triggering, as it increases my own anxiety. You may find yourself more triggered by angry outbursts, or foul language, or gossip. When we are triggered, our Inner Child is feeling unsafe, and we are more likely to be reactive.

Difficult Behavior Defined

Someone who is occasionally hard to get along with is not considered a difficult person. When I first started my career in health care as an aide, I worked with a woman who was snappy, abrupt, and sometimes condescending. As I had just started in the department, I assumed this was her personality. As I continued to work there, though, I discovered that she was going through a divorce, her house needed serious renovations due to poor workmanship, and one of her children was mentally ill. None of these situations was going away overnight, and it had affected her disposition at work, which I learned was not her usual behavior. After most of her life circumstances had resolved, she was much more pleasant, and I really liked working with her. If I hadn't been told what she had been like before her life became challenging, I would have given her a wide berth and missed out on all of the times we enjoyed together.

The person you may be labelling difficult may just be having a bad day/month/year. Check in with yourself: a) Is it you reacting?, and b) Is it situational? What can you say in the moment that might ease the tension? Most people are reasonable when you are open and honest. Difficult people will consistently not respond to reasonable requests. Difficult people have frequent, recurrent behaviors that make them difficult.

So, what does a "difficult" personality actually look like?

In *Coping with Difficult People*, Robert Bramson identifies difficult people and categorizes them based on their problematic behaviors. Here is a summary of these types of people:[1]

1. ***Hostile-Aggressives***—bulldoze over people, make critical remarks, and throw tantrums in order to get their way.

2. ***Complainers***—constantly find fault in everything and everyone but rarely do anything about it, either due to feeling apathetic or refusing to accept the responsibility.

3. ***Silent and Unresponsives***—are mistrustful and withdrawn from others, and reply with one-word (or no word) responses.

4. ***Super-Agreeables***—are supportive in the present but don't always follow through, usually because they have overcommitted in an attempt to please everyone.

5. ***Know-it-All Experts***—superior, condescending, pompous, they claim to know everything about a topic, and cause others to feel inferior to them.

6. ***Indecisives***—stall or procrastinate, won't commit to tasks as a way to avoid work or disappointing people, often don't make a decision until it is made for them.

Why Difficult People are Difficult

"He's not yelling at me, he's yelling for himself."
– Stacey Holloway, "How to Deal with Difficult People"[2]

Difficult people have usually led hard lives. There is a high chance they experienced abuse or trauma, and their problematic behavior is a form of protection. They weren't exposed to healthy coping mechanisms, and therefore do not know how to implement them in times of stress. They are stuck in their Inner Child ego, and react instead of respond. Shame is often at the root of their actions, and they lack a healthy self-esteem to cope with being accountable. Difficult people need to feel a sense of power in a life they often feel powerless in. When this is compounded with getting away with their behavior in environments that don't effectively deal with it (which is *rampant* in health care), it only encourages the behavior to continue.

Difficult people often lack insight into how their behavior affects others. While it may seem obvious to us that the tension in the room could be cut with a knife, a difficult person is often unaware of this. They lack the empathy that many of us HCWs possess, which is something that we, being gifted in this department, have a tough time imagining.

Using Our Superpower, Empathy

Understanding why someone acts the way they do can empower us. It gives us insight into the other person's behavior, helping us empathize with them, and moves us forward so we can exact change with their cooperation. Often, difficult people feel misunderstood. By taking time and energy to understand a difficult person, they will be more likely to respond to you when you ask them to alter their behavior. By shifting our perspective from judgement to curiosity through our superpower of empathy, we can begin to make real, lasting change. When we seek to learn instead of defend, we open up a bridge to allow there to be more understanding on both sides. Even difficult people deserve our respect, even if they do not necessarily reciprocate. By denying them this, we are effectively stooping to their level. There are ways to deal with difficult people that do not compromise our integrity.

Some questions to help understand the difficult person:

1. How much do you know about the person's life and background? Are there areas you can identify that may be contributing to why they are difficult today? What additional information would you need to know to validate this? If you were in this person's shoes, how would you be acting?

2. How accurate is your perception of the person/situation? Do other people tend to agree with you/identify the same issues with this person?

3. Have you ever given this person the benefit of the doubt or are you assuming negative intent? This does not mean you approve of their behavior or pretend it doesn't exist, and it definitely does not mean you can't take further action at a later time. Giving the person the benefit of the doubt means you are willing to consider the possibility that you don't have all the facts. You might not be able to see the big picture, and you assume they are not being intentionally difficult.

We're all human. I believe that if I was born with your genetics, with your life experiences, and if I was in your shoes right now, I would be you. I try to remember this when I am dealing with someone who is challenging, and ask myself how I would want someone to approach me when a conversation needs to happen.

Personality versus Behavior

Behavior can be changed by making a different choice. Personality, as we learned in the previous chapter, cannot be controlled by choice i.e., we can't change our past experiences or upbringing—which shapes the people we become. By defining the problem as a person, we can't do anything to change it. By defining it as a behavior, we can do something about it. By naming specific behaviors as opposed to personality traits, we shift the problem to something we have the power to do something about (e.g., someone raising their voice as opposed to being an angry person).

Left unchecked, difficult behavior can cause chronic stress, lower morale, and decrease our self-esteem. While it is important for us to have empathy for the people with difficult behaviors, it does not mean we need to tolerate it.

Putting Ourselves First

We can't change people who aren't willing to change. The only behavior we can change is our own. You get the behavior you tolerate. If you treat them differently, they will behave differently. When I first started scrubbing for procedures, I dreaded scrubbing in with a surgeon who had a reputation for being difficult. Instead of allowing the reputation to intimidate me, I introduced myself before the case, indicating that I was new, and that I would do my best to work with him, as he had a much different set-up from the other surgeons. I was pleasantly surprised when he showed me respect back. He took time to explain why he preferred things his way, and he was attentive during the case – I never had a problem with him after that. Sometimes, we need to give people a chance before assuming the worst.

Enabling in health care is serious issue. Many of us are conflict averse, and therefore we tolerate behavior that other fields of work definitely wouldn't. Changing our attitude not only gives us our power back (because we cannot control anyone else), it also diffuses the energy of a situation and leads to less conflict. YOU always have the choice. YOU have the power.

Using our superpower of empathy, we can change our reactions, our perspective, and the way we talk to ourselves. We can overcome the difficulties we experience at work with shifting our power back to ourselves. The difficult person doesn't have the problem of dealing with a difficult person—WE do. We can't control them but we can control how we react to them—which starts with our own inner work.

Why We Allow Difficult People to Take Advantage

When we deal with difficult people, we often initiate a stress response, and we will fight, flight, or freeze (or fawn, for the people-pleasers). Our Inner Child feels unsafe and will often act out in whatever way kept us feeling safest when we were children.

How can we prepare for stressful situations/conversations before they occur? By being aware of our triggers. Triggers are anything we react to instead of respond to. They often stem from childhood and are wired in our brains as a stress response to stimuli. Knowing what our triggers are can help us identify them when they come up and, with practice, reprogram our brains from that kneejerk reaction.

There is new information available about our nervous system and polyvagal theory. Stephen Porges has done extensive research around reconditioning our nervous systems in response to perceived threats, as most of us have some form of triggering in our systems. I encourage you to look into this if it calls to you.[3]

Examples of triggering behaviors:

- Tone of voice (e.g., yelling, whining, sarcasm)
- Specific words (cursing, aggressive speech)
- Context of comments (racist, sexist, suggestions of incompetence, stupidity, threats, oppressive)
- Actions (pointing, invading personal space, slamming doors)

How to Interrupt the Kneejerk

By grounding ourselves, we take ourselves out of our reactive brains and back into our bodies. Pausing to do a grounding technique gives us the time and space to interrupt the synapses that are firing and prompting us to fight, flight, or freeze. There are a variety of grounding techniques you can use in the moment. The basis of each of these is to get you out of your head and into your body. Here are some suggestions, but there are many more out there. Pick one that works for you, and try it out the next time you are in a conflict situation.

Breathe—the best way to interrupt a reactive response is to focus on our breath. This immediately grounds us, causes us to go inward, and has us focus on our bodies. You can either take deep breaths, do box breathing (breathing in and out for four counts each), pursed-lip breathing, or another breathing technique that you prefer.

54321—name 5 things you can see, 4 things you can touch, 3 things you can hear, 2 that you can smell, and 1 that you can taste.

Acupressure—pressure points on your wrist, the web of your thumb, or the outside of your hand.

Affirmations—have a go-to phrase that works for you. Keep it simple and encouraging. "I am in my body," "I am safe," or "I am calm," are easy examples.

Anger

"It's okay to be angry, it's not okay to be mean." – Unknown

We all have a different anger threshold, and some people live closer to their threshold than others. It seems that anything will set them off, and walking on eggshells around them causes us our own significant stress.

Often, the workplace discourages us from venting our anger. Obviously, it's never okay to yell or throw things, but we are hard-pressed to find healthy ways to express our anger in the moment. Like other emotions that are deemed unprofessional (e.g., crying in front of a patient), we suppress our anger because it is frowned upon. We then carry it with us, and don't express it in a healthy way (for example, going for a run after work) because the moment has passed and our brains think we're over it. Well, our bodies know better, and if we don't find a healthy outlet to express the anger we feel, it builds. This is why many people who are labelled "difficult" always seem to be at a closer threshold than others—they haven't found a healthy way to cope.

When difficult people show anger, it is really a cry for help. They have a need that has gone unmet, and they feel trapped. Expressing anger is the best way they know how to get a need met (often the need to control the situation)—and it usually works.

People-pleasers have a difficult time with anger. As many of us were parented not to express our anger at all, we do not have coping mechanisms for our anger, and are, ironically, the angriest inside. It is interesting that people-pleasers get triggered by angry people. It may be a mirror for us not expressing our own anger in a healthy way. By learning healthy ways in which we can express our anger, we can be models for those around us for following suit. Making the statement "I am angry" may seem obvious, but it can be very impactful, especially in the workplace, where we tend to suppress it the most. Engaging in a physical activity that you enjoy is another way to channel anger out of our bodies—bonus if it's in nature.

Nonviolent Communication

In his book *Nonviolent Communication*, Marshall Rosenberg discusses how we can be taken away from our natural state of empathy when we judge others.[4] When we make value judgements about other people, we alienate them, and are less likely to connect with them. Using Nonviolent Communication (NVC) can help us be more empathetic and connected to people, even the "difficult" ones.

When we make observations instead, this can lead to a discussion that gets us closer to a solution. The most common reasons conversations get off track is either the need to be right or not asking enough questions. Conflict is not a contest. Resolving conflict is rarely about who is right—it is about acknowledgment and appreciation of differences. Instead of saying "You procrastinate" (a value judgement, open to interpretation), you can offer an observation, such as "You took thirty minutes before you started that task."

Stating how we feel to someone has proven to connect to that person, but we often get mixed up in saying what we think instead of how we actually feel. "I feel that you don't listen" isn't expressing how we feel; it is saying what we think. Getting to our core feelings can feel vulnerable, but it more often than not produces connection, even with people who are seen as difficult. "I feel frustrated/sad/hopeless when you don't listen" can connect to someone deeper than the previous statement, especially as they are less likely to feel defensive about their actions and more concerned with how their actions are affecting the people around them.

According to NVC, judgements of others are an unhealed expression of not meeting our own needs. We are responsible for taking action for our feelings.

We can:

1. Blame ourselves
2. Blame others
3. Tune in to our feelings and needs, or
4. Tune into the feelings and needs of others

In hearing the phrase, "You disappointed me," we can choose to:

1. Accept the judging statement and beat up on ourselves (e.g., "I'm such an idiot, why did I do that?"),
2. Blame the other person for being disappointed and attack them ("You expected too much of me, you're too critical."),
2. Express our feelings and needs (e.g., "I feel hurt that you would say that because I put in a lot of effort."), or
3. Tune into the feelings and needs of others (e.g., "Are you feeling sad because I didn't succeed in completing the task?").

By focusing on our needs and feelings, it becomes easier to have compassion for others, as they, too, could have feelings and needs that have not been addressed.

Steps you can take to diffuse the situation with a difficult person (adapted from *Fierce Conversations* by Susan Scott):[5]

1. *Use your superpower, empathy*—ask yourself why they are being difficult. What would you be feeling if you were in their shoes? Taking the time to understand the person will help diffuse the situation and allow you to speak from logic instead of emotion. Ask yourself how you can address it so there is less anger on both sides. What are you winning if you win this argument? Sometimes our ego wants to be right so much, we run over others, and ourselves.

2. *Pick a good time*—ensure it is private, that you are less likely to be interrupted, and both of you are calm. If one or both of you is/are emotional, it's not the time.

3. *Seek permission*—keep a mild and open manner—conversations often end how they started. "Are you open to talking about …? When would be a good time?" This shows your respect, the topic is important to you, and you are seeking permission about going ahead. This is less likely to cause them to be defensive than "we need to talk." In every situation, there needs to be at least one adult, and the only person you can rely on to be that adult is you. The angry person has much more practice arguing, you won't win.

4. *Don't assume the person will react*—you may be pleasantly surprised. However, do plan for how you will handle it if they do. Our superpower of empathy causes us to take an educated guess on how people will react, and while we are often right, we aren't always. We have to give people a chance. You also might learn insight into their perspective, something you didn't see. Remaining open during a critical conversation is imperative for us to get through the other side.

5. *Keep it brief*—according to Scott, that means under a minute. This is for two reasons: it keeps us from getting into too many details and justifying ourselves, and it also keeps them from zoning out (formulating their defense, usually, and not actually listening to us).

6. *Use collaborative phrases*—recognize you both could be contributing to the issue. Validate them when you can, and exploring alternatives ("Is it possible …") or offering choices ("Could we try …") can help you both reach an understanding. Don't use confrontational language or lip service. Blaming ("You always …"), dismissing ("Whatever"), and condescending phrases ("I'm sorry you feel that way …") won't get you anywhere. Use your superpower of

empathy and speak in a way that mirrors how they do to establish rapport. If they deny their behavior, say, "I had a different experience." That being said…

7. *Speak from the heart* — I once had a manager who was very well-versed in "manager-speak". He had very obviously been prepped on what to say to employees when they came to him with issues – so well, in fact, that I felt like I was speaking to a robot. I left the interaction feeling unheard and more frustrated than when I went in, even though he said "all the right things". There was no heart connection in it, and it didn't resolve anything. Often, getting at the heart of the matter quickly (e.g., "I'm upset that you raised your voice") can get us further than eye-rolling professional jargon ("Can we circle back to…").

8. *Clarify what is at stake*—tell them why this is important, and what will happen if the behavior continues. As with setting boundaries in the preceding chapter, the most important of these is following through on your consequence. If you don't, it signals to the other person that you aren't to be taken seriously. If you state a consequence to the difficult behavior, STICK to it.

9. *Indicate your wish to resolve the issue*—that you're with the person, that it is Us versus The Issue and not You versus Them.

10. *Invite them to respond*—actively LISTEN. Give them a chance to air their perspective. Resist the urge to interrupt, even if you vehemently oppose what they're saying. Their view is as legitimate as yours, and you don't have to agree to make progress. It's not your job to enlighten them to a different point of view. Remember, we often have gone a long time without acknowledging these issues—you are suddenly telling them you're not okay with something that they long thought you were okay with. They are likely to feel blindsided, even if a part of them knows that your request is reasonable. If there is something you don't understand, you have a right to have it explained to you in a respectful manner. By showing genuine interest in the other person's knowledge, you will gain their trust.

While you can listen, remember that you are driving the conversation. They might try to deflect or blame. Remember what your intention is, and keep steering the conversation to the topic you identified.

11. *Resolution*—how can we move forward? Make an agreement, and hold each other accountable to what you both agree on. The person doesn't have to change, and in fact, you can't make them. But if they want to continue having a relationship with you (working or otherwise), they will alter their behavior.

You have a right to be treated with respect, so do not allow inappropriate behavior. By taking the above steps, you can respond more professionally, politely but firmly.

Strategies for Specific Difficult Behavior Types

1. *Hostile-Aggressives*—let them calm down, don't try to engage with them when they are in the heat of their response. Be firm, and call out the behavior that is inappropriate, not them. Don't argue with them, even if they try to bait you.

2. *Complainers*—acknowledge the complaints they are making without disagreeing with them or encouraging them to complain more. Don't try to solve their problem—chances are, they don't actually want a solution, they just want to gripe. Ask questions that may help them reframe the situation. If they continue to complain, and you're feeling bold, you could ask them, "How do you want this discussion to end?" as it may wake them up. Because their script is mostly unconscious at this point, sometimes they need to be jolted out of it.

3. *Silent and Unresponsives*—try asking open-ended questions to see if it opens them up. Be patient for a response, don't fill the silence with talking. Be sincere, and encourage them that you would like to hear what is on their mind.

4. *Super-Agreeables*—create a safe space for them to be open and honest about what they truly think. Ensure that they will commit to what you are asking them to, and not just going along with it because they don't want to upset you.

5. *Know-it-All Experts* — don't challenge their knowledge. Use questions to explore alternatives to their statement. Be prepared on the topic at hand, as they will likely use your ignorance as ammo.

6. *Indecisives*—listen to the issues the person has with making a decision, and don't try to influence them either way—they need to be able to make concrete choices on their own. Ask relevant questions that may help make things clearer for them.

When a Difficult Person Crosses the Line

Calling someone out who has compromised your safety or ability to work is not being a drama queen. You have an obligation to stand up for yourself and your integrity. We don't need to tiptoe around difficult people. It is important that we honor ourselves and our needs and decide what we will and will not tolerate from others. It is more likely that a difficult person will cross your boundaries than the average population, so be clear about the boundaries you set with them, and *stick to it*. A difficult person will also be more likely than most to take advantage of you not following through.

It is normal not to recognize when someone has crossed the line right away. It is perfectly okay to bring it up at a later time. One tactic that difficult people use in this situation is that by the time you bring up the issue (say it is a week later), they don't recall what happened. This may be true, but it is not an excuse to let them off the hook. You are perfectly in your right to address an issue that happened a while ago that you needed time to process. Using specific examples may help the person remember the situation.

When to Ask for Help

Sometimes, we don't feel we are able to deal with a difficult person on our own. Sometimes it is wiser to involve management or administration when interacting with someone who is deemed difficult. Obviously, the ideal is to talk to the person directly, and your superior may ask you why you haven't done so. It is perfectly acceptable to say you didn't feel safe doing so alone. Once the dust has settled after an altercation, if you are still feeling emotional or overwhelmed, you should seek outside counsel.

There are effective conflict management options that you have available to you, and your manager can help you with this—you don't have to do it alone! If it is your manager who is the difficult person, he/she also has a manager—don't be afraid to escalate (despite the world shaming the Karens for escalating, there is a time and a place to do so—don't let the current trend dissuade you).

When to Let Go

Sometimes you can try all of these strategies and the situation still does not get any better (or it gets worse). Perhaps the difficult person was reprimanded and now treats you with cold indifference. It is up to you to decide if you want to continue putting up with this or if your mental health would benefit more from leaving. It's not losing or giving up, you are honoring your needs, and perhaps a change of job is necessary for you to keep your sanity. This is okay, too. Take the time and reflect on what is right for you. You have choices in every facet of your life—your relationships, where you live, who you socialize with. Don't feel trapped or obligated to stay if you truly don't want to. Do what is right for you.

The world will always have difficult people in it wherever we go. Having empathy for their plight, the skills to confront them when necessary, and the wherewithal to know whether we need to bark or bow out will serve us in navigating these situations.

EXERCISES

1. Look back to the types of difficult people listed. Who do you work with that fits into these categories? Make note of the strategies listed to help work with these people, and make a conscious effort to employ them the next time you have an issue crop up.

2. Make a list of things that make you angry. Is there a theme? How does that transpire in the workplace? What triggers you when you are at work? What activities can you do to help channel your anger?

3. What strengths do you have dealing with these situations (think of your personality type)? How could you use your strengths to deal with these situations?

CHAPTER 18

Toxic Workplaces

"You sit in shit too long, it stops smelling." – Jennifer Lewis

I was a brand-new grad nurse. I had finished my final clinical in the NICU, and I was eager to start my new life. Moving out of my parents' place, buying a new car, and having a steady, full-time income, I was excited to be finished with school and start my new career and new life.

I was trying to adjust to caring for very sick newborns, shift work, and managing my new life living on my own, paying bills, rent, etc. It was all very exciting but also overwhelming. I had never cared for the micro-preemies at my clinical placement, so getting used to fragile, 500-gram intubated newborns as a new nurse was very stressful.

It was also probably stressful for my colleagues to try to do their jobs while having to babysit a new nurse. No one had said anything directly to me, but the overall tone I felt was that new nurses didn't have enough experience to be working with such a fragile population. Indeed, there were many days that I felt I was in over my head as some of my babies crashed within minutes, and I didn't feel competent to take care of them on my own. Luckily, I was always near more experienced nurses, and I relied on their expertise when I didn't know what to do.

I know some of them resented so many new nurses on the unit at one time. They had hired ten new people to our unit when I started, and most of us were new graduates. While there were valid concerns with hiring so many brand-new nurses, the unfortunate reality was that there were also many vacancies to fill. While I could understand more experienced nurses' wariness, it was also a fact that they were chronically short. And running short on a unit with critically ill newborns was much different to running short on a medical unit. Having experienced nurses as hires would be ideal, but it was also imperative to have the positions filled so the unit could run.

This left a lot of onus on the experienced nurses to carry our team. Not only were these nurses expected to care for critically ill newborns and be on top of their game at all times, dealing with ventilators, inotropes, pressors, and stressed-out parents, but they also had to support and come to the aid of new nurses coming in. As a new grad, I couldn't fully appreciate at the time how much they had on their plates—I was just doing my best to keep my babies alive. I didn't have the capacity to understand what it must be like to be an experienced NICU nurse having all of that on their shoulders. I did my best to be as helpful as I could, recognizing how much I needed their support.

But I was also afraid. I was afraid to ask questions, afraid to mess up, afraid to admit when I didn't know what I was doing. While I was buddied with nurses for a shift, the overall atmosphere I felt was one of the aforementioned wariness. Most of them watched me like a hawk and were quick to point out if I made an error, no matter how small. This, while understandable, did nothing to instill confidence in me or my abilities.

So instead of feeling prepared when I was on my own, I felt overwhelming pressure to perform perfectly. Which meant not asking questions in case I looked stupid. Which is really, really scary that I felt more damage would be done by asking a question than screwing up. Most of the time, I was able to suck up my courage to ask the question because I knew my babies' well-being meant more than my ego. But the energy it took to do this on a regular basis became draining. On top of dealing with stressed-out, worried parents, I didn't always feel safe to rely on some of my colleagues, as I worried what their reactions would be. It was a pretty isolating first few months of my career.

This only intensified away from the bedside and in the breakroom. I was out of high school now and felt it would be safe to make conversation with my new colleagues. I was a new nurse, struggling to feel competent, and I needed to be accepted by these women. I felt on edge any time I was at the bedside, and desperate to be shown even a shred of kindness. I figured my best bet to achieve this would be at the lunch table, where the topic of conversation was a bit lighter, something I thought I could handle. Little did I know, it wasn't safe to talk here, either. The group that day were discussing head bands, and how to keep hair out of the way when working out. "You can get ones that have rubber on them which work really well!" I chimed in, smiling, trying to get in on the conversation.

The entire group sitting at the table actually stopped talking and turned to look at me, silently. There was a brief pause, and the conversation continued as if I hadn't said anything. I looked down at the table, ashamed. I was sorry I had opened my mouth, and vowed not to engage in conversation with this group again.

I held on to the belief that there was something wrong with me for far too long in that department, long after I had left it. While my decision to leave this job was mostly due to shift work, I also didn't have any love lost between my colleagues on the same line as me. While I was new and obviously wasn't as adept at my job as they were, I also wasn't nurtured or given an environment where I could safely grow. I carried shame of not being good enough—as a nurse and as a person—because I felt I was surrounded by people who insidiously caused me to feel that way. This feeling of not being good enough affected my mood, my morale, and my performance, as I was often so flustered that I would make more mistakes than usual. As a new nurse, it is absolutely expected that I wasn't going to know everything, but the environment I was in prevented me from growing as a new nurse in a healthy way.

Now that I have been away from the situation and am able to look back on it, I realized I should have spoken up. I could have confided in someone who may have been warmer (and there were plenty of those nurses there, too). But the truth was I felt so much shame and questioned my abilities that I just internalized it all—it didn't even occur to me to ask someone for support or guidance. I was so afraid of looking stupid, or asking something that would cause people to think I wasn't competent, that I suffered alone with this ordeal. Sadly, this is all too common, especially among new nurses. My self-esteem had taken such a hit that I didn't believe I deserved better than that at the time.

There were many other elements contributing to this. Being a large unit, it felt impersonal and unwelcoming. The scheduling also contributed to that fact, as lines were created to make it easier for the unit to function. Working with most of the same people all of the time created a cliquey environment, as you often didn't see people who were opposite to you. The unit, like many in the hospital, had a high turnover. Perhaps many of the staff who had been there a long time didn't have enough energy to invest in new people who may not stay, despite the fact that this probably increased the turnover as new staff did not feel welcomed. Finally, the personality types that are drawn to ICUs tend to be more Type A, so the atmosphere feels less nurturing than one with more balanced personalities dispersed through it.

Management was also an issue at that site. Not having many interactions with my managers (there were four, and none of them knew my name, as there were hundreds of staff working on this unit), I can't speak to specific problems. I do know there was little respect and a lot of animosity for these managers. Witnessing the condescending tone that one of them put out in a staff email, I raised my eyebrows at how unprofessional she was. Luckily, I left the department without having to interact with her.

Upon leaving the department, I later encountered other nurses who had worked there. They confided in me that their experience in the department was similar, that it was a cliquey unit and that they felt unsupported. I stayed there for nearly two years trying to stick it out, unhappy but feeling like it was my fault that I wasn't feeling more accepted. Since I was quickly welcomed at my new job, I knew that it wasn't my issue.

Was it right for me to try to stick it out? Perhaps if I had stayed on a little longer, I would have felt more accepted. I would have proven that I wasn't part of the high turnover statistic and received more respect for my dedication. I was hired with ten other staff as part of a hiring incentive, and by the time I left, only two of the originals hired with me remained. I can see why people aren't as invested in such a large unit to get to know others. Yet I wonder how it would affect retention if more effort was given to welcoming new hires.

On the other hand, should I have left sooner? Where is the line between trying to fit in, or making changes to an unhealthy environment, or simply walking away? Obviously, we can't just up and quit if we aren't liking every single job we apply for. But we also shouldn't have to put up with environments that aren't fostering our growth.

While I can't tell you what is right and what is wrong, as every person and every situation is different, I can give you some information on what constitutes a toxic workplace, what can be done to improve it, and invoke self-reflection on whether or not it's worth it to stay.

Toxicity Defined

Toxicity is defined as "the degree to which a substance can harm humans or animals."[1] Some things in life are toxic to us right away—the venom from a snakebite, for example. But the sinister part about toxicity is that we don't always realize something is toxic to us until we are too far immersed in it. Like the frog who got into a pot of water, only to be boiled alive because he had adjusted to the increasing heat, we sometimes can't see the danger until it is too late.

Toxic workplaces are an example of the ever-increasing burner. We seem like we have adjusted, but our bodies haven't. Our chronic pain and illness, our underlying anxieties, and our sense of hopelessness are all signs that the heat is increasing.

We know our workplaces are becoming more toxic. In fact, it is much more common than we realized, even outside of health care. It can exist on an isolated basis between individuals, within a team in a department, or it can be widespread throughout an organization.

With our current health care settings, the water is a full rolling boil. We are taking care of sicker people, we are doing it with less staff and less resources, and we are receiving little to no external support. Our advancement in technology has provided a wealth of new procedures and treatments for patients, and we are now seeing more chronic conditions than ever before. There is an onus on the health care system to "fix" it all. The pressure we have on us as health care professionals is more demanding than ever, and we are trying to do it with less. We can't see how toxic our workplaces are because all of them are. It's like telling a fish to sense the water—it can't, it's all it has ever known.

The Effects of a Toxic Workplace

Spending twelve hours a day in an environment where we feel undervalued, unappreciated, or even bullied has long-term effects on our psyche as well as our body. Reactions to a toxic workplace can vary; some people become anxious, some become angry, some remain in denial. Most of us, however, feel that we don't have the power to do anything about it, and we just suck it up.

Sucking it up long-term has detrimental effects on our bodies. The symptoms of being in a toxic workplace over a long period are similar to those of PTSD:

• fatigue	• insomnia
• tense, achy muscles, more prone to injury	• issues with digestion
• being in a state of constant fight or flight	• anxiety
• depression	• weakened immune systems
• chronic illness	

The problem with toxic workplaces is that we don't always pinpoint our health issues within our work environment. We've been in the environment so long that we can't know if it is the culprit, or if it's something else—our mattress, our diet, or our germy children. And, as it is easier to buy a new mattress than to get a new job, too often we focus on treating the symptoms instead of the big picture.

Toxic workplaces create a cycle of more toxicity. HCWs already have demanding careers, what with shift work, coerced overtime, and conflict in work-life balance.[2] When staff leave, this causes more strain, with even more workload and overtime now expected. The cycle continues, as the remaining staff are unable to maintain this for long and eventually burn out (and leave, either on sick leave or for another position). Additionally, according to the World Health Organization, this discourages the next generation of potential nurses and allied health from entering the field altogether, which only perpetuates the cycle more.[3]

Signs of a Toxic Workplace

So far, we have discussed issues at length around difficult people, bullying, and interpersonal conflict. How do we know when it is a toxic workplace and not just a toxic person?

When most people have the same issue as you do.

There will always be negative people, and there will always be positive people who can work serenely in any environment. But when the majority of people are living primarily in stress, apathy, or fear most of the time, there is an issue.

Signs of a toxic workplace include:

- sick calls
- lack of communication
- gossip, cliques, rumors
- favoritism
- making it challenging to make a complaint (difficulty navigating the system, excessive form-filling, etc.)
- tattling
- taboos/punishment for speaking up
- lack of appreciation
- disrespectful behavior being tolerated
- blatant hypocrisy
- high turnover
- low morale
- narcissistic/absent leadership
- overly restrictive systems
- hypervigilance with tasks for fear of being called out
- intense pressure to finish all the work
- us versus them mentality
- pessimism
- scapegoats getting blamed

The Female Element

According to the World Health Organization, women are exposed to more actual and perceived stressors.[4] We are more likely to be caregivers outside of our careers, and therefore experience more pressure to fulfill all roles required of us (colleague, mother, spouse, cook, cleaner, teacher), with a kinder, more nurturing demeanor.[5] This leads to toxicity showing itself in different forms. There are several reasons why women have a more difficult experience with toxic workplaces than men do:

1. **Women take things personally**—growing up, boys are rewarded for their actions (look at the truck Billy built, look at the goal he scored!), whereas girls tend to be rewarded based on their behavior (she is so sweet, she is so well-mannered). This creates conditioning when we get older that causes women to base our self-worth on our personality, whereas men tend to focus more on their accomplishments. This is why we tend to take things more personally when we do something wrong. We have been raised to judge our self-worth by "being good".

2. **Women are more likely to be people-pleasers**—tying in with taking things personally, we also tend to people-please, as it rewards the "good girl" part of our brains. This adds to toxicity in the workplace as it causes us to seethe silently when we feel underappreciated or used (because a good girl doesn't complain!). We then become fatigued and passive-aggressive in an attempt to balance the over-giving.

3. **Women are more likely to bully in covert ways, avoiding reprimand**—gossip, cliques, and other forms of covert bullying are more likely to be executed by women. These forms of inappropriate behavior are more difficult for a manager to address as they are less concrete.

The Three Areas of Toxic Workplaces

When we think of what constitutes a toxic workplace, we often think of negative people and domineering managers. However, according to Paul White, a psychologist and Kathy Schoonover-Shoffer, an RN, both of whom have done extensive research in the area, it was discovered that it is often more to do with an overall sick system—and there are many elements that contribute to this. When the foundational structure of an organization is not built well, unhealthy behaviors by people typically follow.[6] It is often not the people, but the system, that is the issue. Their studies revealed that there are three primary areas that are common in a toxic work environment: toxic systems, toxic leaders, and toxic colleagues.

Toxic Systems

"It is more cost-effective today for an employer to send its employees into the workplace with inadequate safety protection, knowing that serious, long-term injury will likely result, than to provide adequate safety protection."
— Michelle Gorton in Intentional Disregard: Remedies for the Toxic Workplace[7]

Let that sink in.

We as frontline HCWs often aren't privy to the concerns of people who allocate resources for our health care system (e.g., CEOs, etc.). While we are aware that finances are heavily focused upon, we don't often see how things look from their perspective. Similarly, with most of those roles having been out of scope for a long period of time (or having never actually set foot in a hospital), they are out of touch with the reality that we are facing today. This leads to a toxic work environment. The stakeholders who make the decisions do not understand how their decisions actually affect the bottom line, because they have never actually worked there. This seeps into other aspects of daily life on a busy unit, affecting the employees and the patients.

There are several aspects of toxic systems that contribute to an organization's overall poor function:

1. *Poor communication patterns*—are the classic characteristic of structural problems in a toxic organization. This can occur between employees, employees and

managers, manager to manager, etc. In the health care setting, it can involve patients, family members, nurses, health care aides, physicians, and all other allied health care workers who we interact with in a day. This contributes to confusion, misrepresentation, and ultimately leads to bad decisions being made.

Lack of communication is the most common (and most problematic) form of poor communication. When individuals avoid interaction or assume they know the information at hand, it causes errors in understanding and costly mistakes.

Inaccurate messages are also problematic in the workplace. By giving partial information or omitting details (either for brevity or to avoid discipline), we potentially put ourselves and our patients at risk.

Indirect communication is also problematic. When we communicate through other people, we open up to the possibility that important details may be lost through the other person. This is extremely common in the hospital (e.g., getting a report on a patient when their bedside nurse is on break), and can have disastrous consequences for the patient. Yet the system is built in a way that makes it difficult to operate with proper communication, and we HCWs do our best to make things work.

2. *Policy not being followed*—within a health care system, there are many policies and procedures related to patient care, federal laws, union collective agreements, etc. When any of these policies are not being followed (either by an employee or a manager) on a regular basis, it can lead to a toxic work environment. The reasons policies are not followed can be due to a lack of adequate training, lack of accountability from management, fear of conflict (again, as an employee or a manager), or negligence—when staff feel overworked and underappreciated, they are less likely to follow policy, either due to time/personnel restrictions, or resentment.

3. *Lack of defined rules and responsibilities*—as busy hospital units often have many different roles and tasks, there can be overlap in who can do what role. When it isn't clear who should be doing what, it breeds contempt and blame when tasks don't get done. This can also be confusing and frustrating for patients, as when they ask questions, they can be given different answers by different team members.

How to Improve a Toxic System

The idea of one person improving a sick system seems daunting. One of the biggest barriers to changing a sick system is the perceived limited power we feel in which to make change. We become frustrated and apathetic, and resign ourselves to the fact that nothing can be done. However, we DO have the power to make an impact, and we can improve our daily work lives. How?

By putting ourselves first. We need to stand up for ourselves. While our focus may be the patients and their safety, if we are not safe, then they are not safe. If we have shoddy PPE, they get shoddy PPE. It is natural for us to want to advocate for the patients, but first we have to advocate for ourselves. No one is advocating for us. We need to put our safety and our well-being above our patients. Only then can we be assured that the patients will be getting adequate care, because we are able to give it when our needs are met and we are safe. By each individual focusing on their own needs and safety, we can begin to change the culture that has become so contaminated.

One of the best ways to improve organizational culture is to have a heathy work-life balance. Two of the most important factors to work-life balance are autonomy and flexibility in scheduling[8]. How can you achieve more autonomy and flexibility at work? Start small. Of course, we would love to work when we felt like it and have full control over our daily practice – and in health care, this is actually possible. What are some small ways you could introduce more autonomy over your practice? Is there a process that you can see needs to be streamlined? How about your schedule, is there someone who hates day shifts that you could trade with? Get creative. We may not be able to fix all of the issues in a toxic organization, but making small changes that affect our autonomy and flexibility can make our work lives more enjoyable.

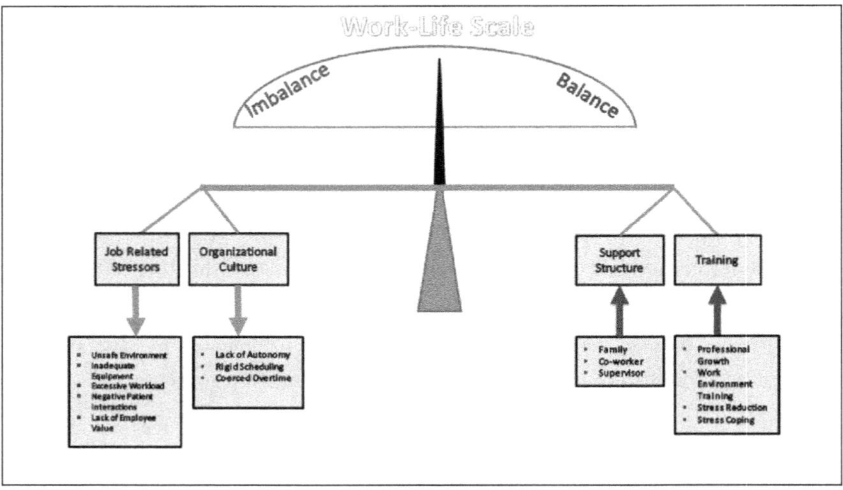

From M.M. Varma, A.S. Kelling, & S. Goswami, "Enhancing healthcare quality by promoting work-life balance among nursing staff," M.M. Varma, A.S. Kelling, & S. Goswami, *Journal of Hospital Administration*, (2016), 5(6), 60. Used with permission.

Other things one person can do:

Commit to direct communication—the single most important action an individual can make is to communicate directly with those around her. This includes going through the correct channels of communication (e.g., giving report directly to the person taking care of the patient), and speaking to those directly involved when an issue arises (e.g., going to a colleague to discuss a miscommunication instead of your manager right off the bat).

Clarify individual responsibilities—often, we are at a loss as to who should be doing what on a busy unit, and we all try to pitch in. By having more clearly defined roles in a department, we can become a more cohesive unit. If required, ask for a staff meeting to discuss what is unclear. Clarify what needs to be done, who is responsible for each action/task, set a date to review actions taken, and identify who should be notified if there is an issue.

Collaborate proactively with colleagues—this helps encourage a flow of communication. When you feel like a team, you speak with each other more often and efficiently. This sense of teamwork also aids morale and allows the tasks to be accomplished more evenly.

Toxic Leaders

"Shit rolls downhill." – Every entry-level employee

Toxic leaders can be anywhere in the organization hierarchy—for nursing, this can be a charge nurse, a nurse manager, a director, and above. Leadership at any level affects all of us, and having a toxic leader in any position will influence how we do our jobs. While they are only one person, they can be devastating to a unit. They affect staff morale, can suppress positive change, and cause unnecessary stress to those they interact with. Most of us have come into contact with a toxic leader at some point in our careers. The way we adapt is either to accept the behavior (and be at risk for developing toxic behavior ourselves), or quit.

The greatest challenge we have in addressing a toxic leader is that they are widely tolerated by most people in the department.[9] Staff feel powerless to change, and so accept it, however grudgingly. And higher-level management are certainly not going to investigate a toxic leader unless there are direct concerns to be addressed. With health care jobs being as portable as they are, we simply leave when things get too much, which does nothing to create a culture of change in an environment that so desperately needs it. The belief that going to another job will only lead to more toxicity is correct—because we haven't done anything to make any lasting change.

Our greatest power starts with ourselves. Recognizing that we do, in fact, have the power to make change will course-correct any apathy or frustration that we have with our situation. There are steps we can take, and we do not have to tolerate toxic behavior—we just don't. Making the perspective shift that you do not have to tolerate what you do not deserve will serve you in your career and in life. You deserve to be treated as a professional, and as a human being. Focusing less on the toxic leader and more on your needs and power can make a huge difference. Putting ourselves first does not just mean in terms of the patient, it also means our colleagues and leaders.

Another power we have is our superpower of empathy. Positions in health care are often run like a hierarchy without the proper steps in place to ensure positions of power are fully qualified to run that way. Nursing sets a blazing example when it comes to this. New grads are lucky to have six months under their belt before being thrown into charge nurse positions. Often times, with staff shortages, younger and younger staff are assuming this role. We do it because it is what needs to be done, but there is little support or education around this leadership role.

Nurse managers are exposed to the same fate. Oftentimes, they are ill-prepared to run a department. Nurse managers are some of the least-trained supervisors for their positions. They often don't have prior leadership experience, and it can be difficult for them to obtain while they are in their roles. They also don't have a lot of support, as most of the time, they are the only manager on a unit. And on some units, they aren't even nurses. If you have been unfortunate enough to report to a manager who is not the same profession as yourself and tried to explain something to them that they cannot fully understand, you will know how frustrating it can be. Sometimes toxic managers are really just the product of a toxic system. Yet that doesn't mean we don't have the right to act on inappropriate behavior.

Characteristics of a Toxic Leader

Toxic leaders can be difficult to identify. Some of the traits may include: [10]

Self-centered—toxic leaders can be ambitious, and may lose sight of anything that doesn't relate to their goals. These goals can either be for the department or for personal gain. When important issues come up that don't relate to their goals (e.g., staffing ratios), they minimize the importance of these issues, or delegate to someone else to deal with. This also might look like not following policy or collective agreements. They are rigid in their thinking and hide their weaknesses and failures from staff and their own supervisors. They take credit for accomplishments made by other staff, and will blame others when something goes wrong.

Controlling—toxic leaders must be in control of everything at all times, giving very little autonomy to staff. In order to maintain control, they micromanage, withhold valuable information from staff, and force others to follow their vision of the unit. They rarely listen to other staff suggestions for how to improve the department, and will point out holes in their suggestions to deter staff from implementing them. They may be manipulative, searching for followers to do exactly as they request, and reward these people in their inner circle by showing favoritism. This leads to a unit that has very little room or ability for change, and people wanting to create a different work environment are thwarted either through refusal to discuss, or by covert "punishment" (e.g., giving undesirable assignments, changing shifts around, etc.).

Disrespectful—condescending tone, making critical comments, and correcting/putting down staff in front of others are all examples of how toxic leaders disrespect their colleagues. This can be subtle, such as making snide comments covered up as jokes, or more aggressive, such as through bullying, threatening, or raising their voices to staff.

Absent—toxic leaders may try to avoid dealing with issues by simply neglecting them. They may be avoidant with communication (not responding to emails), or they may try to brush off significant concerns raised. They also have a tendency to leave before shit hits the fan, seemingly knowing when the splatter is coming. Their ability to move from department to department creates a trail of damaged units in their wake.

Inadequate emotional intelligence—many toxic leaders embody this characteristic, unfortunately. The drive that many leaders have to advance their careers is often rewarded by being as impersonal as possible. Many toxic leaders lack the self-awareness and social skills that are required of a sound leader. They may not be aware of others' emotions or how to handle them, or they may lack empathy for their employees' concerns (not everyone has our superpower, even in health care).

How to Deal with a Toxic Leader

Leaders of any kind possess positional power and authority on a unit. It can seem daunting to create positive change with a supervisor or manager at the best of times, let alone when they have a toxic personality. As a staff member, you can quietly lead from the middle and be just as effective. You have the power to make subtle changes that will improve staff morale but not contribute to the toxicity of the unit. Here are some suggestions when dealing with a toxic leader:

Use your superpower, empathy—as previously stated, many of our leaders (supervisors, managers, educators) don't have official education backing up their position. Many are overworked, and many do not have a lot of support. They may not be able to effectively deal with all of the issues our units are dealing with as they are tied to meetings for the majority of the day. Like us, they rarely receive praise or appreciation for their roles, and their toxic behavior may simply be the only way they know how to cope. One thing you can do (that may shock your manager—in a good way!) is compliment her on where she is doing a good job. She probably never hears this. While she may not be contributing to the health of your unit, she is still a human being, and she is doing her best with what a toxic system has dealt her. This appreciation can open up a dialogue that may steer your conversation (and possibly, your relationship) in a healthier direction.

Recognize that they are inward-focused—toxic leaders tend to be ego-centric. They will internalize anything they deem as a threat, and will most likely be defensive when you come to them with concerns. Having this awareness will allow you to approach the situation from a different perspective.

Be up to date with policies on your unit—don't give a toxic manager ammunition. Know your roles, responsibilities, and policies related to the concern you are bringing up. Don't count on them to know the information for you; your lack of knowledge will make it easier for them to discount you.

Document, document, document—have everything that pertains to the situation in writing. Ask your leader to give you information in writing, and keep track of specific instructions given, decisions made, etc., in this format. This not only protects you from any issues that might arise with your manager specifically, but it also protects you if litigation occurs on the unit. If you have communicated your concerns to your manager about a situation that goes to court, you have proven your accountability if you do become implicated in the circumstances. If you are in any face-to-face meetings, send a follow-up email with the main topics covered and request verification. It might look something like this:

Thank you for meeting with me today to discuss (blank). To clarify what was discussed so we are both on the same page, we agreed on (blank, blank, and blank). Going forward, we will be doing (blank). If something comes up around this, the immediate action I will do is (blank). Do you agree? Did I miss anything?

It's okay if you don't discuss everything in this email, as it gives you a chance to add any points that you may have forgotten to discuss in the meeting. It also provides you a paper trail if anything comes up that you need to look back on, or if you are required to escalate the situation.

I also recommend keeping a journal of the situation if you feel it may escalate.

Sometimes our memory doesn't cooperate, and if you are required to take the matter further or to another party, they may ask you to remember specific facts (dates, specific words used, etc.) For example, if you are being bullied, keep track of all of the times your manager or colleague performed the bullying behavior, what was said, etc., as we often forget these specific details, and it will come in handy if you are contemplating escalating the situation. This is something I wish I had done when I submitted a complaint, as I had to recall details for the claim that caused me to relive the bullying, re-traumatizing me in the process. If in doubt, write it out.

Contain your emotions—ensure that you are not having a conversation (or sending an email) when you are in the throes of your emotions. Your Inner Child has a right to be upset, but don't let her take the steering wheel by sending an emotional email before dealing with those emotions (she unfortunately knows how to type). Make sure you have let yourself feel them first. You are more than entitled to feel every bit of anger and frustration, and once you have given yourself an outlet to properly feel them, you will be much calmer and able to express your thoughts more clearly. You will be more likely to say something constructive, and less likely to shoot your mouth off (not that I have personal experience, or anything …). If you become emotional in the middle of a conversation, you are perfectly within your rights to take a breather, or to request to speak about the issue at another time.

Avoid criticizing the leader or making personal attacks—this will only add fuel to the fire, and will make you appear less credible. Instead, come up with a strategic plan with which to overcome the issue at hand. By being rational and calm, the leader you are dealing with will be more likely to mirror this.

Seek an unbiased opinion—when we are dealing with toxic people, sometimes it is difficult to tell if what we are experiencing is right. Is this acceptable? Like the frog in the boiling water, we can't always decipher what is okay and what is inappropriate when we are so close to it, especially when we have been tolerating subpar conditions for such a long time. When I tell my non-nursing friends stories of what I am dealing with, they widen their eyes in disbelief. Their reaction is a wake-up call that I shouldn't be putting up with this. Toxic leaders can lead you into gray areas of morality and ethics. Asking a trusted friend, or better yet, someone without any personal bias (a counselor, a coach), might help you decide if what you are dealing with requires further action.

Request support from staff—if others on your unit are having the same issues, ask for their support in the matter. This may look like asking for a staff meeting, writing a letter and having them sign it, or having others accompany you to third-party meetings if the situation escalates. I also recommend not having meetings alone—

bringing a colleague or a union rep will eradicate any chance that they misconstrue your words, as you will have a witness to bear them.

Seek outside counsel—this may include your manager's manager, your union representative, or an external consult. If you are unable to rectify the issue with your leader, you may require outside, unbiased influence. Your documentation and support from other staff may help you out with this. Also, having statistics on staff turnover, sick calls, and overtime may be beneficial, as a director may want to know if the manager in question is affecting the unit financially.

There are many workplace resources available to you, including HR, consulting services, and counselors that specialize in workplace matters. The Canadian Mental Health Association website (cmha.ca) has a ton of resources for mental health in the workplace, and have advisors that you can contact regarding workplace issues. You might be eligible for employee assistance programs that entitle staff to a limited amount of free counseling.

There are also consultant agencies that can be contacted that specialize in toxic environments. If your unit is really toxic, it might be worth looking into, as the staff you are bleeding out may be costing more than hiring such a service. The level above your manager might be willing to expense the cost if they are losing significant funds due to staff leaving/absenteeism.

You are never alone, and you always have the power to make a change.

Toxic Colleagues

A third key component in a toxic workplace is toxic colleagues. There are many reasons colleagues may be toxic, and it may not be directly related to their professional lives. Their personal lives may be taking a toll and affecting their ability to work. Financial issues, divorce, chronic illness, substance abuse—all of these can play a factor in a colleague's ability to function at work.

If you suspect that something bigger is going on than meets the eye, using your superpower to empathize with what they are going through will help you decide how to handle the situation. How would you want to be treated if you were going through something like this? If you feel called to reach out, do. You may be the lifesaver that they need to get help. Our empathy is often our guide when navigating through situations like this.

While we can cut our dysfunctional coworkers some slack for a while, it isn't sustainable in the long run to carry their load for them. If you have reached out with little response, or if you don't feel this is the right thing to do, there are steps you can take to help the situation.

Characteristics of a Toxic Colleague

Much of this was discussed in the chapter on "Dealing with Difficult People," but the common characteristics of toxic colleagues are summed up here:

• don't take responsibility for their actions	• blame others, make excuses for their actions
• dishonest, withhold or alter information	• gossiping, passive-aggressive or bullying behavior
• tend to avoid management and belittle those who seek management involvement	• make the same mistakes over and over again, refuse to learn from them
• are inauthentic, either falsely sweet or project an attitude of "toughness," or act differently around different people	• don't handle stressful situations well
• "shirk the work," make arising issues your problem to deal with	• make you feel guilty for not helping them
• create drama wherever they go	

How to Deal with a Toxic Colleague

The difficulty with dealing with dysfunctional people is that we often blame the individual, not the behavior. When we shift the focus from the person to the problem, everything shifts. Looking at how we contribute to the situation will help us when we need to interact with the colleague in question to resolve the issue.

You can't change the person – the facets of what makes up an individual—their personality type, their childhood wounding, and the situations they may be going through presently—all affect who they are. You can't change the person, but you can change what you tolerate.

Do not take responsibility for what you did not do – a toxic person is not able to take responsibility for their actions, and so will likely blame you for whatever has occurred. Do not accept this. Resist the urge to become defensive. Recognize that this person is acting out of integrity; you do not have to sacrifice your own. If a situation arises that may require management involvement, write down everything that occurred while it is fresh in your mind so that you have documentation to back up your account. Stick to the facts—use language that denotes what actually happened, omitting conjecture.

Set boundaries – if you are working with this person on a regular basis, set aside a time (when you are calm) to determine what you will and will not tolerate from them. The next time they violate your boundaries, inform them that they have done so, and explain the consequences. If you have tolerated this behavior from them for a while, they may be taken aback that you are "suddenly" enforcing a boundary. This is normal. They are probably not aware of their behavior, and will deem your reaction to set a boundary out of proportion. Stick to your boundary, and follow through with it if they violate it again.

The Vital Component to Stopping Toxicity: Our Response

"When you replace 'Why is this happening to me' with 'What is this trying to teach me,' everything shifts." – Dr. Rutvi Punjani

While we tend to focus on external factors in a toxic workplace (toxic leaders, colleagues, and systems), the key component to the health of any workplace is our response. Our attitude, our behavior, and what we say to others impacts us and those around us. And like a brooding person affects everyone they come into contact with, so does a happy, cheerful person.

It is easy to fall into Victim mode on the Drama Triangle (my job sucks, no one does anything to make it better, my manager is a nightmare!). And that's okay! We have all been there and will be there again. Recognizing that we are on it is ninety percent of the work. Now you can decide how long you want to stay there.

Working in a toxic environment can be overwhelming. It can feel like so much is wrong and it's disheartening to feel that we can't make a difference. But we *can*. One person can make a huge impact on a unit, whether we are aware of how we are influencing others or not. Think of the time a stranger smiled at you and complimented you. That person probably made your day and didn't even know it.

Working in a toxic environment, it can be easy to sink down into a funk. With many negative people around us, it is easier to just be negative. In fact, it can feel like it's bonding. But when it's at the expense of our bodies and our mental well-being, it is not healthy for us. Being the positive person in a room full of negative ones can seem challenging. But, as misery loves company, so do we attract what we are. If someone makes a jeer at your positivity, it means it's working—you are repelling the negative people away from you! Good job! Keep it up, and you will find that the only people who want to be around you are the people you want to be around.

Some practical things you can do as an individual in a toxic work environment:

• be authentic	• don't engage in negative conversations; it is perfectly acceptable to walk away from them
• turn negative conversations into positive ones	• clarify your roles and responsibilities
• set healthy boundaries on what you are willing and not willing to do, and **keep them**	• practice with integrity. Do what you say you are going to do
• if you need support, seek counsel from someone you trust	• document any decisions made or interactions that may escalate

What Healthy Workplace Culture Looks Like

For those of us that have never worked in a healthy work environment, we might not know what we are striving for. Having never worked in one, I didn't know what I was trying to achieve when I was making change in my department—I just knew I wasn't ok with how it was. Although many of us regularly experience an unhealthy work environment, recognizing what is healthy and visualizing this for our workplace will give us hope and give us a guide for what we need to work on.

Signs of a Healthy Work Environment

• sense of unity, sense of purpose	• commitment to values such as honesty and integrity
• generosity	• negative behaviors such as dishonesty actively and openly discouraged
• celebration of differences	• compassion for others in good times and bad
• fairness, justice	• fun, a sense of joy

While not everyone may subscribe to these values all of the time, you can make it a mission to contribute to more positivity on your unit. Food days, small gifts for people who have been doing a great job, recognition for those who help you out—it doesn't have to be big. But the ripple effect that one person can create in a department can extend to others for days, and be reached even outside the workplace. Ever had a co-worker or patient compliment you? I bet you took that home with you to your family. Just as negativity is contagious, so is positivity. And guess what? We have the power to choose. A little appreciation goes a long way, and giving in this situation feels as good as receiving—I promise!

Knowing When to Leave

Sometimes, you can do all the right things, and it still doesn't make a difference. I had a co-worker who had dealt with a toxic colleague in her previous position. She went through all the right channels, and had support of everyone in her department, including his medical governing body. The physician was forced to take anger management, and altered his behavior, much to the delight of the rest of the team. But he still harboured a grudge against my co-worker and found covert ways to demean her, ways that she couldn't prove. She still dreaded working with him, and despite having gone through the process, she decided that she needed to find another place to work. For her, it wasn't worth it.

Sometimes, we just need to move on. There is no failure in doing what is best for us. And if we don't feel we want to go through a whole process of dealing with a toxic manager or colleague, or if the environment is too much, that is okay.

I remember a nurse who worked in our department for only a few months asked incredulously, "This is what happens here!?!" She was gone within a month. It opened our eyes to the fact that things weren't right in our department and started a dialogue for the possibility of change. Sometimes leaving makes a bigger statement than toughing it out.

You have to do what is right for you. If you love your job apart from one person, then don't let that person ruin your life. You have options, it is up to you whether you choose to use them. You always have a choice.

One thing you can do to help you make that decision is looking at your values. Based on the list you created in the earlier chapter, how does this situation relate? Are you consistently compromising your values for this job? Do you value compassion, but finding yourself lacking it for others? Do you value honesty, but find you are lying to your partner, your friends (or yourself) about how difficult your job is?

What actions do you need to take to realign yourself with your values? Does it involve a simple conversation with your manager? Or is the situation much more complex? You always have options.

If you are contemplating leaving your current position, there are steps you can take that will help guide you.

1. Ask yourself: What do I want to change about my current situation?

2. Look at your limiting beliefs. What's *stopping* you from making a change?

3. What options are open to you? What possibilities are out there?

4. Decide what you will stand for, and what you won't.

5. Think about what steps you can take to improve your workplace, or what steps are required to find another place to work.

It can be scary looking for another job, especially if we have been at our current one for a long time. When I was contemplating leaving my department, this had a compounded effect, as I deemed most of my colleagues family. I wasn't just leaving a job, I was leaving a home.

But I also had to realize I wasn't growing. I was stagnant and becoming more resentful of this fact as each day passed. Growth is super important for us as human beings; we feel in a rut when we aren't growing. This doesn't just pertain to work, but we do a tremendous amount of growing in our careers.

Breaking up with a job can be like breaking up with a bad boyfriend: you don't realize how miserable you were until you're out of it. It might be the best change you ever made. Opportunities might arise from this change that you never dreamt of. You might meet new people, or have a chance to advance in your career that you didn't have at your previous job. If you are thinking about leaving, there is a good chance that something inside you is telling you to go. You always have the power to choose.

EXERCISES

1. Think of someone you work with who always goes over and above what they are expected to do. Think of some small way you can show them your appreciation. You can get them a coffee, a card, or you can just tell them how much you appreciate them. This will not only make your co-worker's day, but will give you a boost of happy chemicals as well.

2. If you are thinking about working somewhere else, but the idea of leaving where you are seems daunting (you feel at home in your current job, you haven't updated your resume, the idea of interviewing seems scary, etc.), you don't have to do everything at once. Start by simply browsing for jobs, seeing what is out there. If you see something, it really doesn't hurt to apply—you might not get an interview, and if you do, you can always turn it down. You have nothing to lose by going to an interview, and everything to gain—including interview experience. You can apply to jobs that are out of your scope, or even out of your career field, just to get the interview experience. By making small steps, you can let your feet get wet and see how it would feel if you were offered another position. Then you can truly know if it would be the right move for you.

CHAPTER 19

Leaving Work at Work

"I'm not okay, you're not okay, but that's okay." – Elizabeth Kubler-Ross

We were staying overtime again, as usual. I was on call with a fantastic technologist, Carmen, and I had a wonderful nurse, Jenny, who was on a later shift coming over to help me out. I didn't know how fortunate I was to have these people with me that day.

My patient was bleeding internally, which is usually deemed an emergency, yet we hadn't been able to get to him right away.

I went out to speak with the patient—he was a big man, over 300 pounds. The unit had sent him down unmonitored and therefore I assumed he was stable. He was lucid but agitated. He was sitting up in bed, asking when we would be getting to him. I replied the radiologist was coming right out to consent him.

As my colleagues and I were preparing the room, the radiologist went out to consent the patient. I heard him calling out to us, and we ran out to see what was wrong.

There was blood—everywhere. The entire hallway was covered in blood. The patient had vomited hundreds of milliliters worth all over our back hallway. I questioned if we should call a code, and the rad replied that he would contact the ICU but to get him on the table *now*.

We quickly brought the patient into the room. He was still conscious, but diaphoretic and even more agitated. He told us he was incontinent of feces, and then his eyes rolled back into his head and he lost consciousness. Jenny and I yelled to Carmen to call a code, and we proceeded to start emergency care—getting oxygen, attempting to start another IV, which was subsequently lost as he was so diaphoretic that he just sweated them away.

The code team—always miraculously present within a couple minutes—came to take over. The patient still had a pulse and was breathing, but this quickly changed. CPR was started within minutes of them arriving, and we worked on him efficiently. We were lining up to take turns doing compressions—he was so large that this was incredibly challenging, and I wasn't strong enough to compress as deeply as I needed to and was soon replaced by someone else.

After what seemed like hours but was probably only thirty or forty minutes, they called the code. Everyone grimly congratulated each other on doing a good job, and the code team started packing up.

"Hold on a minute," I asked, exhausted. "Where is this patient going?" We were an interventional suite, not a unit, so the patient needed to be brought back upstairs.

The code team members shrugged. "Normally if he made it, he would go up to ICU, but he didn't make it."

Carmen was on the phone with the inpatient unit he had been sent down by. They were refusing to take the deceased patient because his bed had already been transferred to ICU. They had already brought his belongings to ICU as soon as the radiologist had called up.

"You'll have to bag him and tag him yourself," a code team member replied, and walked away.

It was eight p.m., we were already three hours overtime, we were still on call and could be paged back at all hours of the night. The patient was covered in blood and feces, and our operating room, his stretcher, and the hallway were covered in blood. Looking back on it, I still get angry with myself for not insisting one of the two areas take the patient. We were exhausted, still in shock, and not thinking clearly.

One of the girls on the code team was helpful enough to go and get a death bundle for us, as we didn't have them in our department. She kindly explained what needed to be done, as we didn't have deaths very often.

Just as we were finishing cleaning up the patient, the ICU phoned to inform us that a family member was on her way down to see him. Our eyes widened in horror, and we madly began mopping and wiping down surfaces that were covered in blood. We hurriedly went to clean up the room, the hallway, and the stretcher, as everything was soiled. We couldn't get everything, but it looked more presentable when the family member arrived.

We waited in our control room as she said her goodbyes. When she had her time, we phoned security to escort the body away and went home to try to get some sleep, as we were still on call and could get paged back at any moment.

Think I left work at work that day?

While hopefully not all days are traumatic for us, we still have situations that we take home and think about on a regular basis.

When I went home, all I thought were "what if" questions: What if we had gotten to him sooner? What if we had called the code earlier? What if I had been stronger so I could have done CPR better?

These thoughts, none of them helpful, still come to me as I reflect back on that day. As a nurse, obviously my focus was what I could have done better for the patient, and I naturally do this, even if it means scolding myself and holding myself accountable for things that were outside of my control.

Psychological Detachment

Having busy, chaotic workloads, health care workers are susceptible to taking things personally and ruminating about it at home. Remembering things we should have done but forgot while eating dinner with our family, cursing ourselves for making that med error, or questioning what we could have done better all swirl around our minds as we try to wash away the day and enjoy time with our loved ones.

Being able to have a healthy work-life balance involves not taking work home with you. Known as psychological detachment, it is defined as "the extent to which an individual disengages from work-related matters during leisure time."[1] Being able to do this improves our well-being, as well as our ability to do our jobs.

HCWs deal with serious, stressful, and tragic situations every day. The typical advice for not taking work home with you is not always helpful for us. Suggestions to use humor, watch a favourite show, or phone a friend to vent are sometimes not feasible. Try meditating after work when one of your long-term pediatric patients on your unit suddenly crashes and isn't expected to recover. And while our friends and family members obviously want to support us, they can't really understand what we are going through when we have a tough day.

This can be isolating for us. I had a roommate who used to complain about how difficult his day was, and I would look at him sardonically and say, "Yeah, but did anybody die?" I was using it as a joke, but in truth, I found I couldn't relate to him when he complained about an employee missing a delivery order. However significant his work tribulations were to him, I just couldn't relate.

This is part of the reason why so many HCWs have friendships with each other outside of work. This is not only positive, it is necessary to establish bonds with people in the field, as otherwise it is difficult to find support. Having someone who *gets it* is imperative to maintaining mental health if we are to thrive in the career that we are so passionate about. While it is also healthy to have friends who aren't in our career field, we nonetheless get validation from the friends who are.

There are so many reasons why we think about work outside of work. Similar to certain fields such as the police force or the military, we actually take on the persona of the job. Ever talk to a cop outside of his working hours? You can usually tell he's a cop. And with health care workers (nurses, in particular), we have certain characteristics that make us easily identifiable. We are nurturing and naturally giving. We go out of our way to help others, even outside of work. It is difficult to turn it off; it's just how we are.

Which is why it is so difficult to leave work at work. We are caring throughout the day, so how do we "turn it off" when we get home?

One thing we have on our side is that we have clear physical boundaries with our jobs—when we leave the hospital (or clinic, or residence), we are off. Our assignments don't continue at home like they do for teachers or managers. We don't usually work from home, so there are clear environmental cues that allow us to turn work off as soon as we walk out the door.

Tips and Tricks to Help You Leave Work at Work

1. *Change out of your scrubs before you leave the hospital*—not only for hygienic reasons, but this signals to your brain that your shift is over. The sooner you end your work day (before you even leave the building), the sooner you can transition to "home" mode.

2. *Visualization*—have a mental image that you visualize as you walk out the door, like you are walking over a bridge and away from work, leaving all of its stressors in the building. With practice, this will help solidify that work stays at work, and it will be easier to turn it off on your drive home.

3. *Listen to a podcast or audiobook on your way home*—this involves more attention than passively listening to the radio, so it will be more difficult to focus on your shift if you need to pay attention to the storyline of a good crime novel.

4. *Have a ritual you do as soon as you get home*—showering is a great thing to do, as it helps reset you mentally as well as physically. My friend Kristin boils the kettle for tea as soon as she walks in the door—it helps her relax and it gives her a chance to sit down and decompress before attending to after-work activities.

5. *Schedule something for right after your shift ends, if you can—a workout class, a massage*—this helps you physically and mentally end your work day and launch right into something else. Bonus if it is something that is good for you. Exercise helps alleviate stress, and a massage will help relax you. What matters is that you are doing something for you, and not thinking about what happened at work.

6. *Not venting to our spouses*—this is a tough one. This effectively takes work home with you as soon as you open your mouth. We all do this, and it's necessary from time to time, but resist the urge to habitually vent about your day to your partner, roommate, etc. If you are still thinking about the situation the next day, talk to a colleague at work about it. The more you discuss work problems when you are not at work, the harder it is to establish those boundaries. It may seem like bonding with your partner, but they are only receiving your side of the story. When you vent to your spouse about a colleague, you are dragging them into your drama. You could work out a spat that you had with a colleague and your spouse could still be upset about it. This does not help you leave things at work, or bond with your partner, or help your relationships at work.

So much of what we do at work our families don't fully understand anyway. When we consistently vent to our families about our jobs, we are cutting into the precious time we have with them. It also causes us to relive the experience the more we talk about it, keeping our bodies in that past, unpleasant moment. We all need to vent sometimes about work, but make an honest effort not to make it a daily occurrence.

7. *Turn off social media, dings, etc.*—these, however insignificant they seem, are mental stimulants that cause you to perk up every time they ring off. If you are feeling anxious and are trying to feel calmer outside of work, this doesn't help. Unless you are expecting an important call, turn down your ringer volume, and absolutely turn off audio notifications from your email or social media—you'll see it when you see it.

8. *Laughter*—it interrupts that thought process that has you ruminating over your day. Even if you don't feel like it at first, put on something you find funny. For me, it's the skit with Richard Simmons on *Whose Line is it Anyway?* Without fail, I will laugh every time at him being the prop for the cast in his tiny shorts, no matter how gloomy I am in the moment. I may not be 100 percent after, but I feel better, and that's a start.

9. *Think of what went right*—it is human nature to zero in on our mistakes, but do we ever grant ourselves the same attention with all of the good things we do in a day? How holding the hand of the little girl who was scared helped her get through her blood test, or how you retrieved a warm blanket for a patient who was shivering in the hallway? For the traumatic event that occurred above, instead of thinking about what went wrong in that scenario, I focus on the fact that I had amazing colleagues with me that day, that I managed to get an IV, that we were able to make the area presentable for the family member. Don't just think about all of the things you did, actually write them down. This will not only get you out of ruminating, but it will provide a visual for you to see all of the good things you do in a day, things you take for granted because you do them all the time. How many people can say they cheered up an oncology patient while they received chemo? Or comforted a family member in their darkest hours? We need to be reminded of the amazing things we do on a regular basis because it is so normal for us. It's normal for Beyonce to kill it onstage, yet that doesn't stop her from owning it, every single time. Normalize celebrating your wins, especially when it feels like you failed.

If you still can't turn it off:

1. *Identify what it is that's still bugging you*—this is probably your Inner Child who is feeling inadequate, so ask her what it is. Is she feeling like she messed up? Is she feeling scared? Talk with her (aloud or silently) and ask her what she is feeling. LABEL it. Often naming it helps us uncover what the real issue is. Tell yourself you will commit to fifteen minutes of ruminating/worrying/ catastrophizing, then, consciously do something else.

2. *Ask for a debrief at work*—chances are, if you lose sleep over something that happened the day before, it would be helpful to talk to someone about it. After the above situation happened to us, my manager suggested we do a debrief. It

seemed a bit unnecessary after a few days, but it actually really helped to get together with members of the code team and discuss how I felt and what could have been better. It was validating, and it gave me the closure I needed to begin to move on.

3. *Talk to a counselor/therapist*—they can offer you a more objective perspective than a debrief at work can offer, and can also provide ongoing support.

And you know what? Some days, you're just going to take work home with you, and none of these suggestions will help, and that is okay. Some days, you just need to survive. Accepting that this is okay and you are safe to feel this way is what you might need in that moment. We save lives for a goddamned living, of course there are going to be days when we are not okay.

It's okay to not be okay.

EXERCISES

1. Think of a time where you had a really awful day. What did you need most in that moment? Was it cheering up? Was it acceptance? Was it validation? The next time you have a bad day, make a conscious effort to ask yourself what you need most in the moment, and gift yourself just that. Ask for support from others if you need to take a night off from other responsibilities.

2. Write out a list of activities you enjoy, and keep them somewhere you have access to. The next time you have a bad day, go through the list and pick one activity you'd like to do. Sometimes, when we are down, we know we need to get ourselves out of a funk, but we feel a bit scattered. Having a list of things written will help give you direction if in the moment you forget.

CHAPTER 20

Letting Go

"Letting go will teach you the art of being soft and humble,
yet powerful and free." – Alexandra Vasiliu

Some things in life we just can't control. Over the years, I have met this lesson many times, and yet I still sometimes fall back into my old patterns.

When my mother was at the height of her physical and mental illness, a couple years after my father had passed away, I was at the end of my rope. My mother, while allowing me enduring power of attorney as it meant I could sign things for her when she didn't feel like it, was nonetheless paranoid that I was stealing from her. She was impulsive, irrational, and prone to mood swings, more intense than ever before. Her disability check was the only income she had, yet she would make extravagant purchases such as first-class flights, offering to take people on tropical vacations. She let her health benefits lapse and was paying $800 a week for her medication. She still had a mortgage payment for the large house she lived in. If her spending continued, she was at risk of losing her home and not being able to afford the medications for her epilepsy, chronic pain, and stomach issues. Her mental illness, coupled with her argumentative nature and clouded by substance abuse, meant I couldn't make her see reason, and she only allowed me to make decisions on her behalf if it suited her mood at the time. The situation was a ticking time bomb, both in reality and in my head.

When she suffered her second stroke, I knew I had an opportunity to do something. While she was admitted, I asked for a psych consult, a mini-mental, and a MOCA to determine if she was capable of making her own decisions. Even with her substance abuse (both alcohol and oxycontin), I knew there was more to her cognitive impairment than this. Despite being fatigued from all of the caregiving I had been doing for her, I was grimly aware of the fact that I would be able to make the "right" decisions for her once they deemed her incompetent, something I was sure they would do. I was mentally selling her house and finding her assisted living, selling her furniture, and seizing control of her finances so that they would last out her lifetime (she was only fifty-five at the time).

The hospital was very supportive of my concerns, and we would regularly collaborate. It was a tricky situation for everyone. One day after a family conference was held, the physician looking after my Mum took me aside. He regretfully told me that they could not deem my mother legally incapacitated. I was incredulous at this. I recounted all of her financial fiascos, her substance abuse, her strokes. She was forgetful, often leaving the oven on or falling asleep with a cigarette in bed. She was a danger to herself and others!

I did my best to explain this to him. He waited for me to finish, smiling patiently. He nodded in agreement, stating he knew that she was in a bad way.

"And her MOCA? She bombed it!" I cried indignantly. How in the world could this be happening?

Again, he smiled at me kindly. "I know she did," he stated quietly. "I feel for you, I really and truly do. But your mother does have periods of lucidity, and with that, I can't take her rights away from her. Once we take them away, they can't be given back. Your mother is one of the many who slip between the cracks in our system, I'm afraid."

I was still looking at him like he had three heads. "But how can you say that, with everything she's done? She's a danger to herself!" I repeated defiantly, knowing I had already lost the fight.

He smiled wistfully at me. "Sometimes in life, we just have to accept that some people are going to make bad decisions, and there is nothing we can do about it." He apologized again and excused himself, leaving me bewildered and wondering what the hell I was going to do now.

That physician gave me the biggest wake-up call I had received during this entire ordeal. While I felt responsible for taking care of my mother now that my father was gone, I couldn't MAKE her do anything, even if I knew it was for her own good. Her mental state obviously in question, I thought I was doing the right thing, even though it was slowly destroying me. My relationships with my friends, partner, and coworkers suffered immensely during that time. I was exhausted, bitter at being dealt this situation in my twenties when I should have been enjoying some of my best years. I was looking for places to find control in a life where I felt like everything was out of control.

Being in command of the situation gave me power when I felt powerless to make any change. This need to control was an attempt to keep me feeling safe. I had already watched my father suffer from cancer, helpless, and despite having the knowledge, resources, and connections, it didn't change the outcome. I had felt shame and sadness that I didn't do more. I now had a mother who was spiraling towards a similar fate, and despite there being a lot of animosity between us, I felt I needed to honour my father's dying request to take care of her. I fell into a similar trap with her, believing that if I could just find the right information, reach out to the right people, or simply say the right thing, it would change the situation. It was too painful at the time for me to process how ill my mother was, and instead of allowing myself to feel the uncomfortable emotions, I charged into (fruitless) action.

So much of life is out of our control, yet we search for ways to try to overcome this fact. Whether it is a person's viewpoint, the flow of the unit, or how a system is run, we have the power to make a real change in any of these if we choose to. The trick is knowing when and where to execute the power we have to change.

This book is all about empowerment—my intention for this book is to open the reader up to her own power, her own worth, her own destiny of change. These are the elements that are in our power to change. Why talk about letting go?

Because mastering the art of letting go gracefully will allow you to accept things as they are, before you try to make change in areas that you deem necessary to uproot in your life—whether that be an altercation with a colleague, a dispute with a manager, or deciding whether to leave a current position. All of these lie within your control. What about these issues requires you to accept what you can't control?

Resistance to Letting Go

> *"Red flags don't feel like red flags when they feel like home."*
> *— The Holistic Psychologist*

Sometimes, we want to let go of something that doesn't serve us—a job, a relationship, Ben and/or Jerry—but we feel resistance. We don't always understand intellectually why we keep choosing to hold on to people and situations that cause us to feel unhappy or stuck. In his book *Letting Go,* Dr. Hawkins attests that much of the world is conditioned to buy into negativity.[1] Our negative belief that things never get better, they only get worse, is programmed into us by our parents and teachers, and perpetuated by what we see on the news every day.

As an '80s baby, one of my favourite movies was *Labyrinth* (David Bowie's tight pants not withstanding). In one scene, Jennifer Connelly's character takes her on-point brows down a wrong turn and falls into a tunnel of "helping hands." They ask her which way she wants to go, up (back towards the castle she is conquering) or down. She elects, since she's pointed that way anyway, to go down. "SHE CHOSE DOWN!" they cry gleefully as they send her into the abyss. I would yell at the TV each time I watched this scene, bewildered at why she would ever choose to go down (ironically into a dungeon where she was meant to forget her purpose).

Unfortunately, many of us "choose down" because we are already heading in that direction. It takes a lot of energy to turn the ship around that has been cruising on "negative" for most of our lives. Holding on to pain serves us in some way, whether we are conscious of it or not. It may keep us righteously angry and grant us someone to blame, or it may keep us in a rut because it is too scary to move on.

Much of the pain we choose to hold on to is due to fear of uncovering what is underneath. It feels better to be angry at someone for hurting us than it does to just feel hurt. Negative feelings are hard to sit with. It feels safer for us to bitch and complain about our working conditions than it does to go through a formal complaint process, or *gasp* find another job. To feel these feelings or make different choices leaves us feeling vulnerable—it is easier to be angry or apathetic.

And this is what keeps us stuck.

Don't get me wrong: We do not deserve to have others hurt us, or to be dealing with the conditions that we HCWs are living with. But we need to accept "what is" before we can do anything about it.

The Power to Choose

People make positive changes every day. The world is filled with people who improve their lives, despite the arduous events we face. It is negative programming that causes us to believe that we are unable to change. We have a choice whether we want to keep seeing the world in a negative light, and buy into the negativity, or if we choose to see things from a more positive (but still realistic) perspective. Through questioning our thoughts, by examining our beliefs, we can slowly start to turn the boat around and begin paddling downstream instead of working hard to go uphill. We have the power to change our thoughts and choose better ones— what thoughts do you choose to believe?

You are free to choose your beliefs. If you desire to let go of negative beliefs/people/situations, it begins with your power to choose. Limiting beliefs such as "I'm too old" or "I'm not smart enough" or "It's like this everywhere" keep us from choosing happiness. Our programming (much of it unconscious) can be changed when we decide to look at it. We run these programs because they were what was introduced to us at the time our beliefs were developing– it's time for a reboot in our thinking.

If you are feeling resistance in changing how you are thinking, look closer. What is it you (or your Inner Child) are afraid might happen if you let go of what isn't good for you? Is she afraid of feeling pain? Is she afraid of being abandoned or rejected?

When I decided I needed a change from diagnostic imaging, the job I was in for twelve years, a lot of emotions came up. I had felt stuck in a rut, but I didn't want to face it because it seemed scary to leave. What if I hated my next job? What if I didn't get enough hours? What if following my passion failed? I stayed in a job that I wasn't passionate about for too long, for the wrong reasons, because it brought up fears that I would not be financially secure and I wouldn't have emotional support (two things I experienced as a child that I was afraid to experience again). I complained and blamed because it was easier than the alternative. I resisted the potential to realize my dreams, and I didn't know why—until I decided to look at *why* I was resisting.

According to Hawkins, if you are experiencing resistance to a potential change, this is a good thing.[2] Our Inner Child is trying to keep us safe by tricking us into believing we aren't capable, it's not working, we're not good enough. It means there are fears coming to the surface that need exploring—we can't change what we are not aware of. Feeling resistance is a marker to tell us something is there for us to examine.

The Benefits to Letting Go

As human beings, we are meant to evolve. Staying the same is not good for our brains, our bodies, and our souls. Letting go of what no longer serves us allows new things to come in. When we fully let go, we experience benefits in many aspects of our lives (adapted from *Letting Go* by David Hawkins)[3]:

Problem-solving—when we let go of the negative thoughts and beliefs we have been carrying, we can see things more plainly. What used to be a block is now a path. When we decide to let go of the belief that we are too old to start a new career, for example, a world of opportunities opens up to us. Suddenly, we can apply to work in a different hospital, go back to school for upgrading, or change careers completely. As soon as we decide to let go of limiting beliefs, we can see things more clearly, and we can make steps to improve our lives.

Emotional growth—when we are not in touch with our emotional intelligence, it affects our cognition. Often, when we have not processed our emotions, we make irrational decisions. The longer we hold on to unprocessed emotions, the longer we continue to stay in situations that are not good for us. I stayed in a job that was stunting my growth because I was afraid, and I continued to choose that situation despite knowing it wasn't what was best for me. Once we process the emotion, things that seemed like a big deal no longer seem to be as scary, and we make different choices as a result. When I accepted my financial and emotional fears of making a career move (and a geographical one), the changes seemed less daunting. While it wasn't easy, it has provided me the growth that my soul was hungering for. How do you imagine you would grow as a person if you made that change you have been toying with?

Lifestyle—when we let go of the limiting beliefs that keep us stuck, we do things we didn't think we were capable of doing. If you were afraid to join a fitness class because you thought you wouldn't be able to keep up but chose to participate regardless, you move a step forward in evolving. Your life can transform before your eyes. Suddenly you are now saying yes to all of the opportunities that you would have said no to before, and your life can completely change. Doing things that we used to avoid out of fear can shift our lives and fill them with the joy we have been seeking. We start doing things we want to do, not just the activities we do out of obligation.

Relationships—when we let go of thoughts and emotions that we no longer need, we become more relaxed, and more loving. When we let go of negativity, we see the world from a lighter, kinder place—and the people and situations shift as a result of it. Our relationships improve as we become who we were longing to be.

Steps to Letting Go

1. *Accept that there is something to let go of*—if you are in the early stages of grief or anger, it might not be something you are ready to do just yet—and that is okay. Our inability to handle discomfort sometimes makes us want to rush through things before we have actually processed them. Give yourself the time and space you need. You will know when you are ready to let go.

2. *LABEL it*—name the feeling. Accept that it is there. What is it that you are holding on to? If it is a grudge, what are you resentful of? What is at the heart of the matter? What about the fact that your manager is piling work on you is really bothering you? Is it that she didn't listen to your concerns? Do you feel that he doesn't care? Is someone else being shown favoritism? If it was a little girl who had this happen to her, what would she likely say is bothering her? That she is feeling left out? That she has hurt feelings? It might sound childish, but naming the pain in the simplest language often gets at the heart of the matter. This is where the wounding is, and why you can't let it go. Be present with the pain (as opposed to numbing it or stifling it) as long as you need to be. Express it through creativity. Then, lovingly let it go.

3. *Journal*—write down what the issue is, connect to your feelings. If it feels right, address it to your Inner Child and see what it is that is really bothering her—the root of the matter. Letting it all out on paper gets it out of our minds and helps us straighten out our thoughts.

4. *Meditation*—set an intention to face what is bothering you and hold it in your awareness. If feelings or thoughts come up, sit with them. Face it, sit with the discomfort. I promise you, if you commit to this, the feelings will often subside.

5. *Visualization*—get creative. See the pain in a human form and see yourself sitting with it. Or putting a Band-Aid on it. Or visualize yourself cutting the cord between you and the issue you are having.

6. ***Create an affirmation when it keeps coming up***—if you have something you are having trouble letting go of, it is likely to keep coming up. This doesn't mean you haven't let it go. Remind yourself of how far you have come, and repeat a phrase each time it does, such as, "This is just a reminder, I have let this go," or "I have overcome this." Pretty soon, when it does come up again, you won't react to it anymore. Since we can't control what happens to us, we can only change how we respond. When we change our response, we know we have truly changed.

7. *Nature*—putting distance between yourself and whatever is bothering you can help, and there is no better place to do so than in nature. Find a quiet spot that you have easy access to, even if it's just your backyard. Notice the details of the trees and flowers. I don't always solve my problems being in nature, but I always feel a bit better after being in it.

8. ***Try to see the bigger picture***—what lesson can you take away from this experience? What won't you do again? By being conscious of this, it will be less likely that there will be a repeat occurrence. I know this can be hard, especially if you have been really hurt, but if you are open to it, it will give you purpose.

9. *Music/dancing*—music helps us get out of our heads and into our bodies. It is healing in and of itself. When you are feeling stuck, find a song that makes you feel like dancing and notice how you feel after you do it—it can give you a temporary reprieve, which gets us off the hamster wheel.

10. ***Be compassionate with yourself***—sometimes we are hard on ourselves for not forgiving. You are now compounding not forgiving yourself with not forgiving yourself! Letting go is some of the hardest work we as humans can do. Be gentle.

Being Open to What Is, and What Will Be

The way through to letting go is first accepting "what is." Accepting what is will help guide you through all aspects of life. Deciding to change from a place of acceptance versus not accepting is the difference between a leisurely stroll versus running uphill: you get to the same place in the end, but your energy and resolve are completely different. Accepting what is includes your personal life, your relationships, your children, your friendships, your hobbies, your religion, etc. Accepting what is will catapult you into making new choices and forging new paths. Deciding to change from a place of acceptance versus fighting with yourself is the difference between walking with a child hand in hand versus dragging them kicking and screaming. It requires so much effort to change what we are shaming ourselves for, as opposed to giving ourselves grace.

Accepting what is doesn't mean accepting that it is okay. Like our resilient cancer patients who face a serious prognosis, they don't deny that they have cancer. But they also don't sit idly by, either. Accepting what is with grace and humility is the first step to making real change. This is something that is deeply personal, deeply spiritual, and not an easy path to walk. Knowing yourself is the best way to know what you want and what you don't want. Being open to change will shift your life outside of the box you see yourself in right now.

From Melody Beattie's book of meditations, *The Language of Letting Go*:

"Today, I will let go. I will stop trying to control everything. I will stop trying to make myself better, and I will let myself be."[3]

Letting go of focusing on the problem produces a major shift in our consciousness. When we stare at the problem, the problem just gets bigger. When we HCWs put ourselves first instead of putting all of our energy into fixing our health care system, solutions come to us. Just because we don't know how to make something happen right now doesn't mean it's not possible.

I was miserable when I was dealing with my mother's health issues, but I felt like I had no choice. I couldn't accept her the way she was, and being fixated on the problem did not help one iota. I wasted a lot of precious time and energy focusing on "fixing" her instead of having the courage to look at my own life and decide what I needed to make me happy. I won't get my twenties back. It has given me more resolve to stop wasting my life trying to fix people and situations that I cannot change, and to focus my energy on doing what makes *me* happy. Don't do what I did. Don't deny that the problem is there, but don't live in it.

Creativity

Be open to exploring new possibilities. There may be things in your life now that you can't change, but being open to opportunities will help you through this. If you have always dreamed of moving to a tropical island, explore what it would look like if you made it happen. I'm not saying jump on the next plane, but daydream what it might look like. Would you live in a mansion? A cute hut on the beach? Would you be working in the health care field, or would you want to try something else? Successful, happy people daydream on a regular basis, and have always done so. From Albert Einstein to Elon Musk, these people tapped into their imagination and emphasized the importance of it. Allowing our minds to wander is therapy in itself, and may spark an aha moment that leads you to something life-changing— for the better.

Perhaps your dreams involve doing something other than health care. Explore that. Don't just shut the idea out. Your higher self is the quiet voice that you hear when you are still, when you fantasize, and this is where great ideas come from! Ever heard of shower thoughts? These occur when our mind is truly relaxed. Allow that Inner Child to dream, to imagine, to play. Don't shut down a possibility just because it doesn't seem rational. Many successful people in the world started with an idea or a dream, and made it a reality. You don't have to be the next Steve Jobs to benefit from this activity. What could you see in your life if you didn't have restrictions put upon it? And know that making a change doesn't have to mean forever. Sometimes we try things and they don't work out – that's okay, at least we tried, and aren't sitting around wondering what if. Toying with ideas can lead to changes, but we have to be open to being open.

There is a reason psychologists and coaches ask their clients what they would be doing if money were out of the picture. What would you do? Explore that! It doesn't mean you have to up and quit your job, but creativity is something that all of us possess, all of us were meant to dive into. Something not necessarily for anyone else, just for you. Maybe you like to paint old furniture, or experiment with gardening. Who cares if it's successful? It opens up new pathways in our brain that have been dormant (maybe since kindergarten) and enriches our lives. What areas of life have you not explored yet, that working full-time-plus hours hasn't allowed you to explore before?

Our world is shifting its perspective rapidly. People aren't buying into the need to work our entire lives to save for a retirement that we may or may not get to. Losing both of my parents young taught me the valuable lesson to enjoy my life and do the things I want to do *now*, because tomorrow may never come. I didn't want to live my father's life of working every day and not stopping to enjoy life until it was too late. I want to enjoy the life I have now. We have no control over our final days, nor do we know when they will come. Why are we living lives for tomorrow? Live for now.

Find joy in everything you do. Find love everywhere it may be, whether it is enjoying a joke with a colleague, or a cup of coffee before you start your shift. Enjoy every moment that you have. We were put here to find joy in our lives. Like a canvas, we are the artist, we decide where to put the paint. What life do you want to create? *You* are the creator of your life!

Loving What Is

Loving what is will help you accept what you cannot change, and give you a clearer perspective for what you value most. This will help you shift from the problem to the solution. Navigating what you will accept and what you will not accept is easier than focusing on the problem. While this book has given you tools to help guide you throughout whatever situation you may be experiencing, at the end of the day, you decide what you want in your life.

If a career in health care is your passion, your dream, your gift to the world, then you will find a way to make it work, even in these tough times. Loving what is will help you accept the little details of the day, whether it be a crabby patient, a difficult colleague, or a heavy workload. But you must decide from within if this is your destiny. You will see a shift once you begin to accept what you cannot control. It will help align you with your next step, whether it be a conversation with a manager or a resignation letter.

EXERCISES

1. Think of a situation that is difficult for you. How have you been trying to control the outcome? What have you been doing that seems like an uphill battle? As difficult as it may seem, imagine letting go of that situation. Picture yourself simply allowing the unit to run the way it is, accepting the people involved as they are, and the situation playing out in a way that involves no action on your part. How does it feel to simply accept the situation as it stands? Is it scary, do you feel like you need to be "doing" something? Or does it bring up other emotions (sadness, for instance) that things are the way they are? Let yourself feel into any emotions that come up.

2. Take the situation that came to mind and go through the steps of letting go as listed above. In your journal, notice what insights and feelings come up as you move through the steps. Once you have completed them (and they don't need to be done

in any particular order, nor do they all need to be completed), notice how you feel about the situation now. Does the process of letting go seem less daunting, less emotional now?

3. Do something kind to nurture yourself as you move through this process—whatever is most nurturing for you. One of the hardest things we do in life is let go of things that are no longer serving us—make sure you are giving yourself empathy and compassion, as well as getting enough support.

CHAPTER 21

Energy Management

"I believe depression is legitimate. But I also believe that if you don't exercise, eat nutritious foods, get sunlight, get enough sleep, consume positive material [and] surround yourself with support, then you aren't giving yourself a fighting chance." – Jim Carrey

While it is important to have information and tools that you can use to maintain a healthy life in the health care field, you need to give yourself a fighting chance. While in the above quote Jim Carrey was referring specifically to depression, it can be applied to anyone at any time.

Our energy levels can become drained very quickly from the work that we do. Our jobs are physically, mentally, and emotionally challenging. We are constantly assessing, intervening, moving, transferring, and being emotional support for our patients, families, and coworkers. Our energy can be all over the place—unable to get off the couch after a long, tiring day, or go-go-go all day at work and then at home and not being able to shut it off when we are trying to sleep. Managing our energy levels to maintain balance is something we could all benefit from.

How can you know if your feelings of stress or overwhelm are related to something physical or emotional if you are not eating right, getting enough rest, or having some amount of physical activity in your life? Eating healthy and getting enough sleep and exercise will place you at baseline. If you are not getting all of these, you are not at baseline. This means you are not able to cope with life as well as what you could be. And most of us are not operating at our actual baseline.

Barriers to Taking Care of Our Own Health

The pandemic has taken a lot out of us. I witness in myself that I am still not sleeping well, not eating right, and not exercising as much as I would like. I'm not taking care of myself when I need to be taking care of myself the most. And this is when it is the hardest to get out of the cycle.

HCWs have a lot of barriers to maintaining our energy levels, more so than the average person. A 2021 study of new graduate nurses found they encounter the same issues experienced nurses have when it comes to healthy eating and exercising.[1] Four main barriers were identified to maintaining a healthy lifestyle for new graduate nurses:

Time—working overtime, changing shifts last-minute to accommodate the needs of the unit, and working twelve-hour shifts makes it difficult to meal plan. It is also more challenging to engage in physical activities due to fatigue, more time needed to sleep, or preference for spending time with loved ones instead.

Shift Work—irregular schedules impede our ability to get quality and quantity sleep. Challenges around rotating schedules cause eating schedules to be off, snacking to maintain energy and fight off exhaustion, and reduced motivation to eat healthy foods. Being physically active is hindered by difficulty participating in group activities and sports due to a rotating schedule.

Work Environment—working without breaks/short breaks causes us to choose foods that are quick and easy, but not necessarily nutritious. It also makes it challenging to find time to drink water (and time to pee).

Work Culture—having unhealthy food choices at the workplace or potlucks can make it difficult to say no to, for willpower reasons as well as a desire to fit in.

It's frustrating when we go to our doctors with complaints of fatigue or mood imbalances and they first recommend more sleep or exercise—but it plays a pivotal role in our energy level, mood, and immune system. I notice right away when I have not been exercising, because I am crabby and more likely to feel anxious, which plays a factor in my sleeping patterns, which affects my decisions to eat healthy … and it becomes a vicious cycle.

I know self-care activities can seem difficult to do in the moment, especially when we are at the point of exhaustion that many of us are in. But doing these activities can actually make us stronger. Self-care can help health care workers cope with stressors (e.g., staffing concerns) at our place of work more effectively.[2]

For those of us who haven't been taking care of ourselves properly, it can seem very daunting to completely overhaul our lives. The idea of starting to exercise, eat healthy, meditate, learn yoga, and find a counselor all at once because we want to really change ourselves can be discouraging. It's our black-and-white, all-or-nothing thinking that keeps us procrastinating. How do we get off the cycle? By making small changes.

The One-Percent Improvement Strategy

In James Clear's book *Atomic Habits,* the author asserts how making tiny changes consistently makes a big impact in our daily lives. Although this information is nothing new, the exercises and tips he gives in order to actually stick with it are very motivating. How do you eat an elephant? One bite at a time.

Clear recounts how, in 2003, Dave Brailsford took the British cycling team to victory in the 2008 Olympics, winning sixty percent of the gold medals.[3] Before Brailsford, the British cycling team had been renowned for its poor performance, failing to win the Tour de France for 110 years. They were so well known for this that one of the top bike manufacturers refused to sell bikes to the British team for fear that it would hurt their sales. By implementing small, one-percent improvements in every aspect of their training, from the bike seats to the cycling shorts to the quality of their sleep, they were able to improve so dramatically that they set nine Olympic records by 2012.

How do small changes make such a big difference? By being easy to do, we set ourselves up for success. The hardest part of starting a new habit is creating the habit itself. By starting small and creating the habit, whatever it is (going to the gym, meditating, asking for help), it becomes ingrained in our subconscious (much like going to the fridge for a snacky snack when we get home from work can become a habit).

Clear demonstrates how doing something daily for two minutes—just two minutes—can create lifelong, lasting habits that lead to dramatic changes in our lives. If you want to cultivate an exercise habit, try going to the gym every day for two minutes. That's the trick, though, just two minutes, then leave. Anybody can do anything for two minutes. This creates the habit, and you will eventually find that you are looking forward to the habit you've created.

In the way of energy management, the suggested tips of maintaining healthy energy levels require dedication, which can be achieved through creating healthy habits. Yes, we know we should be eating right and exercising, yet we aren't doing it. Overhauling your life all at once will set you up for failure. Starting small, no matter how trivial it may seem, is truly the best way to form a daily healthy habit.

Plan, Execute

Make a plan of the goals you would like to achieve. Be thoughtful about why you want to achieve them. I recommend setting an intention for health and wellness as opposed to losing weight (e.g., "I want to go to the gym to get stronger and have more energy" instead of "I want to lose ten pounds"), and set small, achievable targets related to this goal. Start working on them one at a time. Make sure the goals are specific (e.g., "I want to go to the gym three times/week").

Once you have written down what you would like to achieve and have specified how you are going to achieve it, have a plan in place for when, not if, you don't meet a goal. Slip-ups are inevitable, and it's okay to cheat on your diet or skip an exercise class once in a while. Catch yourself when you start to slip … what is the first thing to go? For me, it's meditating. I notice that if I start skipping my morning meditation (more than once a week), I will also start getting lazy with exercising, which leads to eating less than optimally, and … you get the picture.

I had a colleague who was a svelte lady in her sixties. She attributed her healthy weight to weighing herself once a week. If she went up a pound or two, she would cut back that week on sweets or carbs, and her weight would go back to baseline. We have so many habits that we would like to achieve, and it is easy for us to fall off the wagon and not realize it. The trick is to catch it before it gets out of hand.

Keep a journal of your habits. You will start to notice patterns in your behavior, which will highlight what triggered you to miss your goals (e.g., walking by the donut shop every day on your way to work), and you can alter your behavior to set yourself up for success (walking on a different street from said donut shop, for example!).

Motivation plays a very small role in actual success. Research has shown that the people who stick to their goals the most have to use their willpower the least—they set themselves up to succeed. People who have successfully kicked their addictions don't hang out with the same people they were using with, nor do they go to the same places. Self-control is supposed to be used on an as needed basis, not all of the time. If your environment is requiring you to use self-control more often than not (e.g., having tempting foods in your pantry), then look at how you can change your environment to help you succeed.

Tips and Tricks for Energy Management

Prioritizing Your Tasks

When we have a lot to do, everything can seem overwhelming. When I was consumed with all of the tasks of dealing with my mother's estate, it all seemed like a huge mountain to climb, whether it was researching lawyers or simply making a phone call. Even the smallest task seemed too big to handle, and it was. I had too much on my plate, and every little thing that came up sent me into a torrent of tears.

The reason we feel unable to make decisions when we are under stress is backed by science—our brains don't function as effectively as they would if we weren't, and we aren't able to see things as clearly. I was definitely under this fog—I couldn't make any decisions, let alone good ones. I was paralyzed by overwhelm. My memory was impaired, and I felt like I was treading water, barely keeping my head up. Sound familiar? As HCWs, we live this every day if we are on a busy unit and have responsibilities at home. This is our normal—only it isn't "normal" to be under stress all of the time, we've just managed to cope. We have a million and one things in our heads, and we somehow manage to keep it straight—most of the time.

One thing that helped me and still does to this day when I have a lot to do is making a list of tasks, prioritizing them, and ticking them off one by one as I complete each task. My Inner Child loves making lists and gets great satisfaction from crossing each one off—it makes her feel productive and in charge, and it definitely helps her feel less anxious.

The reason this works is similar to why journaling works—it gets all of the information out of our head and onto paper. We are mentally purging all of the things that we are trying to remember to do, and we immediately feel lighter once we don't have the added stress of having to remember it—it is all out on the table for us to see.

Most of us are visual learners, and getting all of our tasks written down helps us see things better. It may seem unimportant to write our tasks down, but I promise you, it is effective. Not only will it help us see everything on one page (hopefully only one!), but it also gives us a chance to really clearly look at which of these tasks are truly important—and which probably aren't.

We can take this a step further and categorize our tasks by urgency and importance. At work, most of our duties may truly be important and urgent, which is why I recommend you try this for your home activities at first. Once you have gotten used to using this tool, you will be able to categorize your work activities easier. Try this at home and see how your life shifts once you recognize which of your daily tasks truly need to be done. When we are overwhelmed, everything seems urgent, but is it?

The Eisenhower Matrix

U.S. President Eisenhower used this concept when he served in the military, enabling him to make quick but rational decisions as he served his country, first in WWII, then as president.[4] The model helps us decipher what is important to us, what needs to be done now, and what can wait. It can also help us figure out what WE need to do versus what we could possibly ask another to do.

Urgent and Important Activities

Of all of the tasks we do in a day, which are truly important, and which are truly urgent?

This is where emergencies and unforeseen situations will crop up. This can also be where some of our tasks that were left until the last minute occur. With proper planning, that can be avoided. If you schedule time to handle unexpected issues, you will stay on top of things.

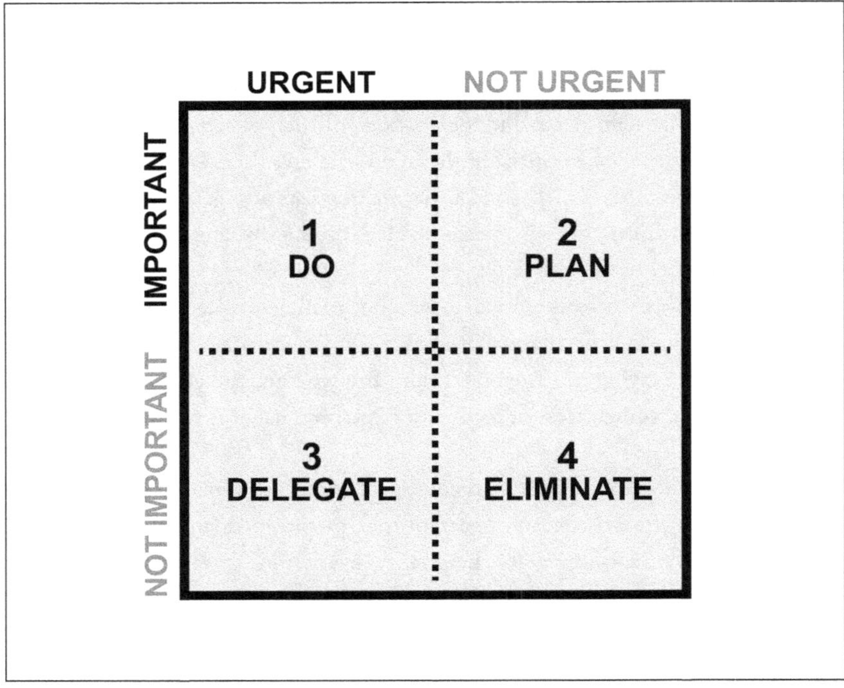

Important but not Urgent Activities

These include the tasks you set to achieve your goals (personal or professional). I like to place my daily self-care activities in this category—it reminds me that my health and well-being are important in the sense that I will deteriorate without them. This action alone shifts your perspective to what is valuable in your life—you.

Your me-time that you schedule into your planner also belongs in this category, such as seeing friends/family, or taking a course to further your education. These activities fill your cup, and will keep you in optimal well-being.

Not Important but Urgent Activities

"Your emergency is not my responsibility." Ever have a family member who left something to the last minute, then needed to be bailed out (looking after their kids, for example)? This is the category that can seem the hardest to deal with, as the issues at hand *are* urgent (your family member having to go to work and needing childcare does need to be dealt with). But we fall into a trap here, because these urgent tasks do NOT have to be done by us. These are the real obstacles in having a balanced life, but are also where you can make the most change to your time. You feel guilty for not being able to help someone who has a problem on their hands, but at the end of the day, this is not our responsibility. These tasks need to be delegated or rescheduled. This may be difficult at first, but delegating is an important skill for us HCWs to develop.

Not Important & Not Urgent Activities

These are just a distraction. Have you ever found yourself doing something because you didn't want to be doing something else? In university, I must have had the cleanest bathroom in the city … because I didn't want to be writing my paper. In our heads, we can come up with all sorts of things we could be doing when we don't want to be doing something else (scrolling on our phones instead of doing something that is better for our health, for example). Categorizing it allows us to see what we are unconsciously doing—trying to distract ourselves. Cancel, ignore, or set aside these activities, as they do not help you in balancing your life.

All of the above-mentioned steps will help you to concentrate on your activities and keep the clutter out of your mind.

The Art of Delegating

One skill that will help you in preserving your energy is delegating. While it may take time to recognize what is truly important and valuable in our lives, we have immediate commitments that we can't necessarily just drop. If you have taken on too much and you don't know where to start, delegating is a great skill to develop.

Delegating is an imperative skill to have when we have a lot of things on our plate—and it is important to be able to do it at work and at home.

Delegating is something a lot of us aren't used to doing. Or perhaps we aren't used to doing it at work, but are okay doing it at home, or vice versa. If you are adept at getting your kids to do their laundry but lack the confidence to ask a co-worker to do a set of vital signs on your patient while you are busy doing something else, ask yourself why that is. The same question can be asked if you are okay asking for help at work, yet feel guilty asking your spouse for help with the dishes.

Asking yourself why you feel uneasy will lead you to address the real, underlying issue. For example, I dreaded asking a colleague for help, because I knew if I did, I would be met with either a flat-out no (fear of rejection), or a litany of excuses, complaints, and exasperated sighs (fear of guilt). Once I was armed with this knowledge, I could rationalize it more clearly in my head. This is where self-parenting comes in handy. By identifying what my Inner Child was afraid of, I could parent her and resolve the underlying issue.

Inner Child: If I ask her to help me, she'll just say no (fear of rejection).

Inner Parent: And then what?

IC: It means she doesn't like me.

IP: Okay, well, it probably doesn't mean that, she is probably just really busy and feeling tired. But if she doesn't like you, what does that mean for you?

IC: It makes me feel sad. And scared, because if she doesn't like me because I ask for help, then other people might not like me, too. And then I will be alone (fear of abandonment).

IP: Ah, I see what you are really afraid of now. I can tell you that she doesn't dislike you, and people won't dislike you just because you ask for help. And if they do, then those people are not the people you want to be around! It is okay to ask for help. You are safe to do so. And you are never alone, because I am always here for you.

You will notice that when I do self-parenting, I speak in a way that a child would understand, because it is a feeling we have that is at a child's level. Consciously, we don't think people dislike us because we ask for help. But a subconscious part of us (one that was likely rejected for asking for help when we were young) feels unsafe asking for help, because that hurt hasn't healed. It seems silly to us on an intellectual level, but by honoring the part of us that wants to be heard, we are more likely to deal with the issue and heal it so we can move on.

Why is delegating so hard to do?

We're not used to it—most of us have lived our lives being fairly independent. We care for our patients, our families, and our friends. We are used to giving, not receiving. It makes sense that we would feel uncomfortable asking for help, and it is this discomfort that causes us to avoid doing it—we are avoiding feeling uncomfortable. With practice, this feeling will ease up, I promise!

We feel guilty—this comes especially at work. Asking our already busy coworkers to help us doesn't seem to make sense—we are all busy! Adding to their workload just makes us feel worse. But getting in the habit of asking for help will give others permission to do the same. Your coworkers probably don't want to burden you either, yet we are more effective as a team. Asking for support will not only help you feel more comfortable doing so, but it will promote a sense of cohesiveness with your colleagues.

We are afraid we will be told no (or hear complaints)—we all suffer from a fear of rejection to some degree, this is normal. Asking our coworkers or family members for help can be intimidating, especially if they are not likely to say yes. If your colleagues and families are used to you doing most of the tasks for them, it is not likely they will jump for joy if you delegate something to them. But the more you do, the more they will get used to it, and it will become the new normal. Don't ask, don't get!

We are overwhelmed and unable to see things clearly—sometimes we have so much on our plate that we don't even know where to start in asking for help. I completely get this. Make a list, or use the Eisenhower matrix to get it out of your head and onto paper. Even if you are unable to change anything at that time, you will feel calmer and more in control simply by offloading everything that is in your head.

We are perfectionists—ever asked someone to load the dishwasher, only to do it for them because they didn't do it right? Some of us type-As like to have things done in a certain way, and we would rather do it ourselves because we know we will get it done properly. As we saw explored in the Perfectionism chapter, this is effectively shooting ourselves in the foot. Not only are we denying someone the chance to help (and grow), but we are piling more onto our plates because we can't give up control. We need to be open to the other person not doing it exactly right—they're not going to get better at it if we keep doing it for them!

We don't want to seem weak—asking for help is pretty much the strongest thing we can do. Yes, it makes us vulnerable. Yes, it puts us out there for rejection or judgement. We fear we will be seen as someone who doesn't have their shit together, and as an HCW that can seem really scary to admit. If we can't take care of ourselves, how can we take care of others?

By asking for help, you ARE taking care of yourself. It is one of the hardest things to do, yet most of us want to help. In fact, most of us feel good when others ask us for help, because we genuinely want to help our loved ones. In health care, we often don't want to seem weak or disorganized because we want our patients and colleagues to respect us. Being honest and genuine in your asking for help will allow others to see the real you, and give them the opportunity to honor you and your request.

Tips and Tricks for Delegating

Plan ahead—once you make a plan, it is easier to execute—I will do x, you will do y. At work, it may seem silly (and admittedly, isn't always possible) to take time out to do this when you are already busy. But by taking that extra five minutes after report to plan your day, it will be easier to see which tasks you need to do, and which ones can wait or be delegated to someone else. This makes it easier when it comes to the time to ask for help, because you already have a plan in place, and your subconscious is executing the plan.

This will also be imperative when you begin saying no to extra tasks being asked of you—when you have a plan and know what you are doing in a shift, you can figure out more easily what you can actually add on to your day and what you can politely decline. At my previous position, we used to start and end the day with a quick "huddle" that made sure everyone was on the same page—it didn't take long, but things definitely ran smoother when we did it. We were able to see what work we had left, what needed to be added, and what could wait until the next day. Stopping for a few minutes might seem like we are wasting time, but it is actually granting us more—as well as a clearer mind, to boot.

Practice—like with anything else, it is easier to do something when you have practice doing it. If you need help asking for help/delegating, practice on small things first, things people will be unlikely to tell you no for (e.g., pass the salt!).

Be patient with yourself and others—the first time you delegate something, it will almost certainly not be done the way you would have done it—nor as quickly. Yet if we keep doing the tasks that others could be helping us out with, others won't have a chance to improve at doing the task. Yes, your husband might not fold the laundry the way you do, and it might take your teenager twice as long as you to clean the kitchen. Being patient with others (and not critical) will help you and others get the job done.

The same can be said at work. You might chart an assessment differently than somebody else, yet this is no reason to avoid asking for help. That being said …

Pick the right people—obviously you need to trust the person you are delegating to. Being selective about who you choose to help with what task will set you up to succeed in delegating appropriately.

Play to others' strengths—perhaps they are better suited to doing a task than you are. Don't like vacuuming? Maybe someone doesn't mind it as much as you do. Prefer to chart over performing wound care? I'm sure someone would be happy to trade you tasks!

Explain why you are delegating—people will be more likely to help you if you explain why you need the task done. Include when (Mr. Jones missed his pain medication, is having 10/10 pain, and needs his narcotics now), what you are doing instead (because obviously you are delegating a task that you aren't able to do for a good reason), and why you chose them (you know that patient well and I trust you to take care of my patient while I am with another patient).

One percent—make small changes. Try delegating once a week at first, then once per day. It will become easier as you go along, and more likely to stay a skill you are comfortable with.

Diet

As we are in health care, I don't need to tell you why our diet is important—we have the background to know what happens in our body when we eat healthy food as opposed to junk.

As someone who has struggled with weight and food all of my life, I can tell you I know how difficult eating "right" can be. There is so much out there on eating certain foods, buying organic, vegan, gluten free, and it changes all of the time.

With shift work and having busy families, it can be challenging to eat healthy. Sometimes quick and drive-thru-able is better than nothing at all. We sometimes just have to do it to get by, which makes total sense. Sometimes, as with the pandemic, situational reasons contribute to not eating right, including depression.

If you want to make the drive-thru an exception rather than the rule, I recommend working with a nutritional coach or dietician. He or she can help you if you don't know where to start.

If you know what you should be eating and just aren't doing it, make a plan for the week. Shop based on that plan (and don't buy anything else), and then execute. What has worked for me is having a day where I do all of the food prep for the week (the day before I go back to work). Chopping vegetables, putting out lunch meat, and portioning it for healthy serving sizes saves time. I'll make a big pot of soup and have that for part of the week. Slow cookers/Instapots are a dream, too, as you can throw a bunch of vegetables in with your protein source and let it cook for you while you are at work. Making more than you need and freezing what you have left is also a time-saving option. With COVID, we now have more delivery food services than ever. They may be more expensive, but if you are eating out more than a couple times a week because you don't have the time/energy to cook, they may actually save you money—they will definitely save you time and energy (which is just as important).

I would also encourage you to look at priorities: this is the only body you have. If you do not have time to make the food that nourishes you, your body will make time later—and not in the way you want it to. Nothing is as important as your body, and feeding it right will keep your body healthy the longest. We want to be able to take care of our patients until we retire, not become one of them because we didn't take care of ourselves.

One percent—again, if you're trying to do too much at once, you will likely not succeed. Implementing small changes until you are used to it will set you up to keep them as lifelong habits. For example, for week one, put more veggies on your plate. Week two, if you drink soda every day, eliminate it for one day out of the week. Small changes make a big impact once you stick to them.

Water—we all know the benefits of drinking more water, but I wanted to stress it here because it has a major impact on our energy levels and brain function. Dehydration can cause headaches, decrease our immunity, and cause constipation. Jacque, my nursing instructor, used to look at us with narrowed eyes if we were less than cheerful and ask us if we were pooping—because if you're grumpy, you're probably not pooping enough!

Sometimes, it can be hard to get our eight glasses—or whatever your body says is right for you. Either we don't have time to drink during a busy work day, or it causes us to go to the bathroom too much, or we simply don't like the taste. It can be a challenge, but the benefits—feeling clearer, having more energy, not to mention skin that looks a-MAY-zing—outweigh the nuisances.

If you don't feel you have time, having a water bottle and taking sips between patients here and there can help. Also, setting a timer every hour when you are first getting started to remind you to drink can help—if anything, you will get so annoyed by the timer that you will want to drink more often just so you don't have to listen to it!

If you are worried about having to pee too often, I hear you. I scrubbed in for cases that could last hours—there've been times where I was literally praying for the case to end so I could go to the bathroom. The first few days you start drinking more water, you will notice an increase in times you go. Your body quickly adjusts to the amount you give it (it is probably begging you for more), so within a few days you probably won't be voiding much more than you do now. I recommend starting to drink more water on days off when you don't have to worry about it as much.

One percent—start gradually. If you only drink two cups of water a day, set a goal to drink three a day for a week and increase from there. This will give your body the time to adjust gradually and will set the habit of drinking more.

Caffeine is a Lie

Ah, the only addiction that is socially acceptable. My love, my joy, my home. To sip on a cup of coffee while perusing the newspaper, a latte in a café as the rain drizzles down, a sweet cup of joe in the winter hanging out by the fireplace. Can you tell how much I love coffee? So can everyone else … and they could tell when I hadn't had it. Which is why I shocked everyone (including myself) when I gave it up.

I had to give it up for my Therapeutic Touch course, as it disrupts forms of energy healing. As I began to do more treatments (sans my one true love), I realized how much it affected me in general. I noticed the longer I went without the coffee, the less anxious I felt. I was calmer, more grounded, dealt with overwhelm better.

And I started to notice I was sleeping better, also. Having been through a lot of stress over many years, I never woke up feeling refreshed. For the first time in eons, I started waking up feeling like I actually got a good night's sleep, despite always having eight hours. I actually had more energy without it! WTF!

Now, I know I have declared my love of caffeine, and you are probably saying to yourself, "Self, that's great. She was addicted to coffee and felt better without it. She probably drank a ton a day. I only drink one cup, so it's no affecting me!"

Well, Self, I can tell you you're wrong. My love affair with java started at eight a.m. and ended before eleven. I had one, count it, *one* cup of coffee a day. I may have had more on vacation or the odd pick-me-up if I was working on call, but the majority of the time, it was only one cup. And I drank it before the afternoon. So I can tell you that if it affected me, and I noticed a change by eliminating one cup a day, you might be affected by your one cup, too.

In his fascinating book, *This is Your Mind on Plants*, Michael Pollan does a deep dive into the history of caffeine. According to Pollan, ninety percent of us ingest it regularly (children getting it through carbonated beverages).[5] Few of us think of it as a drug, much less an actual addiction (we joke about it, but I think many of us know it's true). It's not baseline, it's an altered state. It just happens to be an altered state that most of us share. Caffeine made the modern world, influencing global economics, the slave trade, science, and politics. In Europe, public coffeehouses (which women were not permitted to enter—we had tea) were where books were written, policies were developed, and governments were overthrown.

Pollan, abstaining from caffeine himself for the book very reluctantly, recognized his own withdrawals. He suffered from writer's block while writing the very book he was researching, noticed he missed the smell, the culture, and how it affected his daily routine. But he also noticed he was sleeping "like a teenager again, and wak(ing) feeling actually refreshed." Despite the benefits, he ironically admitted he would be "rejoining the ranks of caffeine-dependent as soon as I can."

People on caffeine are "faster, not smarter." It improves our focus and ability to concentrate, affecting linear thinking, but negatively affects our creativity. We may be better at tasks, but we lose our enjoyment from a rich, fulfilling life. It is a psychoactive drug, and because it makes us more productive, it is completely embraced by society.

Caffeine is an adenosine antagonist. Adenosine levels gradually rise throughout the day, signaling us to sleep when our body needs to. Caffeine binds to these receptors—the adenosine doesn't go away, and once caffeine is out of our system (a twelve-hour quarter-life, meaning it is still affecting us at midnight if we had a cup at noon), we feel the crash. Symptoms of caffeine withdrawal include headache, fatigue, lethargy, and difficulty concentrating. Caffeine simply hides or postpones the exhaustion by blocking adenosine, leading us to feel more tired than what we would be if we didn't have it. And what will we do when we wake up exhausted? Reach for another cup of coffee. The energy the caffeine has given us is stealing it from our sleep later that night, and as this carries on, the compound interest it takes from us regarding our health as we continually have poor quality sleep is more than its worth, even if it is declared the liquid black gold of the white-collar worker.

Matt Walker, the author of *Why We Sleep*, is alerting the public to a caffeine-fueled health crisis, stating we are not getting enough quantity and quality sleep. Caffeine itself might not be bad for you (we hear studies touting its benefits of decreasing the risk of cancer, type-2 diabetes, etc.), but the effects of it stealing our sleep far outweighs those benefits. Decrease in quantity and quality of sleep is related to increased risk of Alzheimer's, stroke, obesity, heart failure, depression, anxiety, and suicide.[6] The shorter you sleep, the shorter you live. As many of us in health care are already taking years off of our lives with shift work, we are at even more of a disadvantage. And caffeine, while it may be appearing to help us with this lifestyle, is actually doing us more harm than good. Even people who claim they can have a cup of coffee and fall right asleep are decreasing the amount of REM they are entering "by fifteen to twenty percent."[7]

Caffeine is the enemy of sleep. In Pollan's book, Bill Dement, a legendary sleep researcher, replies, "True, but it's also the friend of the waking!"[5] Even sleep researchers are hooked.

It makes me wonder how much of our anxiety is exacerbated by it. Almost all of my colleagues drink coffee—an addiction that would be argued as necessary with the long hours we hospital workers put in. Yet I also noticed that many of us are high-strung, and some of us have a generalized anxiety disorder. I wonder how many of us would have less symptoms of anxiety if we were able to give it up.

Now, I didn't give it up completely—I switched true loves from bold and beautiful to decaf. So I'm getting a touch of it. And I'm not saying you need to do this, but if you do struggle with difficulty sleeping or anxiety, it might be worth trying. Once I got over the hump (and the caffeine-withdrawal headache) after a few days, I was in the clear. I get to enjoy the taste of the coffee I love without the side effects of caffeine.

One percent—if you are balking at the idea of giving up caffeine, fair enough. But if you drink multiple cups a day and want to cut down, again, one percent—go slowly, as your body has gotten used to the caffeine, and you will likely notice side effects. If you drink three cups a day, try having one day a week where you only have two—on a day off, as it may be easier then. Do this for a few weeks until you are used to it, then gradually add a day a week where you only have two. It seems easier to go faster, but you will keep your results if you go slow. Or, you know, if you want to tell me to suck it…

Exercise

I know, I know. For those of you who exercise and love it and make it a part of your life because you love it, bully for you. My friend Camille is an example of someone who loves exercise and has the gains to prove it.

For the rest of us: working out sucks. Seriously. I can't stand being out of breath, or the pain of doing too many push-ups. After a long shift, the *last* thing I want to do is go to the gym, surrounded by proof of my lacking dedication – go run somewhere else, Marathon Man.

But for serious, I struggle to exercise. It is not something I like to do and will make any excuse not to go, which is compounded by the fact that I live in a tundra and it is much easier to stay inside six months of the year. It has been a lifelong experiment of finding types of exercise that I like. Once I am in the habit of something, I can usually stick to it. Dancing is something I enjoy, so '90s R&B in my living room, it is!

If you are like me and struggle to be active, I hear you loud and clear. It can also be trying to have the energy to do so when we have such an active job—our feet complain as much as our mouths do at the end of the day. I am by no means perfect, but I know when I am exercising regularly (getting my heart rate up), I have more energy, my mood is significantly better, and my jeans actually fit (thanks for keeping me in pants for the past three years, leggings!).

Again, setting a goal and sticking to it will help you achieve a more active lifestyle. While I am the first to admit I don't meet my goals with exercise as often as I would like, I do know that I am more active than what I would be without them.

Finding something you like makes a huge difference—if you're not into running, don't run (unless it's like Phoebe from *Friends*). Find an activity that gets your body moving that you enjoy, and think outside the box if you need to. If jumping on a trampoline works for you, go for it. Your Inner Child would probably love that!

One percent—start small. Like, really small. Like, if you are a couch potato like I was, start by walking around the block. That's it, that's all you have to do in the beginning. Which helps, because sometimes, now that I am more active, a walk around the block is all I will do—but it's better than nothing. Gradually increase the time you are active to twenty minutes—and really, that's all you need.

Sometimes, I don't have twenty minutes—so I break it up throughout the day. I sneakily squeeze it in at work! I will do stairs on my break, squats when I go to the bathroom, and jog on my walk home instead of walk. I set a goal to do x number of lunges in a day, and if I haven't done them by the time I get off work, I'm doing them before supper (which I hate, so I'll do everything in my power to avoid that).

As it is my least favorite activity, I try to get it done first thing in the morning. If I don't, there's a good chance I won't do it at all. I either go for a jog right out of my house, or do a workout in my living room—if I have to go somewhere to exercise (the gym, for example), I will find more excuses not to do it.

You probably will find some form of exercise that you enjoy (hopefully more than I do), so if you do, it will be easier to stick to.

Sleep

I'm a pretty light sleeper, so it is imperative that I go to bed at a time that allows me to get eight hours, as it is likely I am not sleeping the entire night. Most of us are probably not getting nearly enough sleep with young children, shift work, and all of the things we juggle in a day.

Yet again, it is our body that suffers. Sleep deprivation can cause drastic effects in our mood, immune system, and energy levels. Chronic sleep disturbances can lead to severe illness, weight gain, and inability to function in our professional lives. Getting enough sleep is necessary for us to survive.

Try telling this to a shift-worker who has a baby at home.

Again, I get it. For some people, eight hours isn't possible. End of story. Period.

But what could you do to get more sleep? Better quality sleep?

If you are chronically busy running around and sacrificing sleep in the process, something has to give. And it will probably be your body. Take a good, hard look at some of your tasks that you have set out for yourself in a day, a week—do all of these things actually need to be done? If so, perhaps some of them need to be delegated, whether that means asking family members to help out or paying someone to do them. Nothing is more important than your health.

For me, I couldn't handle the shift work. I would be awake post-night shift after three hours and couldn't get back to sleep. I would go in chronically sleep-deprived to care for critically ill babies. I tried everything to adjust to it, it just wasn't for me. Luckily, my unit had the option of eight-hour day-evening rotations.

Some people really love shift work, others, not so much. I encourage you to find what works for you, not what you tolerate. If you love nights, maybe a colleague would be willing to do all of your day shifts so neither of you are switching back and forth. Maybe you need to find a job that is only days—which is what I ended up doing, barring being on-call.

Health care workers have it tough when it comes to sleep—it is a part of the job. But it doesn't have to be the norm. You can find something that works for you, you don't have to stick it out just because everyone else is, which is something I thought I had to do as a new grad.

Tips and tricks that have worked for me:

Have your bedroom be sacred—do nothing in it but go to sleep. Don't eat in it, watch TV, or be on your phone. This will signal to your body that when you crawl into bed, it is time to sleep and you will have an easier time doing so. Once I implemented this, I started falling asleep so fast after getting into bed that it takes me months to finish the book I'm reading, as I can only get through a few pages a night! Blackout blinds and ear plugs may also be helpful if you are sensitive to light and noise.

No screen time—limit your screen time in the evening and eliminate it completely two hours before going to bed—the blue light keeps us awake. I know this may be tough for those of us attached to our phones, but it makes a big difference. Speaking of phones …

Device notifications—turn them off. Do you really need to hear when you have a new email at ten p.m.? The constant dinging we hear causes us to be alert—each little beep derails us from winding down at the end of the night. I actually have my phone on silent most of the day—I found the noises made me anxious. You might not be as sensitive to noises as I am, but they are having an impact on your psyche. I also noticed how emotionally charged I would get about Facebook posts, and if I was reading something unpleasant (which is most of FB, let's be real), it would cause me to ruminate and I would have a harder time getting to sleep. So go on a social media diet right before bed. If you are having a tough time breaking the phone habit, the one percent can be applied here, too. Track the amount of screen time and decrease it gradually.

One percent—again, it comes down to habits. If you are in the habit of staying up late when you have to work early, and toss and turn if you go to bed too early, try going to bed fifteen minutes earlier than you would normally for a week. Or, if you want to get up earlier to be more productive, try setting your alarm for fifteen minutes earlier.

Alternative Healing

When we think of holistic healing, what often comes to mind for health care workers are modalities that might help our patients. While some of us might be curious and are exploring alternatives from allopathic medicine, holistic activities in regards to ourselves is less established, in practice and in the literature.[8]

While many of us are concerned about public health in Canada and worry about the effects that private health care might have here (witnessing what our counterparts in the States experience), we also have to concede that our own system isn't working. Patients can be on wait lists so long that they get diagnosed with life-threatening conditions due to a lack of access—we are seeing this on our medicine units every day. A simple knee surgery becomes a knee replacement. Primary cancers become metastatic. Booked routine procedures become emergency surgeries. Working in diagnostic imaging, I can tell you that we saw patients falling through the cracks every day.

As we mourn for our patients who the system has failed, we also need to get curious about what else is out there—for ourselves as much as for our patients. "Alternative" healing has been around longer than Western medicine. While some Western purists may eschew alternative forms of healing (Eastern medicine, energy medicine), there is no denying these forms of healing have been around a lot longer, and just because science hasn't quite caught up to how they work, it doesn't mean they don't. Tai Chi/Qi Gong has been established for centuries, and I can attest to its effectiveness in restoring my energy and mental health after a long shift.

Some alternative healing is being explored and accepted in hospitals. I have been trained in Therapeutic Touch, which is a form of energy healing, and I have met several nurses who practice this in their workplaces. I know some physicians are becoming more open to these modalities, as a friend confided in me that her father's physician was practicing Reiki on him in conjunction with his Western treatment.

One type of alternative healing treatment that has been studied in people with PTSD is Emotional Freedom Technique (EFT). This technique combines cognitive behavioral therapy with acupressure or tapping. The patient might make a statement that acknowledges their pain and that they accept themselves while tapping on acupuncture points. A study in 2017 found this technique helpful for war veterans struggling with symptoms of PTSD.[9] I also have found it very effective for my own trauma. As many of us in health care surely are experiencing PTSD due to the pandemic, this is one type of holistic healing that can help us overcome our stress and burnout as we attempt to move on with our lives.

While most of us practice allopathic medicine, it is important for us HCWs to explore other alternatives. Health and healing are ever-changing, and we owe it to ourselves to be open to other forms of healing that we may not have been educated in.

Meditation

I am mentioning this here because it is important for energy management, but I will go into more detail in a later chapter because I find this practice pertinent to my well-being.

I used to think meditating was for monks. And even as data came out to support its health benefits, I scoffed. It was for anxious people (I was anxious, I just didn't know it at the time), or hippies. It was one of those things that you heard was good for you but didn't bother to try.

When I first started out, it was boooooooooring. Oh, Mylanta, I had a hard time with it. If you are someone who is in your head a lot and ruminates, I'm not gonna lie—you will find it challenging. But I can also tell you it is the absolute best thing for you if you worry or are anxious. Even if you aren't, it has its benefits, but it is especially important for those of us who worry a lot as it affects our energy levels.

You see, the more we ruminate, and get stuck in our heads, the more tired and drained we will feel at the end of the day. All that stewing takes up an exorbitant amount of energy, and it gets us nowhere. Meditating is the best tool we have of combatting the monkey chatter in our heads. We will feel more energized, less anxious, and more in control, because we are able to allow our thoughts to pass by without attaching our well-being to them. There are many books and apps out there on meditating, but it really is something we can do anywhere, anytime, for free.

But what is meditating? Do you think you already know? Because I thought I did, until I started actually doing it. I thought it was literally sitting upright with my legs crossed and saying "OM." Which it can be. But it can also be so many other things. Just like with exercise, there are many forms of meditation that you can try that might work better for you.

I thought it was quieting your mind, making your mind "go blank," when actually, it's more like watching your thoughts. It's normal to have thoughts when you meditate, it's not getting attached to them when they come up that is the work. And if you do, that's okay – the work is in going back to center, each time. Don't beat yourself up as a beginner. It can take years to master—I've been doing it steadily for five years and I am nowhere close to being an expert.

There are many different types of meditation: walking meditation, guided meditation, etc. It can also be an activity—anything that you lose track of time over. Scuba divers love the water because they focus on their breath and let go of everything happening at the surface—that's a form of mediating. Painters who lose themselves in their work for hours at a time—that's meditating. If you have a hobby where you can forget about your life problems while you are immersed in it (for me, writing), then that is a form of meditation for you, and I encourage you to find hobbies that do that for you. It shuts off the monkey chatter and allows us to just give in to the process.

Once I started meditating regularly (both through writing and sitting), it was a huge game changer for me. I was calmer, more collected, and able to handle the stresses at work better. Things started shifting in a huge way, and priorities in life came into laser focus—I no longer tolerated people or things that would cause me to disrupt this inner calm I had discovered. It is one of the most important tools I attribute to me making drastic improvements in my life.

One percent—try meditating for five minutes a day—that's it. Stop and breathe and watch your thoughts for five minutes, and gradually increase from there. As you get more comfortable, try different types.

EXERCISES

1. What area of your life would you like to work on changing your habits? Don't try to do it all at once: pick a topic (exercise, sleep, nutrition) and implement a one-percent strategy to make a habit stick. If it's exercise, and you are starting at zero, try walking around the block for a week, then walking it twice the next week, and gradually increase as you go. Make the goals specific and measurable, even if they are only one percent—it's still important!

2. Journal how your habit is affecting your energy level—you might not notice right away (or you might—sometimes the feeling of actually starting gives us a boost on its own!). Notice what might have tripped you up if you miss a day, and give yourself empathy—this is a journey, not a race.

CHAPTER 22

Mindfulness and Meditation

"The little things? The little moments? They aren't little." — Jon Kabat-Zinn

For many of us, life is whizzing by. We are running from work to home to sports for our kids, and have little time to actually experience life. When we have so many commitments, we need to be organized and efficient. Life fills up with activities that are meant to be enjoyable, but can start to feel more like tasks and obligations, even the activities that we enjoy, such as seeing friends and family.

Much of that changed with the pandemic. Suddenly, we were forced to slow down. Some of us cried for joy that we no longer had to engage in all of the obligatory events we had subscribed to. Some of us paced at home, feeling like a caged animal. Whether it was a blessing or a curse, the pandemic gave us the space to look at our lives more closely. It gave people awareness into what in their lives was working, and what needed to change. It helped many people be more present, and really value what in life is important.

For many of us HCWs, we were not granted that time or space. When the world was in lockdown, we were gearing up for battle. We did not receive the gift of being able to look at our lives and make changes accordingly. For many people, the pandemic brought about big life shifts. For us, we are only now able to start breathing again as the world begins to move forward. As the health care system is on the brink of collapse in many areas of the world, there is no time like the present to get more present.

Health care workers were facing crisis long before the pandemic hit. Stress is theorized to be the biggest occupational health hazard we experience after musculoskeletal injuries.[1] Depression was on the rise from a 2017 study of nurses and physicians, ranging from twenty-five to forty-three percent.[2] According to a 2018 study, burnout affected half of all nurses, physicians, and other allied health.[3] The fact that half of us were experiencing these symptoms *before* the pandemic should be raising alarms for what the future of our health care delivery system might hold.

While we are still recovering (for those of us who remain in the field), shit is getting real. Since we could not rely on our health authorities or government to protect us during the most traumatic time our workforce has experienced, it is clear that we must rely on ourselves. We need to have adequate tools moving forward if we want to continue to survive working in the shambles of our health care system. The first step is putting ourselves first. Next, we need to develop skills around resiliency to help us continue serving the people we have dedicated our lives to.

The trauma that HCWs have experienced during the pandemic will have lasting effects. Similar to veterans reliving war long after peace has been declared, we are going to be dealing with the fallout of the pandemic's effects long after the virus weakens. We will need support in a variety of ways. Working with a therapist to express the grief and anguish many of us are feeling can be beneficial. However, some of us do not feel this form of therapy helps; it can be a slow process, we don't always have time for regular appointments, and it is costly, even with health benefits. Medication can help, but may have mixed results.

There are many tools out there to support us as we embark on the next stages of the pandemic. One such practice that we can do anywhere, at any time, on our own, is mindfulness. This practice has been around for centuries, but perhaps associated with monks or spiritual gurus, and not necessarily embodied by the general public. As mindfulness becomes more present in our culture, we can glean more insight into how it can specifically help health care workers.

Mindfulness is one of the best tools we have in getting through the next phases of the pandemic. Through mindfulness, we become more present, grounded, and calm. It allows us to accept the world for what it is, and helps us stay focused as we encounter one task at a time. It is incredibly beneficial for staff working in high-acuity, face-paced environments to practice mindfulness. Resilience can be established by practicing mindfulness. Being mindful helps us "reduce the cases of distress, anxiety, fear, and helplessness that occur through the trauma of COVID-19 clinical settings." [4]

What is Mindfulness?

We hear this term a lot—what does it actually mean?

Think of how much of your day is run on autopilot. You get up, shower, brush your teeth, have breakfast, drive to work, do your job, drive home, make dinner, and watch TV before going to bed. All of those things you do is primarily run by your subconscious brain—you have done it so often it has become automatic. Our brains do this to decrease the amount of energy used for certain tasks—reading, for example, as we don't need to sound out each word anymore because we've seen them many times.

But when we run on autopilot for such a large percentage of our lives, it is easy to take most of it for granted. It's only when something major happens—the loss of a job, a marriage ending, or the loss of a loved one—that we wake up and start recognizing what is truly important in our lives.

You don't have to wait for something big to happen to get out of these patterns. Pausing to practice mindfulness for just a few minutes at different times during the day can help you appreciate your life more, without having to make a major change.

Mindfulness is the energy of being fully aware of the present moment. It is to be truly alive with those around you and with what you are doing. According to Jon Kabat-Zinn, the guru in mindfulness, mindfulness is "the awareness that emerges through paying attention on purpose, in the present moment, and non-judgmentally to the unfolding of experience moment by moment."[5]

Mindfulness is the exact opposite of being on auto-pilot. It is a slowing down as opposed to having a short-cut in our thinking. It is being intentional with every-thing that we do—because we have the power to choose. We choose to get up in the morning, we choose to go to work, and we choose to come home and sit in front of the TV because we have been in the habit of doing these things day in and day out. It is really hard to break the pattern, because our brains have gifted us with being on autopilot to conserve energy. So don't beat yourself up when you revert to your old ways of eating in front of the TV.

Like any habit, it takes time and effort to break. It's like driving on a road that has been driven many times—it's easiest to drive within the tread down path, and the more you drive, the deeper the ridges become. It's challenging at first to drive over them. But the more you do, the less deep the ridges become and you begin to form a new habit—it just takes time. Mindfulness helps us be more conscious about our choices and grants us the opportunity to witness ourselves (and perhaps our less-desirable habits).

So how do we start overcoming the auto-pilot habit?

Slowing Down

Does it feel like your life is whizzing by at breakneck speed? Do you feel like your children are growing up way too fast? Did the last ten years at your current job pass in a blink? Chaotic existence is the new norm, and we sometimes feel like we are missing out on life, even though we are experiencing it all.

Being mindful can help alleviate some of those feelings, because we actually slow down and take the time to experience the life we are living. Ever scarf down a bag of chips and wonder how you ate the whole bag? Yup, me too. Slowing down helps us actually enjoy what we are doing. If you're gonna binge on the salt and vinegar, you may as well enjoy it!

Slowing down can be challenging as a health care worker with a family, doing shift work, juggling day care and hockey practice (and the tiny blip that we call a social life). But even with all of this in our schedules, we can find time for being mindful. Whether it is enjoying a coffee while at soccer practice, or listening to your favorite song on your way to work, or a quiet meal outside on your lunch break, the beauty of being mindful is that you don't have to change anything in your routine to do it—you just have to be present for what already is happening.

One Thing at a Time

With so many things we have to juggle as an HCW, it can be difficult to get away from multitasking, especially when our lives have come to depend on us being proficient at it. Yet we can also shoot ourselves in the foot with this, as it can lead to disorganization, forgetting details, or paying more because we've left things too late. Sometimes we don't get ahead by doing more.

One-tasking is the new sexy. Try focusing on the task at hand, and only that task. By tackling one thing at a time, you are setting yourself up to be more efficient, as you can focus more clearly on what you are doing and will therefore perform it better than if you were doing more things at once. You also will find a greater sense of satisfaction at completing the task, and will feel less tense in doing so.

Intention Setting

Intention refers to the underlying motivation for everything we think, say, or do. Intention setting is a powerful tool that helps guide you throughout the day. Ask yourself, "What do I want to accomplish today?" or, "How do I want to feel?" Setting an intention to feel a certain emotion (e.g., light-hearted) will help your subconscious carry out the instructions your higher thought processes want to experience.

Setting the intention: "Today, I just want to let go of the feelings of resentment I have at work." You don't have to commit to doing it all day, every day, but just for today as much as you can. Then, throughout the day, check in with yourself. Be mindful of the intention you set for the day, and remember it when triggers come up. It's okay not to get it perfect, and the more intentions you set, the more your subconscious will help you feel the way you intended to. Pretty soon, your mood will shift to reflect that intention, and your communications and relationships will adapt to reflect that shift.

Mindful Daily Activities

With these activities, try being more mindful as often as you can. No one is perfect, but even if you adopt the one-percent Atomic Habits strategy (e.g., the first five minutes of a meal, when stopped at a red light), you can practice being in the present moment. It costs nothing, you can do it anywhere, any time, and it makes a huge impact on your nervous system.

Mindful Eating

Gone are the days when we had to ration food. It is so abundant and we have such a variety that we forget how imperative it is that we have it—we take it for granted. The pandemic has given us insight (however temporary) of living a life where resources were scarce. We can begin to be more grateful for the food we have, and not mindlessly munching in front of the TV.

Eating is something we do on a daily basis that we derive pleasure from. Being more mindful of what we are eating, how it tastes, the texture, sweetness, etc., will turn eating into a much richer experience.

Before the meal—once you have sat down with your meal, pause before you actually begin eating. Where did the food come from? Was it from a farmer's market, and if so, how much work was put into getting it on your plate? How did you attain the food? What work did you do in order to buy it?

Prayer before meals is something that many people do. If you are not religious, still take a moment to be grateful for being able to eat—there are so many people in the world who do not have this luxury. You don't have to feel guilty about this, just be thankful that your life situation allows you to eat nutritious meals every day.

Listening to your body—rate your hunger on a scale of one to ten, and tune in to your body's sensations: Is your stomach growling? Are you thirsty? Tuning in to your body will ensure that you don't overeat. Aiming to eat until you are at a seven will also assist with not overeating.

While eating—eat in a peaceful environment. Turn off the TV, switch the cell phone to silent, and eat in a place that is meant for eating (i.e., not at your kitchen sink or your living room). If sitting down with the family, it might be more difficult to concentrate on eating mindfully at first. When I first learned to do this, I had to eat alone for the first few weeks in order to really check in with what I was experiencing. I had gone my whole life eating on autopilot. I rarely felt satisfied when I finished a meal, even if it was an indulgent one because I wasn't truly tuning in. Now, when I have a treat, I try not to feel guilty about it. I savour each bite, and I find I eat less because I was fully present for what I was consuming.

Pay attention to the texture, the sweetness, the saltiness of the food, how it feels as you bite down. Choose foods that you actually like, not just ones that you feel you "should" be eating because they are healthy. By eating mindfully, you give yourself permission to eat the foods you truly enjoy, because you won't overindulge in them.

Mindful Driving

Driving can be the time in our day when we are on autopilot the most. It's no coincidence, then, that it can also be the place where we experience the most frustration if we run into a traffic jam or get cut off by irresponsible drivers. We are so focused on getting home to do all of the tasks that we have created for ourselves that anything but smooth sailing will cause us to shift from auto to angry.

Driving is actually a great place to practice being mindful, as we have nothing else to do if we are stopped at a red light (because we are not checking our texts, right!?!). Box breathing is a great form of relaxation for us at any point of the day. This practice involves taking a deep breath in four seconds, holding for four seconds, exhaling for four seconds, and resting for four seconds. This is a great technique for moments of stress and overwhelm, yet in the moment it can be difficult to remember to do. By practicing the box-breathing method at every red light, you program yourself to remember to do this more easily, so that in times of stress it comes more naturally.

Mindful Waiting

No one likes to wait in line, especially not now that we have smartphones and have become much less patient than ever before. Waiting in line can be boring, and it can be tempting to check our phones, get exasperated with the person holding up the line counting change, etc. Instead, use it as a chance to be mindful. Observe yourself as you feel the boredom, notice the irritation as you watch the person ahead fumbling with change. What does it feel like in your body? Is there tension? How is your breathing? Is it shallow, regular, etc.? Use this as another opportunity to box-breathe, or set an intention of relaxing the muscles in your body. Resist the urge to check out with your phone. Notice the person in line ahead of you—maybe they are wearing a nice jacket, you could compliment them and ask them where they got it from, thus making someone else's day and getting more real, in-person connection.

What is Meditation?

"It is indeed a radical act of love just to sit down and be quiet for a time by yourself." – Jon Kabat-Zinn

I decided to dedicate an entire chapter to meditating because I truly believe having this skill in your repertoire will be one of the most powerful you have—if you stick with it.

Ok, let's be real, here. Meditation is effing hard. For anyone who has tried it, it isn't easy. Yet, the benefits are numerous and affect every aspect of your life.

When I first started five years ago, I thought I was doing it "wrong" because I couldn't quiet the chatter. While we can achieve a state through meditation where our mind slows down, this isn't exactly the goal. It's more like watching our thoughts, and not getting attached to what comes up.

When I become still, I hear all of the crap that I don't necessarily hear consciously, but perhaps register subconsciously. I hear my Inner Child being critical ("You're fat.") or fearful ("What happens if I can't make my mortgage payment?"). I hear thoughts saying mean things about others that I would never say out loud ("She's such a slut."), or replaying old stories in my head ("They forgot the camera on my graduation day?!"). And of course, I hear myself planning my day ("Better do the laundry before the weekend.") or thinking utter nonsense ("Will self-driving cars still need windshield wipers?").

What meditating does is not necessarily quiet the thoughts, but it helps us become less attached to them. I could (and still do, that's why it's called a practice) analyze the thoughts I listed above, and feel shame for having them, try to pretend they're not there, or think about how I could change them. But all of that requires energy and just increases my attachment to those thoughts. Think about it: When you hear a toddler say something rude or funny, you figure that they must have heard it somewhere, and are mimicking a parent or something they saw on TV. The same goes for our thoughts—we have been exposed to so much in our lives, and tucked much of it away in our subconscious, that it's bound to come out if we stop to hear it. You are not your thoughts; you are just someone witnessing them.

Meditation helps us to give our thoughts less credence. And if we do get caught up in a thought, that's okay. The present moment brings us back each and every time, ready to start again.

Being Unattached to the Outcome

Much like meditation gives us an opportunity to become unattached from our thoughts, an important part of mediation and mindfulness is being unattached to the outcome. When we sit down to meditate, often we are looking for a specific outcome—to achieve peace, to create resilience, to establish calm. While this can and does happen, sometimes it does not. Much like participating in sports or a yoga practice, sometimes we show up and it all goes south. This happens in life as it does in meditation—sometimes, all we do is sit and ruminate. That is okay—that is why it is called a practice.

According to Kabat-Zinn, focusing on the outcome of an activity can lower our performance if we allow negative emotions to seep in. Whether the activity is doing laundry or applying for a new job, if we allow our emotions to dictate how we see them (e.g., labelling laundry "boring" or focusing on the fear of failing to attain said job), we decrease the likelihood of seeing the results we would prefer to see. Mindfulness negates this by causing us to focus on the activity itself, instead of focusing on the possible (negative) outcomes. When we focus on the process and not the outcome, it reduces the feelings of anxiety and depression and increases the feelings of joy. This, in turn, increases the chance of having the desired outcome.[6]

Society has caused us to only value progress, causing our lives to be chaotic, distracted, and disconnected. Mindfulness nudges us to tune in consciously in a world where we are mostly tuned out. The benefits of doing this are worth pursuing this practice.

Mindfulness is a form of self-care and self-compassion. Instead of judging ourselves for having anxious thoughts (or numbing/distracting ourselves from feeling them), we can just let them be.

The Benefits of Mindfulness/Meditation

Practicing mindfulness and meditation can have a significant impact on our health and well-being. The effects of this practice are visible in Tibetan monks, with reported changes to their EEG, fMRI, and PET scans.[7] According to a review of the effects of mindfulness on nurses, mindfulness "significantly" improves nurses' mental health.[8] There is a decrease in anxiety, depression, pain, and stress in nurses who practice mindfulness. They report feeling calmer, have greater problem-solving abilities, and have increased self-acceptance.[9]

All of us feel pain and inadequacy at times of our lives; it is a part of being human. Mindfulness allows for self-compassion in that it causes us to tune in to these experiences instead of feeling ashamed of them. "When we are mindful, we observe our thoughts and experience our feelings without judgment or applying meaning; we hold our painful feelings as part of our experience; we do not cling to them or run away from them."[10]

There are benefits to making mindfulness a daily practice:[11]

Physical

Our bodies heal faster—research has proven that meditation reduces inflammation at a cellular level. This aids in healing the body from a multitude of ailments, including wound healing, chronic pain and acute injuries. Reducing stress increases our ability to heal.

Strengthens our immune system—people who practice mindfulness have demonstrated increased immune function. Our bodies are working more in sync, and therefore we are less likely to get sick—something that is becoming increasingly more important, and was always important for us HCWs who are around illness and disease on a daily basis.

Better sleep—regular meditation helps us fall asleep more easily, sleep longer, and have a better quality of sleep. As many of us are shift workers, this is incredibly important, as our sleep cycles are already being challenged by our careers.

Psychological

Reduces stress and overwhelm—of course. This is the reason most of us seek out meditation, as many of us suffer from this throughout our lives. It is a tool that helps when we are feeling overwhelmed, as well as keeps us responding calmly when we are not feeling this way.

Increases self-awareness—meditation involves watching our thoughts. The more we meditate, the more thoughts we watch – and sometimes we don't realize that we have certain thoughts or feelings until we become still enough to hear them. Self-awareness is one of the most powerful tools we can cultivate, because without it, we don't know we have an issue. Meditation is a key technique in discovering more self-awareness.

Improves self-esteem—meditation helps us get more in touch with our higher selves, and can give us insight into feelings of unworthiness or feeling unlovable. It also gets us more in touch with our bodies, which can be a place of low self-esteem, especially in women. Learning to tune in to our bodies helps us accept them as they are.

Reduces anger—by helping us acknowledge our feelings and truly feel and experience them, meditation assists us in allowing us to let them go. Feelings often come up in meditation that we were repressing, and by allowing them to come up (and feel them), they are more readily released.

Combats loneliness—humans are social creatures, and many of us fear being on our own for many reasons, including boredom, abandonment, or just being alone with our thoughts. Meditation eases this by dedicating alone time with ourselves. Once we get over the fear of our thoughts and being lonely, we often find we begin to like our own company.

Helps us be more compassionate—with an inner sense of calm and a spiritual practice, practiced meditators find they have more compassion for people. This is something we HCWs have already, but may be stretched at times.

Regulates mood disorders—meditation has been found to help those who suffer from depression, anxiety, and PTSD. As we in health care are becoming more and more plagued by these, this is a tool that can help that doesn't require a prescription or the cost of therapy.

Cognitive

Increases focus and memory—with practice, the monkey-mind chatter we all experience begins to wean, and we become more focused and sharper, even when we are not meditating.

Helps us handle stress at work more easily—with more focus and a greater sense of inner calm, we can deal with things as they happen. We are present and focused on the situation at hand, not ruminating over what could have been done (living in the past), nor anxious about the fallout (living in the future). This helps us think more clearly and come up with solutions more readily.

Variations of Meditation

As stated in the Energy Management chapter, meditating does not have to mean sitting in the lotus position for hours at a time. Nor does it have to mean sitting at all. Any activity that causes you to be mindful, in the moment, is a form of meditation—even if it's high-fuelled! For a race car driver, racing is meditating. He is never as focused as he is going around those turns, and that is what it is all about. Whatever keeps you mindful keeps you in the present, and keeps you getting all of the benefits listed above. Finding the right activity for you is part of the fun. For those of you who have tried meditating and have deemed yourselves unable to do it, I encourage you to keep trying—you just haven't found the type that works for you. There are many apps and YouTube videos that are great resources for starting out.

Seated Meditations

Guided meditation—if you are new to meditation, I highly recommend starting here. Being present can be tough for beginners as our minds and bodies aren't used to being still, and guided meditations offers something to focus on as we get used to it. This involves a voice walking you through a visualization. This could be anything—walking through a forest, different colors of light, etc. Don't worry if your mind can't picture it exactly, what matters is that you focus on the voice and being in the present moment. Don't worry if your mind wanders even with this, it is part of the practice.

Mantra meditation—this involves repeating a word or phrase throughout a meditation. Again, it is helpful for beginners who tend to let their minds wander, as it guides you to focus on the chanting aspect of the meditation. You can use an affirmation of your choice, or there are more formal versions (Japa meditations or the Ho'oponopono meditation).

Binaural Beats—are a perception of sound heard by our brains. Requiring headphones, a slightly different level of frequency (Hz) is delivered in each ear (usually with accompanying music), causing our brains to create a third tone. Studies have shown this helps our brains get into meditative states more smoothly. There are plenty of these type of meditation videos available on YouTube.

Movement Meditations

Walking meditation—involves being mindful about each step we take, noticing how our footsteps hit the ground, the smell of the air, the rustling of the leaves. For those of us that are fidgety, this is a way to meditate that doesn't require sitting.

Yoga—is a mindfulness practice. For those of you doing yoga, you are already engaging in a form of meditation. If you have attended yoga simply for the physical benefits, I encourage you to elevate your practice and really sink into the deeper levels that yoga offers.

Tai Chi/Qi Gong—another mindful body movement practice. These types of movement are slow and focused, and offer an energetic component. The first time I attended a class (it was a fusion of both types), I felt amazing—and I knew I needed it in my life.

1. Pick a meditation practice mentioned above that piques your interest (e.g., explore meditation apps or YouTube videos). Commit to doing this practice for five minutes a day and gradually increase. Journal any insights you have to the effects this has on your energy and mood.

2. Pick a daily activity that you can practice being more mindful while doing (driving, eating). For example, focus in on the details of eating an apple—the freshness, the crunchiness, etc. Practice this for a week and see how different you feel as you move through your daily activities.

3. Think of a situation where you feel attached to the outcome (e.g., winning at a sporting game, being assigned an area at work, etc.). Practice being non-attached to the outcome, and notice how you feel after. Was it easy, liberating? Or difficult? Simply notice the aspects that were challenging for you.

CHAPTER 23

Spirituality

"We are not human beings having a spiritual experience. We are spiritual beings having a human experience." – Pierre Teilhard de Chardin

I grew up in an Irish-Catholic family. While we didn't attend church regularly, the traditions and perspectives of the Catholic church were ingrained in how we were raised. Attending a Catholic school invited more bible stories and ideologies as we grew up. I distinctly remember my high school teacher telling us she was supposed to fast-forward the prophylactic portion of a human sexuality movie we were watching because the Catholic school system didn't allow education on it (like a rebel, she didn't).

By the time I reached my twenties, I had pretty much eschewed everything about religion. I always had a spiritual side, and was never an atheist, yet I couldn't ignore all of the drama circling around the Catholic church, namely the pedophile priests. Travelling to Europe and learning of how corrupt the church had been there, studying the ornate cathedrals built while the people starved, far from being impressed, it made me exceedingly angry.

I was conflicted, because I could see how my religious friends found comfort and community in their various parishes, halls, and mosques. Like I said, I always believed in a higher power, yet I didn't know how it fit in with my life, especially during turbulent times.

I remained curious despite my misgivings, and was drawn to more New Age forms of spirituality. You could argue this had started when I was young and learning about astrology (I am such a Pisces), and my interest in New Age forms of spirituality developed when I turned away from traditional religion. It was more of a passing fascination until I lost my parents.

I was angry, sad, and felt like a victim. I wondered what I had done to deserve all of the pain and stress that I was going through. While I survived the ordeal, I was left with wondering what it all meant. I wasn't truly coping with it, despite how it looked to the outside world.

This was when I embarked on a spiritual journey in earnest. I started reading spiritual books with voracity, and eating up any and all I could get my hands on. Books such as *Love, Medicine, and Miracles* by Bernie Siegel, *The Surrender*

Experiment by Michael Singer, and *Conversations with God* by Neale Donald Walsch helped me through the most difficult times in my life.

I began to change my outlook. Instead of asking why life was happening *to* me, I started asking how life was happening *for* me. Believing in a higher power (and a bigger picture) allowed me to make sense of the suffering I had endured in my childhood and twenties. I no longer blamed others for my trauma, but rather, I felt empowered that I could choose how to look at it. Like Viktor Frankl in *Man's Search for Meaning*, a psychiatrist who survived the Holocaust, I discovered how powerful I was with simply choosing how I wanted to see the world.

This was especially helpful in my nursing practice. I used to see my patients as people I pitied—this was a form of self-preservation. In order to avoid the pain of seeing so many people suffer, I felt sorry for my patients and did what I could to ease their suffering. I didn't see them as capable beings who were on a spiritual journey, I looked at them like victims. I believe many of us view our patients as victims, which does not help them heal, it only enables them to see themselves as such. I now try to see my patients as inspirational, people going through a passage, and instead of feeling sorry for them, I do my best to support them as they navigate it.

Another magical ability I found I had within me was the power to forgive. Having been abused and bullied as a child, I held a lot of resentment and anger in my heart. Diving into the spiritual realm allowed me to learn about the importance of forgiveness. With empathy as my superpower, I really put myself in my parents' and tormentors' shoes. While it does not excuse their behavior, nor does it belittle the feelings I felt while I was being abused/bullied, I was able to forgive. Truly forgive. And let me tell you, the feeling of truly forgiving someone is so effing freeing. It was a weight I'd been carrying around for so long that I didn't know how heavy it was until I let it go.

It also gave me the ability to simply allow what happened in my life instead of trying to control it—and others. I have the power over me—no one else. Being in a state of allowing, I could accept whatever came at me more easily, and was less likely to try to change it. I was also less likely to try to change others or influence their behavior because I thought I was right. While it is an ongoing lesson (some days are easier than others), reminding myself that I don't have control over others gave me a sense of peace that I have never felt before. I found love in my heart for people I used to butt heads with. It is in every aspect of my life, from personal relationships to colleagues to my patients. Realizing that we are all on our own spiritual path and not trying to enable anyone else gives me so much more freedom to enjoy people as they are, not as I think they should be. I will stress, this is a daily exercise for me, and some days I do better than others. All of this empathy I now have would not have been possible without a spiritual practice.

The Benefits of a Spiritual Practice

While undertaking a review of spirituality for health care workers, there is a definite paucity of literature. In fact, all of the studies I found mention this. "Although there has been increased nursing research about the importance of spiritual care in building resilience, most studies have focused exclusively on the spiritual care of the patient and not of the nurse."[1] This could be due to the nature of what spirituality actually means, the blurred lines between religion and spirituality, and the negative connotations that the term "spirituality" has.[2]

Spirituality can be defined as "an individual's essence as a person; a relationship with an infinite being; relationships with others; and the search for fulfillment, meaning, and purpose in life."[3] It can involve religion, but the two terms are not mutually exclusive. For me, spirituality is a relationship with everything around me, that there is something bigger than me in the universe. It is a deeply personal, deeply sacred relationship, and is as unique in each person's experience as each person is unique.

According to the literature, having a spiritual practice can build resilience, reduce emotional fatigue, and reduce workplace stress and burnout.[4,5,6] While more focus is needed in studying the effects of spirituality on the health care worker (and not just the patient), we have the ability to embody a spiritual practice today.

Why am I talking about spirituality in a book for empowering health care workers?

Because we are spiritual beings.

Because health care, when it is in its most healing form, is about addressing people holistically. Because it is where we draw our strength. It is where we accept the unacceptable, live with the unliveable. We witness death, illness, abuse, mental illness, and other forms of human suffering on a daily basis. We question why our pediatric patients succumb to cancer when they haven't even begun to live their lives. We agonize when we see a drug-addicted mom who has the rest of her children in foster care take her drug-addicted baby home. We question the morality of doing every life-saving measure for an elderly patient with a stroke, only to revive someone who will become a human vegetable for the rest of her life. We are saddened and feel useless when we discharge a homeless person back on to the street instead of having the resources to properly care for his mental health and addictions. As we watch our health care system crumble, we anger at the fact that we have been predicting this outcome and no one has listened.

What happens without faith is that we shut it off. We either do not have the capacity to deal with witnessing daily human suffering, or we condition ourselves in order to survive. Humans are extremely efficient at this, and we can normalize almost anything. The poor oncology child who lost their battle with cancer, the suicidal patient who gets discharged without proper follow-up, the terminal patient with a missed diagnosis, each becomes one of many. We see so much that it is not only natural, but necessary to turn it off. Yet there is a small part of us questioning why. Why all of the suffering? Why do we have to work with such limited resources that we cannot give the care these people need?

This is where spirituality came into play for me. After suffering my own loss and traumas, I was desperate to find meaning in it all. I hadn't been able to truly focus on my patients because I had been dealing with my own stuff. Spirituality gave me the strength and courage to look at my own shortcomings, and helped me assess where I needed to find forgiveness, in myself and in others. Finding spirituality has made me a better person, and a better nurse.

What does spirituality look like for me?

I believe we are all more than our bodies, more than our minds. I believe that we were created out of love, and we are here having a human experience. All of our life happenings, our joy, our sorrow, our victories and failings, we are here to experience it fully, to be truly present with it all. If something comes along that I don't necessarily welcome (looking at you, COVID), I ask myself, "What is this here to teach me?"

We might witness and feel powerless in our patients' suffering, but honoring them on their path empowers us to help them the best way we can—providing compassion and care, being a light on their journey where they may be experiencing darkness. We don't have to own our patients' suffering, yet by being a friendly face and listening, we are providing them with more comfort than we know.

Miracles happen every day, and it is those who have determination and a strong sense of faith that cause these miracles to happen. Being a nurse, I am able to see how little we actually know about the human body, how often we send patients home with no solution for their mysterious symptoms. There is still so much we haven't discovered about the human body and how it works, despite our shiny technologies. We have been looking at the body from a fragmented perspective in Western medicine for so long, that now our miracle drugs and cutting-edge surgical procedures are no match against the pandemic of chronic illness. Everything is energy, everything is connected. We need to start looking at people like the whole beings that they are, not just a meat suit with organs.

Spirituality and Medicine

In my search for healing, I came across a book that is the epitome of "woo," Louise Hay's *You Can Heal Your Life*[7]. I've always been open to alternative healing, but this one was too much for me at first—connecting throat issues (like cancer) with not speaking your truth? Get real, lady.

Yet being a nurse, I was curious about certain aspects she described in the book. Relating to chakras, the throat chakra is said to be impaired/blocked when we don't speak up. While I at first was very skeptical, I had to admit I was also slightly curious.

Working in radiology, we place feeding tubes for people with head and neck cancers, and I noticed anecdotally that these patients were mostly men. According to the CDC[8], men are twice as likely as women to be diagnosed with head and neck cancers, and this is "regardless of whether they drink alcohol or smoke tobacco"[9], so why are men so highly linked to head and neck cancers? My own father passed away from esophageal cancer, and with him being a smoker and a drinker, I didn't question where the disease came from. But my father was also the strong, silent type who didn't speak up. He had endured a significant amount of trauma and stress in his life, but it only came out when he was drinking. He also never shared his feelings nor spoke about his past, obviously growing up in an era where boys don't cry. It made me curious, then, that we saw so many men with this disease.

Could it be, that we really are energy, and our emotions being suppressed over and over are causing there to be misalignment in that area? It sounds impractical from a Western, literal sense, yet there is still so much that Western medicine doesn't know (nor does it bother to explore). Someone with an Eastern training in medicine would probably agree with this. And like exploring other religions and having a more well-rounded view of others' beliefs, we should be exploring other forms of medicine in our hospitals. While some allopathic doctors are getting on board, it has yet to catch on in Western hospitals. Knowing that we are bigger than our bodies helps us see beyond the physical, which can assist in our own healing as well as the healing of our patients.

Thankfully, some Western physicians are starting to see the mind-body connection – and put it into practice. Gabor Maté's work delves deeply into this. His book, *When the Body Say No*, gives both examples from his practice and personal life, as well as scientific backing to support this ideology[10]. The practitioners we have that honor this aspect of ourselves can be some of our greatest healers. I truly believe that we help our patients the most, not through the procedures we perform or the pills we administer, but through the empathy that we offer them. The fact that we have lost this technique of healing in our professions due to the overwhelming workload and tasks we are expected to do, not to mention the critical shortage of staff, is one reason why patients are sick—and a major reason why we are burnt out. We are not nurturing in a way that our souls know we should be.

How can we cultivate a spiritual practice?

A spiritual practice can literally be anything. It can be your cup of coffee on your deck, it can be a daily jog or yoga class, or a weekly visit with a loved one. Anything that connects you to something that is higher than yourself can be considered a spiritual practice.

Here are some suggestions. Lean in to what interests you, and leave what doesn't. Generally, our instincts know what we are craving, and if something jumps out at you (even if it's just a little hop), explore it. You never know where it will lead.

Meditation—a way to get in touch with our deeper selves.

Nature—hiking, swimming in the ocean, just being present in nature.

Journaling—untangling our jumbled thoughts and invoking insight into our daily experiences.

Breathwork—Wim Hof has been credited with introducing much of mainstream society to breathing exercises that give us numerous health benefits, including stress reduction and lowering blood pressure.

Reading spiritual texts—either religious books/bibles, or whatever interests you in your library/bookstore/Kindle in the spirituality section.

Music—from chanting and drumming to religious hymns, music assists us in our spiritual practice. Whether it be gospel or tribal, find the music that gets you in the zone (sitting still or dancing).

Find your tribe—look for groups that discuss spirituality in the form you are interested in, whether that be a bible study or a bra-burning sisterhood. There are often local meditation groups available by the cost of donation, so look into what is available in your city/town. Find what your heart is speaking in others.

Take a class—yoga, Tai Chi, nature walks, ecstatic dance, spiritual teachings—whatever floats your boat. This is another way to meet like-minded people.

Spiritual Retreats—this helps immerse you in the art of spiritualty long enough to be able to disconnect from your busy homelife and dive deeper into spiritual practices. This can be a yoga retreat, a meditation retreat, a women's retreat, a vipassana (no speaking) retreat, the list goes on.

When we focus on our own spirituality through loving ourselves first, we are able to give from a deeper, humbler place. Developing a spiritual practice is unique to every individual, and sacred. Enjoy exploring what spirituality means to you, and what it means to be a spiritual being. Enjoy creating a spiritual practice, something that is meaningful, and something that is just for you.

E X E R C I S E S

1. Gratitude—what are you grateful for? A gratitude journal, while cliché, is recommended by therapists and spiritual teachers alike—because it works. We can't be thinking about the negative when we focus on the positive. This was a big help for me in some of my darkest days. Even if the only thing I could name that I was grateful for was that I had a roof over my head or food in my fridge, it helped ground me when I was lost in worry. I didn't always feel a hundred percent better, but I always felt at least ten percent better, and that's a win.

2. Explore teachings of another religion/spiritual education—if you have your own religion, and even if you don't, explore teachings of another form that you might be interested in—Buddhism, The Tao, etc. While you might not agree with everything you learn, it offers you another perspective that might just change the way you see things. I have a friend who left the Mormon church, and while he doesn't practice most of its teachings, he still gives a portion of his earnings to other causes he supports because he chooses to. He took what he believed in, and he left what didn't. Take what works for you, and leave what doesn't.

CHAPTER 24

The Patient as His Own Healer

"All of Western medicine is built on getting rid of pain, which is not the same as healing. Healing is actually the capacity to hold pain." – Gabor Maté

You know the patient. The one that forgets his med list and doesn't know what medications he is on, uttering, "My wife usually handles all that." The one who denies having diabetes but you see she is taking metformin. The patient who refuses to move himself in bed, relying on others to reposition him and barking orders while doing it.

The patient on dialysis who brings in fast food for lunch.

The patient who may not say anything, but allows his family members to do the fighting for him.

The patient who hears a grim diagnosis and accepts it without looking into options because, "What's the point?"

These are all examples of patients who have given their power away. They have accepted whatever their doctor has prescribed them, have taken no responsibility in their own care, and have left it up to the health care professionals because "they're the experts."

Only, we aren't.

We are not the experts of our patients' own bodies. While we have extensive knowledge and education surrounding anatomy and physiology of the body, this does not make us experts in our patients' lives. And there needs to be a shift in power.

We know the system is failing our patients. We are suffering burnout now more than ever, and much of it is because we know we are fighting a losing battle. When I began my career as a nurse, I believed that I was making a difference. Now, it is difficult to go to work each morning, knowing that my patients are getting sicker. I cannot help them in ways I wish I could, and it feels like my contributions make no difference. We HCWs have taken on the burden of healing our patients instead of helping them. We feel responsible for their welfare, and are carrying the heavy weight of the health care system's failure.

This isn't our fault.

To add to our burden of working in a failing system, we experience patients, like the examples above, who expect us to do everything for them. These types of patients can be the most frustrating for us to deal with, mostly because they have willingly decided to check out of their own lives. Witnessing these types of patients as they demand more and more resources while not accepting responsibility for their own health adds to the frustration and burnout we are already suffering from as HCWs. We are trying to help people who, in effect, don't know how to help themselves.

Why have patients taken a backseat in their own care?

Medicine has changed so much over the decades. There has been a ton of advancement in the care we provide to patients. New techniques for treating disease, cutting-edge technology, and complex treatment plans requiring the involvement of more than one specialist can create confusion and paralysis for patients who don't know how to navigate the health care system. No wonder our patients rely on us so heavily: navigating health through the eyes of modern medicine is an enigma that even those of us in the system are confused by. In addition to all of the treatment plans for complex disease processes, we are experiencing a polypharmacy pandemic that makes it difficult for patients to take control of their health. With so many medications being prescribed, it's difficult for patients to remember what they are taking, why, and what may be interacting with what. Doctors so freely prescribe medications for the littlest of ailments, and it is causing a health care crisis. As quoted in his revolutionary book *The Body Keeps the Score*, Dr. Bessel Van Der Kolk states, "Mainstream medicine is firmly committed to a better life through chemistry."[1]

My own mother fell prey to this, suffering from migraines for most of her life. Her physician at the time so freely handed out narcotics that she became addicted to them in a very short time. This was, I believe, what led to her untimely death, having gone down the rabbit hole of medication to fix her issues. With each new medication came a new symptom, which was of course given another medication to combat it. She went from being a vibrant, larger-than-life woman to a zombie before my own eyes. She became unable to work, and then unable to get around the house, and then unable to function cognitively. Her migraines took a backseat to the crippling addiction she had to narcotics, and it consumed her. Despite being a nurse and having the knowledge, I was powerless to change her mind about her predicament – nothing else mattered other than numbing the pain. The only time she went out was to go to her family doctor, the hospital, or the pharmacy. I watched her slowly disappear, and there was absolutely nothing I could do about it. It was agonizing.

This is probably why I am so passionate about preventing my patients from going down this path. My mother relied so heavily on her doctor's careless advice that she didn't stop and recognize that she was the star of her own health, not her doctor. And we lost her.

We put much store in modern medicine, yet modern medicine is leaving out a huge chunk of our holistic health. We have gained so much power through the use of drugs that we forget how powerful our mindset is, deeming it "soft" data. Up until recently, schools of healing in every culture, from Indigenous cultures in North America to the Aztecs to Traditional Chinese Medicine, involved all facets of the human being, not just the physical one. One of the radiologists I worked with used to jokingly refer to himself as a "fancy plumber," and he's not far from the truth. We treat humans like backed-up sinks instead of as the intricate, holistic creations that we are.

Many patients suffer under the delusion that their health care providers know best, and we as health care providers are not helping that perspective much. While it may be drilled into our heads to ensure our patients are active participants in their own health, in reality, we see very little of this demonstrated. They give up their power as soon as they walk in the door of their family medicine clinic or hospital. A health scare can be intimidating, overwhelming, and with the added stress of not knowing what is causing their malady, it can be easy for our patients to defer to someone else. There is more and more onus on medicine to find the answer to the everchanging and increasing causes of chronic illness. Our patients' obedience to their health care team causes them to give up their power.

There is also, of course, the fact that it is easier to take a pill than it is to change a way of life. In his book *Love, Medicine, and Miracles*, Dr. Bernie Siegel recounts that, given the choice between an operation and a change in lifestyle, eight out of ten patients will choose the operation because "it hurts less." [2] They don't need to alter their eating habits, or exercise, or even peer into their behavioral patterns. Modern medicine has offered a pill (or a scalpel) to fix what ails our patients, and we health care professionals are more than happy to oblige.

Why do we in health care enable this behavior? There are a few reasons.

The main reason we don't empower our patients is because we don't have time to. When we are busy with charting, transferring, pouring medications, doing rounds, changing dressings, etc., when would we have time to empower them? Our roles have significantly changed over the years, and we are not at the bedside as much as we used to be. Our caregiving is more complex, and our role of nurturer has shifted into tasks—administering meds, doing swallow assessments, drawing bloodwork, and interpreting it. We are so busy looking at screens and charts that we forget why we went into these professions in the first place. The human element of healing is dissolving more rapidly than a sublingual Ativan.

The only comfort I provide in my job on a regular basis is giving out warm blankets. That's it. It's the only nice thing I do for my patients. My other duties have shifted to charting, poking, pushing medications, and transferring.

Another reason we don't empower our patients is because we want to maintain some semblance of authority. We want to educate our patients, and we want them to trust us. We went to school for our professions, and we know more about the human body than the average person. We look to establish rapport by giving them knowledge. We want to be seen as people who the patient can trust and rely on. We should not only be giving out the knowledge we have, but empowering the patient to be accountable for his health in calling him to action. Too often, we do for the patient what the patient, armed with the knowledge we have secured for him, could do for himself.

While we need to empower the patients who have given up their power, we also need to respect the patients who are standing in it. We need to encourage that patients take an active role in their health, and, despite their lack of knowledge, we are not the experts in their care—they are. When a patient has a multidisciplinary team of health care workers active in her health, she knows what is best for her, as we lack experience in fields of health care different from our own. By giving her autonomy, it will inevitably lead to her to being less dependent on us, and we can focus on the patients who truly are totally reliant on us.

Dr. Siegel observed that his patients who were the most likely to overcome their illnesses (some of them life-threatening) were the ones who were the most active in their care (and admittedly, to Siegel, the most annoying). They respected their health care team, but were assertive about their views, and made decisions that they deemed best for themselves. Most of the time, when a patient disagrees with us, we often find them "difficult." But how can we know what is best for them, just because we have medical training? If you have ever questioned a mechanic or made a decision contrary to what a financial advisor may have made, you will know that, despite their expertise, you are the one in the driver's seat. We know what works best for us, even if it isn't always a conventional choice. We need to start treating our patients like people with autonomy, and not just following what we deem the best solution.

In a review of Siegel's book, Dr. A.B.R. Thomson mused about the art being taken out of the science. He attests that physicians' roles are to accept the patients as they are, and to help them with their expertise, however "this may be difficult for us to accept because in medical school we learn all about disease, but we learn little about what disease means to the person."[3]

Another reason we may disempower our patients is because it is easier. We have access to the list of medications and surgical history, so we don't need to hold them accountable for knowing what they are taking and why.

For patients with limited mobility, sometimes it may seem simpler to do the work for them, using our muscles where the patient may be able to at least contribute. There has been an upward trend in musculoskeletal injuries in HCWs, and some of that comes down to the fact that we are too impatient to wait for them to move themselves. This not only causes patients to be more reliant on us, but is a cause for more physical stress on our bodies, which leads to injury and disability. Many of our health authorities require us to complete annual safe transferring courses because our injuries are costing dollars. Despite having the knowledge and annual education in regards to proper transferring, we still aren't doing it.

The Exceptional Patient

Through his work speaking to patients and their caregivers, Dr. Siegel created a group therapy called "Exceptional Cancer Patients (ECaP)." This therapy created a safe space to lovingly confront patients' illnesses and facilitate lifestyle changes and empowerment in their therapies. After years of witnessing certain types of patients who seemed to excel in their healing, Dr. Siegel christened them "exceptional."

The definition of an exceptional patient is one who is resilient, confident, and accountable for his own healing. Some characteristics of an exceptional patient include:[4]

• having a strong sense of self	• demonstrating high self-esteem and self-love
• being self-reliant, but not hyper-independent	• being grounded, not in denial about their illness
• being receptive and creative—when given advice or aspects of care that they may not prefer, they find a way to make it work for them	• having careers they like, and are eager to return to work
• managing setbacks well; they expect them to happen and don't sink into a depression when they do	• engaging in self-care activities such as meditation and getting out in nature

Since we are holistic beings, we need to treat the whole patient, not simply the area affected by disease. Trauma can affect our nervous system, our endocrine system, and our immune system. It is proven to make physiological changes to the brain.[3] Our state of mind affects our entire body system. It makes sense, then, that a positive mindset can heal it.

The Simonton Method, developed by O. Carl Simonton, a radiation oncologist, and Stephanie Matthews-Simonton, a psychologist, is a program for cancer patients that treats them through connecting mind and body. Through use of cognitive-behavioral therapy (CBT), visualization, and mindfulness/meditation, this method treats cancer patients from a holistic point of view. These patients tended to live longer and have a greater sense of well-being. [5]

According to Siegel, much of today's illness can be traced back to an inability to love ourselves. Patients of his who didn't speak up for themselves and neglected their own needs were the "most likely to become ill."[6] He purported that patients need to be assertive for the sake of their healing, and that being afraid to ask questions only causes their health to suffer.

Siegel would ask his patients four questions for guiding treatment, which allowed him to gauge the strength of their will to live, and helped glean their attitudes towards themselves:

1. Do you want to live to be a hundred?

    Most people don't say yes to this without some guarantee of health.

2. What happened to you in the year or two before your illness?

    This explores the psychological factors and possible stressors that contributed to the illness.

3. What does your illness mean to you?

    If it automatically means death, there is much to look into, and what being ill means to the patient in regards to quality of life.

4. Why did you need the illness?

    Sickness gives people the permission to do what they think they wouldn't be able to do without getting sick. It can make it easier to say no to duties, burdens, or jobs. It can allow people to feel like victims. It can make it easier to ask for help, give us attention or love, or it can be an excuse for failure.

The last question is definitely the most interesting (and the most unnerving, I'm sure) for the patient. No one would ever say they brought a sickness on to themselves consciously, but when we dive into what the illness represents (or what it is giving us permission for), it is interesting what can come up when asked this question.

How We Help the Patient Be His Own Healer

Now that we have more information about how to empower ourselves, how can we help empower others? Instead of viewing our patients as helpless victims, where can we encourage them? Where can we give them choices, where can we hold them accountable for their own health? How can this be achieved? By being a co-healer in their health, we give them their power back.

Patients who are considered difficult or uncooperative because they want to know every detail of their health care records are those most likely to get well. They ask a lot of questions and express emotions freely. You know these patients, and yes, they are a pain in the ass. But they also are the ones who are most accountable for their own health, and not simply relying on the health care system to fix them or blindly believing that what we tell them to do is right for them (which, if you've ever made a med error, you will know that they have every right to be questioning us—we're human, too). By encouraging our patients to be their own advocates (and honoring the ones who already are, even if they are "persistent"), we allow our patients to take their health back.

We can also help empower our patients to heal by being direct with them. Many of us are too afraid to ask our patients questions about their illness for fear of upsetting them. We often don't have time to ask them about their personal lives, or how they are *really* feeling.

Being truly seen is a gift so few of us encounter these days, with many of our interactions being superficial, but it provides a deeply impactful experience for our patients. One of the nurses I used to work with, Celia, had a gift for this. She was kind and caring, but she also wasn't afraid to ask patients real, honest questions. It gave her patients the opportunity to be vulnerable, and with Celia's kind demeanor and adeptness in listening, many of her patients received a moment of true healing while under her care.

We are also gun-shy in giving our patients optimism when we do not know the prognosis. We don't want to offer them "false" hope, yet how do we know what the future will bring? Much of that is up to the patient! O. Carl Simonton of the Simonton Method for cancer patients averred, "In the face of uncertainty, there is nothing wrong with hope."[7] Giving the patient hope through granting him autonomy and a positive mindset can be instrumental in their healing. Much like we need to be a calming presence for our children in times of adversity, we need to execute reassurance for our patients. They, like children, need to know we see them as capable of coping with this adversity.

For some patients, this is what they need most desperately from us. While we can't save everyone, it is our role to give them comfort, and giving them hope is something we, while we may feel uncomfortable doing when we see so much death, have the power to do. Just remarking that they, the patient, have the power to choose, and providing them with options, helps give them their power back, even on a small scale. We aren't doing them a disservice by giving them hope if we truly believe in the power they have to heal themselves. We see miracles every day—why can't the patient sitting in front of us be one of them?

Since the illness usually fulfilled some psychological need by the patient, it is important to reframe their perspectives on health. Instead of looking at illness, it is important to shift to an emphasis on wellness. We often focus on disease instead of focusing on health.

Reward well-being instead of punishing illness. Encourage our patients to eat well and be active, acknowledge their hard work, compliment them on their achievements. Start to see them as people on a journey who are capable of healing. This may be difficult with how the world is right now, but we all could benefit from the positivity. Progress is still progress, no matter how small a step.

Alternative Models of Healing

We have been trained in Western medicine to only value Western medicine. There is still so much we do not know about the body, especially in regards to chronic illness. Modern medicine is failing our patients. Eastern therapies, many of them pertaining to energy medicine, are gaining attention and respect among liberal practitioners in the hospital. We can only throw so many pills at people before we realize there must be another approach.

We need to think outside the box in a revolutionary way. By emphasizing the patient as his own healer, we can begin to shift the focus from the patient being a powerless victim to someone who is engaged in his own convalescence. This may be radical thinking from a Western standpoint, but it is not at all new to ancient cultures who have kept their practices alive in the face of modern medicine.

While there is a movement toward more natural forms of healing, it is still important to stress that many of these therapies should be explored in conjunction with allopathic medicine. The exposure of profit-only Big Pharma has contributed to a growing mistrust of Western medicine. As someone who leans towards more natural remedies, I can see the schism widening, and the pandemic has only intensified this.

The us versus them is occurring in our schools of health, when we all desire the same thing: wellness. Each patient is an individual, and can have many types of healing as part of their path. Instead of this or that, we can look at the benefits of this *and* that—for a cancer patient, this might look like chemo *and* Reiki. We do not have to "win" when it comes to which form of healing works—all that matters is that our patients get better.

I recently discovered Therapeutic Touch. Despite it being co-created by a registered nurse, I had never heard of it before. I was intrigued by it, and wanted to learn more.

Developed by an RN named Dolores Krieger and an intuitive healer named Dora Kunz back in the '70s, TT (as it is commonly referred to) is a form of energy healing that emphasizes the patient's power to heal himself.[8] Similar to Reiki, TT uses the therapist as a conduit for balancing the patient's energy field. It is stressed that the patient is the one responsible for his health, and, while he is not actively doing anything during a session other than relaxing, it is taught to the patient that he is the one creating his own healing. The TT therapist is merely a facilitator in helping the patient heal himself. This was different from any other forms of healing I had encountered before, which usually placed the practitioner as the one "healing" the patient, whether it be a doctor or a massage therapist.

Dolores was fascinated by Dora's ability to see energy and help heal others. She was an academic, and performed countless studies and research based on what these two ladies developed. While not intuitive, Dolores felt anyone could learn what Dora was doing, and they both taught TT right up until their deaths. If you are interested, Dolores Krieger's book *The Therapeutic Touch* is a good place to start in learning how TT can help our patients with relaxation and pain control. Thousands of nurses are taught this therapy, and more health care professions need to be aware of its benefits.

TT is not the only literature that exists on patients doing their own healing. As health care workers, we know (and see!) miracles happen. Patients who have been given a grim diagnosis can have a miraculous recovery or remission. Some patients DO take back their power in the face of adversity, and it helps them not only come to terms with the diagnosis they may have received, but thrive in the face of it.

Joe Dispenza is the most current physician stating the importance of the power of our minds to heal ourselves. A chiropractor who was hit by a truck, fractured six vertebrae, and was told her would never walk again, he healed himself with rest and visualizing healing his spine, one vertebra at a time. After committing to doing this work for others, his books, such as *You are the Placebo*, are filled with patients, who, through meditation, visualization, and an intention to take an active part of their healing, are continuing to have miraculous results. [9]

My father had a similar thing happen to him. Right after I was born, he hurt himself seriously at work, fracturing his spine. He was told by his doctor that he would never walk again, and if he did, he would certainly not be going back into construction. Newly married and having a baby at home to support, this didn't sit well with my father. Forever stubborn, he refused to accept this, and proceeded to prove his doctors wrong by not only learning how to walk again, but returning to his job in construction so he could support his family.

What was the central issue? He refused to give up. He refused to accept what someone told him about his ability, and (rather arrogantly) insisted that this wouldn't be the case for him. The power of his mind, coupled with the determination to support himself and his family, allowed him the power to heal. He not only walked again, but he went back to his physical job.

This is nothing new. Athletes are given exercises to visualize winning, and it helps them secure their gold medals. Entrepreneurs visualize the goals they set for themselves and soon make it a reality. Vision boards, while a fun arts-and-crafts activity, have real merit in helping us visualize what we want to accomplish.

The patient has the power to heal himself. What can we as HCWs do to help facilitate this? Give them their power back. It is not healthy to have our patients rely on us as much as they do, and we are witnessing the results of this in the current health care crisis. We are health care workers who are human, and we make mistakes. Not only this, we have little time to truly be with our patients, and so we need to respect that we don't have all the answers for them.

We need to stop doing all of the heavy lifting (literally and figuratively). Our patients are autonomous beings. We can offer knowledge, experience, and, most of all, hope. But it is their journey. Exceptional patients take charge of their lives, and use health care professionals as members of a team, not relying on us to heal them.

EXERCISES

1. Think about a typical work day for you. Where in your practice do you empower your patients? Where might you enable them? Brainstorm ways you can give your patients more autonomy in their care. It might not always be possible due to time constrictions, but endeavoring to find new ways to support our patients may actually help them get better quicker.

2. What alternative healing modalities do you utilize already? What therapies intrigue you? Look into what you are curious about. Is there a way to incorporate these therapies in your daily life? In your health care practice?

3. Look into the works of Gabor Maté, Bernie Siegel, Therapeutic Touch, and Joe Dispenza. They come with a "woo" warning, but you also might find information that empowers you to be an active participant in your own healing, as well as your patients' healing journey.

Epilogue

I have been a caregiver my entire life. I have been a nurse for fifteen years. With a heavy heart, I am in the process of leaving traditional bedside nursing. Some of you reading this might be contemplating a similar option. My passion for health care workers has led me down a path where I want to be supporting them more fully, starting with completing this book. I am excited to see where this new path takes me.

During my parents' illnesses and subsequent passing, I was barely able to keep afloat. It was my coworkers who were the most involved in ensuring I was okay. Pre-made dinners, visits, texts, phone calls, it was this group of people who got me through the most difficult time in my life. My close friends (who were also co-workers) even organized a trip to Chicago for my birthday (I was born on St. Patrick's Day and had always wanted to see the big celebrations they had there— they dye the river green!). When they presented this gift to me (in public, for all the world to see my ugly crying), they told me they had received enough from my co-workers to fund the entire trip within two days of collecting, that's how generous and giving the people I called family for twelve years were. The superpower empathy is especially strong here.

We health care workers are the people who console each other after a traumatic case. We are the people who step up our game when a co-worker goes home sick or has a family emergency. We are the people who we stay late to help out because our colleagues are drowning in work. Even the ones who drive us nuts, we love them because they belong to us, for better or for worse.

We go over and above what is required of us. We do it with grace, with humility. When I felt overwhelmed with the amount of work we had to do, it was being inspired by my colleagues who went the extra mile for a patient that propelled me to keep going. I grew so much during this time period in my life. I have this special group of people to thank, whether it was through supporting me or through being a lesson where I had to stand up for myself. I am sure you have people in your career that have helped you grow, and you are a different person because of them.

For most health care workers, our job isn't just a job. Our coworkers are family. We go through experiences together that our friends and family members just can't understand. We bear witness to intense aspects of being human that most people never imagine. We are amazing beings, and we have a wonderful gift of being able to give. My hope is that by the end of this book, you have received the tools you need to carry on being amazing health care workers before you get to the point of walking away.

And if you do decide to walk away, I applaud your strength and ability to look at your life clearly and make the right choice for you—it isn't easy. In fact, it will probably be the most difficult thing that you do.

Through my career as a health care worker, I have discovered so many gifts that I didn't know I had—my strength and determination (some managers and radiologists might label this as stubborn—potato, po-tah-to), my ability to cheer people on and make them laugh, my ability to lighten the mood when it was needed (an aptly timed desktop photo of Tom Jones in a speedo or a T-rex costume ambush). When I left, I was sad that I wouldn't be able to be this person there anymore. Someone pointed out to me that I get to keep these gifts—they were given to me by this department, and while I was no longer a part of it, I got to carry the gifts with me, and I will be able to use them wherever I go.

What gifts has being a health care worker given you that you didn't have before you entered into your field? Remember that wherever you go, you will always get to take these with you, even if you are not physically there anymore.

I think of my time in each area that I work like high school—I grow and learn lessons and become a better version of myself in an environment that fostered learning. And with each "graduation", I could celebrate that I had learned all I needed to learn. I reflect back fondly of my career so far, grateful for everything that was given to me, no matter how hard the lesson, for it made me who I am today.

Regardless of the path you choose, whether you stay in your unit or field or do something else entirely, you will always have your superpowers. With the tools explored here to help strengthen these, you are unstoppable.

Thank you for showing up, every day. I am so grateful for your dedication, and please know that this gratitude is truly felt from the bottom of my heart. You deserve the very best—and now you know how to give that to yourself. Receiving from those who give with all of their hearts is one of the best gifts to be granted.

Do it for you.

You got this.

Endnotes

FOREWORD

1. International Council of Nurses (ICN), COVID-19 update. *International Council of Nurses*, 2021.
2. J.E. Arnetz, C.M. Goetz, B.B. Arnetz, E. Arble, "Nurse reports of stressful situations during the COVID-19 pandemic: Qualitative analysis of survey responses," *International Journal of Environmental Research and Public Health* 17 no. 21 (2020), 8126-8138.
3. K. J. Foli, A. Forster, C. Cheng. L. Zhang, Y. C. Chiu, "Voices from the COVID-19 frontline: Nurses' trauma and coping," *Journal of Advanced Nursing*, 77 (2021), 3853-3866.
4. F. Hossain, A. Clatty, "Self-care strategies in response to nurses' moral injury during the COVID-19 pandemic," *Nursing Ethics* 28 no. 1 (2021), 23-32.

CHAPTER 1

1. The ANA Enterprise, "Year One COVID-19 Impact Assessment Survey," *American Nurses Association*, March 9, 2021.
2. Ibid.

CHAPTER 2

1. M. Buheji, N. Buhaid, "Nursing human factor during COVID-19 pandemic," *International Journal of Nursing* 10 (2020), 12-24.
2. J.E. Davidson, J. Proudfoot, K. Lee, S. Zisook, "Nurse suicide in the United States: Analysis of the Center for Disease Control 2014 National Violent Death Reporting System dataset," *Archives of Psychiatric Nursing* 33 (2019), 16-21.
3. Ian Bremmer, *Us vs Them: The Failure of Globalism*, New York: Portfolio (2018).
4. Michael Yeo, Anne Moorhouse, Pamela Kahn & Patricia Rodney (eds.) *Concepts and Cases in Nursing Ethics, Third Edition*, Peterborough, Canada: Broadview Press (2010).
5. Ibid.
6. Ibid.
7. Ibid.
8. Ibid.
9. Ibid.
10. M.J. Johnstone, "Whistle blowing and accountability," *Australian Nursing Journal* 13(5), (2005), 8-10.
11. A.A, Grandey, "When 'The Show Must Go On': Surface acting and deep acting as determinants of emotional exhaustion and peer-rated service delivery," *Academy of Management Journal* 46(1), (2003), 86-96.

CHAPTER 3

1. Elizabeth Kubler-Ross, M.D., *On Death and Dying*, New York: Scribner (1970).
2. K.D. Neff, Y. Hsieh, & K. Dejitterat, "Self-compassion, achievement goals, and dealing with academic failure," *Self & Identity* 4(3) (2005), 263-287.
3. J.R. Nelson, B.S. Hall, J.L. Anderson, C. Birtles, & L. Hemming, "Self-compassion as self-care: a simple and effective tool for counselor educators and counselling students," *Journal of Creativity in Mental Health* 13(1), (2018), 121-133.
4. K.D. Neff, "Compassionate letter writing: write a letter to themselves from the perspective of this compassionate friend," *Self-compassion exercises*. Retrieved from http://self-compassion.org/.

CHAPTER 4

1. Dictionary.com
2. Conor Neill, "Understanding Personality: The 12 Jungian Archetypes," (2018), https://conorneill.com/.
3. Susanna Barlow, "Understanding The Healer Archetype," (2021), https://susannabarlow.com/.
4. Galia Benziman, Ruth Kannai, and Ayesha Ahmad, "The Wounded Healer as Cultural Archetype," *CLCWeb: Comparative Literature and Culture* 14.1 (2012).
5. W. Caan, L. Morris, S. Santa Maria, & C. Brandon, "Wounded healers," *Nursing Standard,* 15(2), (2000), 22-23.

CHAPTER 5

1. Royal Society for the Arts (RSA). "Brené Brown on Empathy," (2013), https://www.youtube.com/watch?v=1Evwgu369Jw.
2. T. Wiseman, "A concept analysis of empathy," *Journal of Advanced Nursing,* 23(6), (1996), 1162-1167.

CHAPTER 6

1. Brene Brown, "Definition of Value," *Dare to Lead List of Values,* (2022), brenebrown.com.
2. Neil Greenberg, Mary Docherty, Sam Gnanapragasam, Simon Wessely, "Managing mental health challenges faced by healthcare workers during covid-19 pandemic," *BMJ* (2020); 368: m1211.

CHAPTER 7

1. Better Help Editorial Team, "The 16 Personality Types: Why Knowing Your Type Is Important," (2022), Retrieved from https://www.betterhelp.com/advice/personality/the-16-personality-types-why-knowing-your-type-is-important/.
2. The Myers and Briggs Foundation, https://www.myersbriggs.org/.
3. 16 Personalities, https://www.16personalities.com/.
4. PersonalityHacker, https://www.personalityhacker.com/.

CHAPTER 8

1. Oxford English Dictionary, "ego," OED Online, Oxford University Press, (2022).
2. PersonalityHacker, https://www.personalityhacker.com/.
3. Robert Jackman, *Healing Your Lost Inner Child: How to Stop Impulsive Reactions, Set Healthy Boundaries and Embrace an Authentic Life,* Practical Wisdom Press, (2020).

CHAPTER 9

1. Nancy Levin, *Worthy: Boost Your Self-Worth to Grow Your Net Worth,* Carlsbad, CA: Hay House, (2016).
2. Gabor Maté, M.D., "When the Body Says No: The Cost of Hidden Stress", Toronto: Vintage Canada, (2004).
3. Ibid.

CHAPTER 10

1. Henry Cloud and John Townsend, *Boundaries: When to Say Yes, How to Say No To Take Control of Your Life,* Grand Rapids, MI: Zondervan, (2017).
2. Robert Jackman, *Healing Your Lost Inner Child: How to Stop Impulsive Reactions, Set Healthy Boundaries and Embrace an Authentic Life,* Practical Wisdom Press, (2020).
3. Susan Scott, *Fierce Conversations: Achieving Success at Work & in Life, One Conversation at a Time,* New York: Berkley, (2004).

CHAPTER 11

1. Julie de Azevedo Hanks, *The Assertiveness Guide for Women*, Oakland, CA: New Harbinger Publications, (2016).
2. Erin Salmond, Susan Salmond, Margaret Ames, Mary Kamienski, Cheryl Holly, "Experiences of compassion fatigue in direct care nurses: a qualitative systematic review," School of Nursing, Rutgers University, Newark, Jersey City Medical Center, RWJ/Barnabas Health, Jersey City, and The Northeast Institute for Evidence Synthesis and Translation (NEST): a Joanna Briggs Institute Centre of Excellence (2019).
3. Kasia Urbaniak, *Unbound: A Woman's Guide to Power*, New York: TarcherPerigee, (2021).
4. Ibid.
5. Julie de Azevedo Hanks, *The Assertiveness Guide for Women*, Oakland, CA: New Harbinger Publications, (2016).

CHAPTER 12

1. C. Dall'Ora, J. Ball, M. Reinius, & P. Griffiths, "Burnout in nursing: a theoretical review," *Human Resources for Health*, 18(41), (2020), 1-17.
2. Benjamin Frank Miller, "Compassion Fatigue," *Miller-Keane Encyclopedia and dictionary of medicine, nursing, and allied health*, (1992), cma.ca/physician-wellness-hub/content/compassionfatigue/.
3. C. Dall'Ora, J. Ball, M. Reinius, & P. Griffiths, "Burnout in nursing: a theoretical review," *Human Resources for Health*, 18(41), (2020), 1-17.
4. Benjamin Frank Miller, "Compassion Fatigue," *Miller-Keane Encyclopedia and dictionary of medicine, nursing, and allied health*, (1992), cma.ca/physician-wellness-hub/content/compassionfatigue/.
5. J.E. Davidson, J. Proudfoot, K. Lee, S. Zisook, "Nurse suicide in the United States: Analysis of the Center for Disease Control 2014 National Violent Death Reporting System dataset," *Archives of Psychiatric Nursing* 33, (2019), 16-21.
6. S. Monteverde, "Caring for tomorrow's workforce: moral resilience and healthcare ethics education," *Nursing Ethics* 23 (2014), 104-116.
7. Susan Scott, *Fierce Conversations: Achieving Success at Work & in Life, One Conversation at a Time*, New York: Berkley, 2004.

CHAPTER 13

1. B. Fursland, B. Raykos, and A. Steele, *Perfectionism in Perspective*. Perth, Western Australia: Centre for Clinical Interventions, (2009).
2. R. Shafran, Z. Cooper, C. Fairburn; "Clinical perfectionism: a cognitive-behaviorual analysis," *Behaviour research and therapy* 40 7, (2002), 773-91.
3. Byron Katie, *Loving What Is: Four Questions that can Change Your Life*, Easton, PA: Harmony Press, (2021).
4. B. Fursland, B. Raykos, and A. Steele, *Perfectionism in Perspective*. Perth, Western Australia: Centre for Clinical Interventions, (2009).

CHAPTER 14

1. S. Karpman, M.D., "Fairy tales and script drama analysis," *Transactional Analysis Bulletin*, 7(26), (1968), 39-43, https://www.aconsciousrethink.com/9667/karpman-drama-triangle/.
2. S. Karpman, M.D., *A Game Free Life: The new transactional analysis of intimacy, openness, and happiness*, San Francisco: Drama Triangle Publications, (2014). https://www.listeningpartnership.com/insight/about-the-drama-triangle-and-how-to-escape-it/
3. David Emerald, *The Power of TED* (The Empowerment Dynamic)*, Edinburgh, UK: Polaris Publishing, (2009). theempowermentdynamic.com

CHAPTER 15

1. Susan Scott, *Fierce Conversations: Achieving Success at Work & in Life, One Conversation at a Time*, New York: Berkley, 2004.

---

2. A.B.R. Thomson, M.D., "Love, Medicine, and Miracles," *Canadian Journal of Gastroenterology,* 3(3) (1989), 131-133.

3. Robert Half Talent Solutions, "Two in Five Workers in Canada Have Quit Due to a Bad Boss, Survey Reveals," Robert Half blog, October 8, 2019, https://www.roberthalf.ca/en/two-in-five-workers-in-canada-have-quit-due-to-a-bad-boss-survey-reveals/.

4. Kasia Urbaniak, *Unbound: A Woman's Guide to Power,* New York: TarcherPerigee, (2021).

5. C. Dellasega, *When Nurses Hurt Nurses: Recognizing and Overcoming the Cycle of Bullying.* Indianapolis, IN: Sigma Theta Tau International, (2011).

6. Isabel Wilkerson, *Caste: The Origins of Our Discontent,* New York: Random House, (2020).

7. Ian Bremmer, *Us vs Them: The Failure of Globalism,* New York: Portfolio (2018).

8. Daryl Davis, "Why I, as a black man, attend KKK rallies," TEDxNaperville TED Talk, November 2017, https://www.ted.com/talks/daryl_davis_why_i_as_a_black_man_attend_kkk_rallies/.

CHAPTER 16

1. American Nurses Association, "Position Statement: Incivility, Bullying, and Workplace Violence," July 22, 2015, https://www.nursingworld.org/practice-policy/nursing-excellence/official-position-statements/id/incivility-bullying-and-workplace-violence/.

2. C.M. Clarke, D.J. Kane, D.L. Rajacich, K.D. Lafreniere, "Bullying in undergraduate clinical nursing education," *Journal of Nursing Education* 51(5), (2018), 269-276.

3. C. Edmonson, & C. Zelonka, "Our Own Worst Enemies: The Nurse Bullying Epidemic," *Nursing Administration Quarterly,* (July/September 2019), 43:3, 274-279.

4. M. King-Jones, "Horizontal violence and the socialization of new nurses," *Creative Nursing Journal,* (2011) 17(2), 80-86.

5. Penny A. Sauer, Thomas P. McCoy, "Nurse Bullying: Impact on Nurses' Health," *Western Journal of Nursing Research,* (December 2017), Vol. 39(12) 1533-1546.

6. H.K. Laschinger, C.A. Wong, G.G. Cummings, A.L. Grau. "Resonant leadership and workplace empowerment: the value of positive organizational cultures in reducing workplace incivility," *Nursing Economic$,* (2014) 32(1), 5-18.

7. Soyun Hong, Heejung Kim, Sujin Nam, Janet Yuen Ha Wong, Kayoung Lee, "Nurses' post-traumatic stress symptoms and growth by perceived workplace bullying: An online cross-sectional study," *Journal of Nursing Management,* (January 23, 2021), 29(5).

8. Bessel Van Der Kolk, M.D., *The Body Keeps the Score: Brain, Mind, and Body in the Healing of Trauma,* New York: Penguin, (2015).

9. C., Edmonson, & C. Zelonka, "Our Own Worst Enemies: The Nurse Bullying Epidemic," *Nursing Administration Quarterly,* (2019), 43:3, 274-279.

10. Ibid.

CHAPTER 17

1. Robert Bramson, *Coping with Difficult People,* New York, NY: Anchor Press/Doubleday, (1981).

2. Stacey Holloway, "How to Deal with Difficult People," training workshop, http://www.hollowaygroup.ca/.

3. Stephen Porges, *Polyvagal Safety: Attachment, Communication, Self-Regulation,* New York: WW Norton, (2021).

4. Marshall B. Rosenberg, *Nonviolent Communication: A Language of Life: Life-Changing Tools for Healthy Relationships,* Encinitas, CA: PuddleDancer Press, (2015).

5. Susan Scott, *Fierce Conversations: Achieving Success at Work & in Life, One Conversation at a Time,* New York: Berkley, (2004).

CHAPTER 18

1. Webster's, "toxicity," Webster's Online Dictionary, (2009).

2. Z.C. Chan, W.S. Tam, M.K. Lung, et al, "A systematic literature review of nurse shortage and the intention to leave," *Journal of Nursing Management* (2013), 21(4), 605-613.

3.   World Health Organization. "The World Health Report 2001: Mental Health: New Understanding, New Hope," World Health Organization, 2001, http://www.who.int/whr/2001/en/whr01_en.pdf?ua=1/.

4.   Ibid.

5.   M. Ross, E. Rideout, M. Carson, "Nurses' work: balancing personal and professional caregiving careers," *The Canadian journal of nursing research = Revue canadienne de recherche en sciences infirmieres*, (1993), 26(4), 43-59.

6.   Paul White & Kathy Schoonover-Shoffer, "Surviving (Even Thriving?) in a Toxic Workplace," *Journal of Christian nursing: a quarterly publication of Nurses Christian Fellowship* (July 2016), 33(3):, 142-149.

7.   Michelle Gorton, "Intentional disregard: remedies for the toxic workplace," *Environmental Law*, (Fall 2000), 30(4), 811-842.

8.   M.M. Varma, A.S. Kelling, & S. Goswami, "Enhancing healthcare quality by promoting work-life balance among nursing staff," *Journal of Hospital Administration*, (2016), 5(6), 58-62.

9.   G. Flynn, "Stop toxic managers before they stop you!" *Workforce*, (1999), 78(8), 40-44.

10.   George A. Zangaro, "Recognizing and overcoming toxic leadership," *Journal of Nursing Administration* (2017), 35(7/8), 336-341.

CHAPTER 19

1.   B. Smit, "Successfully leaving work at work: The self-regulatory underpinnings of psychological detachment," *Journal of Occupational and Organizational Psychology*, (2016), 89: 493-514.

CHAPTER 20

1.   David Hawkins, *Letting Go: The Pathway of Surrender*, Carlsbad, CA: Hay House, 2014.

2.   Ibid.

3.   Melody Beattie, *The Language of Letting Go: Daily Meditations for Codependents*, Center City, MN: Hazelden, 1990.

CHAPTER 21

1.   E. Brogan, C. Rossiter, C. Duffield, & E. Denny-Wilson, "Healthy eating and physical activity among new graduate nurses: a qualitative study of barriers and enablers during the first year of clinical practice," *Collegian*, (2021), 28(5), 489-497.

2.   W. L. Awa, M. Plaumann, & U. Walter, "Burnout prevention: A review of intervention programs," *Patient Education and Counseling*, (2010), 78, 184-190.

3.   James Clear, *Atomic Habits: An Easy & Proven Way to Build Good Habits & Break Bad Ones*, New York: Avery (2018).

4.   S.J. Scott, "The Eisenhower Matrix: Make Urgent vs. Important Decisions with 4 Quadrants," Develop Good Habits website, (November 15, 2018), https://www.developgoodhabits.com/eisenhower-matrix/.

5.   Michael Pollan, *This is Your Mind on Plants*, New York: Penguin, (2021).

6.   Matt Walker, *Why We Sleep: Unlocking the Power of Sleep and Dreams*, New York: Scribner, 2018.

7.   Ibid.

8.   D. McElligott, S. Siemers, L. Thomas, & N. Kohn, "Health promotion in nurses: Is there a healthy nurse in the house?" *Applied Nursing Research*, (2009), 22, 211-215.

9.   D. Church, S. Stern, E. Boath, et al, "Emotional freedom techniques to treat posttraumatic stress disorder in veterans: review of the evidence, survey of practitioners, and proposed clinical guidelines," *The Permanente Journal* (2017), 21: 16-100.

CHAPTER 22

1.   D. Bernal, J. Campos-Serna, A. Tobias, S. Vargas-Prada, F.G. Benavides, & C. Serra, "Work-related psychosocial risk factors and musculoskeletal disorders in hospital nurses and nursing aides: a systematic review and meta-analysis," *International Journal of Nursing Studies* (2015), 52(2), 635-648.

2.   C. M. Kuhn, & E. M. Flanagan, "Self-care as a professional imperative: physician burnout, depression, and suicide," *Canadian Journal of Anaesthesia*, (2017), 64(2), 158-168.

3.	H. L. Fred, & M. S. Scheid, "Physician burnout: Causes, consequences, and (?) cures," *Texas Heart Institute Journal*, (2018), 45(4), 198-202.

4.	R.D. Williams, J.A. Brundage, E.B. Williams, "Moral injury in times of COVID-19," *The Journal of Health Service Psychology*, (2020), 46(2): 65-69.

5.	J. Kabat-Zinn, "Mindfulness-based interventions in context: past, present, and future," *Clinical Psychology: Science and Practice*, (2003), 10(2), 144-156.

6.	Ibid.

7.	Ibid.

8.	L. Guillaumie, O. Boiral, & J. Champagne, "A mixed-methods systematic review of the effects of mindfulness on nurses," *Journal of Advanced Nursing*, (2016), 73(5), 1017-1034.

9.	J. Cohen-Katz, S. Wiley, T. Capuano, D.M Baker, L. Deitrick, & S. Shapiro, "The effects of mindfulness-based stress reduction on nurse stress and burnout: a qualitative and quantitative study, part III," *Holistic Nursing Practice* (2005a) 19(2), 78-86.

10.	J.R. Nelson, B.S. Hall, J.L. Anderson, C. Birtles, & L. Hemming, "Self-compassion as self-care: a simple and effective tool for counselor educators and counselling students," *Journal of Creativity in Mental Health*, (2018), 13(1), 121-133.

11.	Matthew Sockolov, "29 Scientific Benefits of Meditation: What the Research Tells Us," One Mind Dharma website, November 15, 2017, https://oneminddharma.com/benefits-of-meditation/.

CHAPTER 23

1.	M. Wallace, S. Campbell, S.C. Grossman, J.M. Shea, J.W. Lange, T.T. Quell, "Integrating spirituality into undergraduate nursing curricula," *International Journal of Nursing Education Scholarship*, (2008), 5, 1-13.

2.	K. Ausar, N. Lekhak, & L Candela, "Nurse spiritual self-care: A scoping review," *Nursing Outlook*, (2021), 69(4).

3.	M. McEwen, "Spiritual nursing care," *Holistic Nursing Practice*, (2005), 19, 161-168.

4.	M. Wallace, S. Campbell, S.C. Grossman, J.M. Shea, J.W. Lange, T.T. Quell, "Integrating spirituality into undergraduate nursing curricula," *International Journal of Nursing Education Scholarship*, (2008), 5, 1-13.

5.	C.H. Rushton, J. Batcheller, K. Schroeder, P. Donohue, "Burnout and resilience among nurses practicing in high-intensity settings," *American Journal of Critical Care*, (2015), 24, 412-420.

6.	K. Ausar, N. Lekhak, & L Candela, "Nurse spiritual self-care: A scoping review," *Nursing Outlook*, (2021), 69(4).

7.	Louise Hay, *You Can Heal Your Life*, Carlsbad, California: Hay House, Inc. (1984).

8.	Center for Disease Control and Prevention -https://www.cdc.gov/cancer/headneck/index.htm

9.	Jun-Ook Park, Inn-Chul Nam, Choung-Soo Kim, Sung-Joon Park, Dong-Hyun Lee, Hyun-Bum Kim, Kyung-Do Han, and Young-Hoon Joo. Sex Differences in the Prevalence of Head and Neck Cancers: A 10-Year Follow-Up Study of 10 Million Healthy People. *Cancers* 2022, 14(10), 2521.

10.	Gabor Maté, M.D., "When the Body Says No: The Cost of Hidden Stress", Toronto: Vintage Canada, (2004).

CHAPTER 24

1.	Bessel Van Der Kolk, M.D., *The Body Keeps the Score: Brain, Mind, and Body in the Healing of Trauma*, New York: Penguin, (2015).

2.	Bernie Siegel, M.D., *Love, Medicine and Miracles: Lessons Learned About Self-Healing From a Surgeon's Experience with Exceptional Patients*, New York: Harper & Row, (1986).

3.	A.B.R. Thomson, M.D., "Love, Medicine, and Miracles," *Canadian Journal of Gastroenterology*, 3(3) (1989), 131-133.

4.	Ibid.

5.	O. Carl Simonton, James Creighton, Stephanie Simonton, *Getting Well Again: The Bestselling Classic About the Simontons' Revolutionary Lifesaving Self-Awareness Techniques*, New York: Bantam, (1992).

6.	Ibid.

7.	Ibid.

8.	Dolores Krieger, Ph.D., RN, *The Therapeutic Touch*, New York: Atria Books, (1979)

9.	Dr. Joe Dispenza, *You are the Placebo*, Carlsbad, California: Hay House, Inc. (2015).

* 9 7 8 1 7 3 8 8 3 9 4 0 7 *